The Occupational Therapist's Workbook for Ensuring Clinical Competence

The Occupational Therapist's Workbook for Ensuring Clinical Competence

Marie J. Morreale, OTR/L, CHT
Adjunct Faculty
Rockland Community College
State University of New York
Suffern, New York

Debbie Amini, EdD, OTR/L, CHT, FAOTA
Director of Professional Development
The American Occupational Therapy Association, Inc.
Bethesda, Maryland

Routledge
Taylor & Francis Group
NEW YORK AND LONDON

The Occupational Therapist's Workbook for Ensuring Clinical Competence includes ancillary materials specifically available for faculty use. Please visit www.routledge.com/99781032956978 to obtain access.

First published in hardrback 2024

First published 2016 by SLACK Incorporated

Published 2024 by Routledge
605 Third Avenue, New York, NY 10158

and by Routledge
4 Park Square, Milton Park, Abingdon, Oxon OX14 4RN

Routledge is an imprint of the Taylor & Francis Group, an informa business

ISBN: 978-1-03-295697-8 (hbk)
ISBN: 978-1-63-091049-5 (pbk)
ISBN: 978-1-00-352527-1 (ebk)

DOI: 10.4324/9781003525271

For Product Safety Concerns and Information please contact our EU representative: GPSR@taylorandfrancis.com
Taylor & Francis Verlag GmbH, Kaufingerstraße 24, 80331 München, Germany.

Additional resources can be found at
https://ww.routledge.com/9781032956978

Dedication

This book is dedicated to occupational therapy students everywhere. May you find joy in your work as you facilitate the ability of others to participate in meaningful occupations.

Contents

The Occupational Therapist's Workbook for Ensuring Clinical Competence includes ancillary materials specifically available for faculty use. Please visit www.routledge.com/9781032956978 to obtain access.

Acknowledgments

I am grateful for the opportunity to collaborate on this book with Debbie Amini. I appreciate her many insightful contributions to this project and truly value our friendship. Her knowledge base and heartfelt dedication to the profession never cease to amaze me. I am forever thankful to Ellen Spergel, past coordinator of the OTA Program at Rockland Community College, for giving me a start in academia. Her wisdom, kindness, and support regarding occupational therapy education have had a tremendous impact on me. I also want to thank Donna Knoebel, OTA Program Coordinator, for her support of this project and expertise in the area of mental health. Appreciation goes to Kathy Babcock, Academic Fieldwork Coordinator, for the tireless job she does to ensure that our students meet and exceed expectations for fieldwork. I also thank Mae Eng and Randy Marti for their knowledge regarding adult and geriatric rehabilitation. My students deserve thanks for providing feedback when completing many of the worksheets. A special mention goes to Brien Cummings at SLACK Incorporated for sharing in my vision for this book and helping to bring it to fruition. In addition, my son Michael deserves recognition for continuing to help me upgrade my technology skills. Finally, special thanks to my husband Richard for tolerating my obsession with writing. Without his love, patience, and support, this book would not have been possible.

Marie J. Morreale, OTR/L, CHT

Thank you, Marie Morreale, my college friend, peer, colleague, confidante, and inspiration, for inviting me to be a part of this exciting text.

Debbie Amini, EdD, OTR/L, CHT, FAOTA

About the Authors

Marie J. Morreale, OTR/L, CHT, has been teaching occupational therapy assistant (OTA) students at Rockland Community College, State University of New York in Suffern, since 1998. As an adjunct faculty member, Marie teaches "Professional Issues and Documentation" and "Geriatric Principles." Over the years, she has also taught several other courses in the OTA program including "OT Skills," "Advanced OT Skills," "Therapeutic Activities," and "Advanced Therapeutic Activities." Marie has made significant contributions to curriculum development and also served as interim coordinator of the OTA Program.

Marie graduated *summa cum laude* from Quinnipiac College (now Quinnipiac University). She has experience working in a variety of occupational therapy practice settings, including inpatient and outpatient rehabilitation, long-term care, adult day care, home health, cognitive rehabilitation, and hand therapy. Marie has been a certified hand therapist for more than 20 years and also served several years on a home health professional advisory committee, consulting on quality assurance issues. Marie has written or coauthored several other occupational therapy texts, including *Developing Clinical Competence: A Workbook for the OTA; The OTA's Guide to Documentation: Writing SOAP Notes* (3rd ed.); and *The OTA's Guide to Writing SOAP Notes* (2nd ed.). In addition, she authored a chapter on documentation for *The Occupational Therapy Manager* (5th ed.), published several occupational therapy articles, and is the author of several online continuing education courses. Marie is active in her church community and enjoys anything travel related.

Debbie Amini, EdD, OTR/L, CHT, FAOTA, received her Bachelor of Science in Occupational Therapy from Quinnipiac University, her Masters of Education in Curriculum Instruction/Supervision from the University of North Carolina at Wilmington, and her Doctorate of Education in Adult and Community College Education from North Carolina State University.

Dr. Amini joined the American Occupational Therapy Association (AOTA) as Director of Professional Development in 2014. Her previous employment experience includes clinical hand therapy practice, directing an occupational therapy assistant program, and working as an assistant professor of occupational therapy in an Masters of Occupational Therapy program.

Dr. Amini has served in multiple volunteer leadership positions with AOTA, including as Hand Rehabilitation Subsection Coordinator from 2002 to 2005; Physical Disabilities Special Interest Section Chairperson from 2005 to 2008; member of the AOTA's Commission on Practice from 2008 to 2011; and Chair of the AOTA Commission on Practice from 2011 to 2014.

Dr. Amini was the "Hands On" department columnist for ADVANCE for Occupational Therapy Practitioners from 1999 to 2011 and "Inside Occupation" from 2011 to 2014. She has authored several articles that have appeared in *ADVANCE for Directors in Rehabilitation*, the AOTA's *Physical Diabetes Quarterly* newsletter, *OT Practice* magazine, and *The American Journal of Occupational Therapy.* She has also written several online courses and textbook chapters. She currently serves on the editorial review board for *The Open Journal of Occupational Therapy* and *Occupational Therapy in Health Care.*

Dr. Amini has presented numerous times at the AOTA, the North Carolina Occupational Therapy Association, and American Society of Hand Therapists annual conferences and has conducted multiple 2-day regional workshops.

Introduction

How to Use This Book

This workbook is designed to help occupational therapy students and new practitioners demonstrate the practical problem-solving and real-life clinical reasoning skills essential for fieldwork and clinical practice. This user-friendly resource helps the reader apply occupational therapy concepts, improve narrative and pragmatic reasoning skills, and measure the attainment of knowledge and skills needed for successful transition to fieldwork and entry-level practice. The variety of assessment methods and learning activities used throughout the text include case studies; vignettes; multiple choice, matching, and true/false questions; fill in the blanks; and experiential activities. The worksheets, learning activities, and worksheet answers are written in an easy-to-read format with topics broken down into smaller units and explained step-by-step to allow for easy, independent study. Thoroughly explained answers are provided for worksheets so that readers can check their responses with suggested best practices.

A wide variety of client conditions, situations, and intervention options are presented for different practice areas. Knowledge and skills are assessed for fundamental aspects of occupational therapy, such as professionalism, ethical decision making, evidence-based practice, evaluation and intervention planning, occupation-based interventions, effective communication, supervision, role delineation, activity analysis, cultural competence, interprofessional collaboration, group process, emerging practice areas, department management, safety, documentation, billing and reimbursement, and more. Many helpful tips are presented to guide the occupational therapist (OT) in proper clinical decision making, professional conduct, and meeting standards of care.

Although the exercises in each chapter are presented in a logical progression, each chapter is fully independent of the others. Thus, the reader can skip around and complete individual chapters or particular exercises in the order most conducive to individual learning needs. Worksheets and learning activities are also useful as role-playing exercises and for studying in small groups. This manual can be used as a companion text for multiple classes throughout an occupational therapy curriculum or as a useful study aid when preparing for fieldwork or the national certification exam. Many of the exercises can also be used to help measure attainment of knowledge outlined in educational standards delineated by the Accreditation Council for Occupational Therapy Education (ACOTE; 2012).

This text originated from *Developing Clinical Competence: A Workbook for the OTA* (Morreale, 2015) and was completely adapted and revised to make it more appropriate for entry-level OTs and occupational therapy students at the professional level. New material was added to reflect the higher-level clinical reasoning skills, knowledge base, and additional competencies required of OTs. The instructional methods, learning activities, and worksheets presented in this book stem from the authors' combined decades of experience teaching occupational therapy and occupational therapy assistant (OTA) students. Because many of the worksheets and learning activities were developed to specifically address common mistakes or difficulties exhibited by occupational therapy students during their academic coursework and fieldwork, this text is intended to help the reader avoid making the same errors.

As the exercises in this manual are completed, the information presented will help the reader to understand important occupational therapy concepts and measure attainment of various clinical knowledge and skills. The workbook is designed to help ensure that the reader will be able to apply clinical decision-making skills appropriately, implement effective interventions safely, demonstrate professional behaviors, and communicate more effectively. Answers to the worksheet exercises are explained clearly and simply at the end of each chapter. However, because it is impossible to present or predict every possible scenario or intervention, it is important to realize that answers are often examples of best practice. It is possible that you may come up with other best practice examples that may also be correct. This workbook is not an instruction manual, and thus it is intended for readers who have basic knowledge of occupational therapy theory and who possess basic technical skills. Readers should seek additional information from appropriate resources to fill in any knowledge gaps that may become apparent when completing worksheets within this text.

Guiding Principles

The specific roles and responsibilities of the OT and OTA in the areas of evaluation, intervention, and targeting of outcomes are delineated in the American Occupational Therapy Association's (AOTA) *Guidelines for Supervision, Roles, and Responsibilities During the Delivery of Occupational Therapy Services* (AOTA, 2014a) and *Standards of Practice for Occupational Therapy* (AOTA, 2010). An OT establishes and directs the intervention plan, supervises and collaborates with the OTA, and delegates responsibilities and aspects of client care for which the OTA demonstrates service competency and is in accordance with state and federal regulations (AOTA, 2010, 2014a). Considering that each client, population, or organization is unique with individual circumstances, OTs and OTAs use a holistic, client-centered approach. A variety of methods and interventions are implemented to work toward the goal of contributing to a client or population's occupational performance, as is described in the *Occupational Therapy Practice Framework: Domain and Process* (AOTA, 2014b) and *Scope of Practice* (AOTA, 2014c). The services that OT practitioners provide are also guided by the *Occupational Therapy Code of Ethics* (AOTA, 2015), relevant laws, facility policies, third-party payer requirements, and evidence-based practice.

Although this book presents sound examples of best practice, an OT practitioner must always use clinical judgment to determine the methods, interventions, or recommendations that are most appropriate for a client's personal situation. OT practitioners must carefully consider the client's medical status and circumstances; specific client factors, contexts, and skills that hinder or support performance; precautions; contraindications; safety issues; available methods; and current evidence supporting clinical practice. It is important to realize that a "standard" intervention for a particular condition, such as a specific physical agent modality, orthotic device, exercise protocol, communication strategy, or adaptive device, may not be appropriate for all clients with the same diagnosis. Also, an intervention plan might delineate more than one device or method as a particular kind of intervention For example, a condition that requires orthotic intervention may necessitate using both a nighttime static positioning orthosis and a daytime dynamic mobilization orthosis.

The scenarios presented are representative of situations commonly encountered in clinical practice. The names and specific details have been fabricated to create optimal learning exercises so that any specific resemblance to an actual person is purely coincidental. It is the authors' intent that this book will be a useful resource to help occupational therapy students succeed academically and become competent, ethical practitioners. Any feedback or suggestions for future editions is welcome.

References

Accreditation Council for Occupational Therapy Education. (2012). 2011 Accreditation Council for Occupational Therapy Education (ACOTE®) Standards. *American Journal of Occupational Therapy, 66*(Suppl. 6), S6–S74.

American Occupational Therapy Association. (2010). Standards of practice for occupational therapy. *American Journal of Occupational Therapy, 64*(Suppl. 6), S106–S111.

American Occupational Therapy Association. (2014a). Guidelines for supervision, roles, and responsibilities during the delivery of occupational therapy services. *American Journal of Occupational Therapy, 68*(Suppl. 3), S16–S22.

American Occupational Therapy Association. (2014b). Occupational therapy practice framework: Domain and process, 3rd edition. *American Journal of Occupational Therapy, 68*(Suppl. 1), S1–S48.

American Occupational Therapy Association. (2014c). Scope of practice. *American Journal of Occupational Therapy, 68* (Suppl. 3), S34–S40.

American Occupational Therapy Association. (2015). Occupational therapy code of ethics (2015). *American Journal of Occupational Therapy, 69*(Suppl. 3), 6913410030. http://dx.doi.org/10.5014/ajot.2015.696S03

Morreale, M. J. (2015). *Developing clinical competence: A workbook for the OTA*. Thorofare, NJ: SLACK Incorporated.

Chapter 1

Communicating Effectively

Occupational therapy practitioners must demonstrate good verbal and nonverbal communication skills and incorporate therapeutic use of self throughout the occupational therapy process (American Occupational Therapy Association [AOTA], 2014b). This chapter presents worksheets and learning activities to help you use therapeutic communication techniques, manage various situations appropriately, and respond professionally when interacting with clients, families, significant others, caregivers, colleagues, and other disciplines. Practical communication tips are provided to help you make a good first impression, explain your role effectively to different audiences, ask open-ended questions, actively listen, and show empathy. Answers to worksheet exercises are provided at the end of the chapter.

Contents

Morreale, M. J., & Amini, D.
The Occupational Therapist's Workbook for Ensuring Clinical Competence (pp. 1-33).

Worksheet 1-1

Initial Client Encounter

Penny Payshent is a 78-year-old female who sustained a right cerebrovascular accident (CVA) 4 days ago, resulting in left hemiparesis. Penny was admitted to a skilled nursing facility for rehabilitation and currently requires moderate assistance for self-care and transfers. An occupational therapist, Jennifer, is performing Penny's evaluation today. Consider Jennifer and Penny's initial conversation that follows. What suggestions would you make regarding the therapist's interaction with the client?

OT: *Hey Penny, I'm Jennifer, your OT. It is nice to meet you. How are things today?*
Client: *Well, my TV isn't working and my breakfast was late this morning. Who are you again?*
OT: *I'm Jennifer, an OT.*
Client: *What's an OT?*
OT: *OT stands for "occupational therapist."*
Client: *Another therapist was already here this morning. I think her name was Mary.*
OT: *Mary is the PT, a physical therapist. I'm from the occupational therapy department.*
Client: *Oh, I have been retired for 12 years. I do not want another job.*
OT: *Of course. Rest assured I am not here to find you a job.*
Client: *What are you going to do to me then? I'm really tired and would like to take a nap.*
OT: *OT is part of the rehabilitation department here. It is similar to PT, except they work on walking and the lower extremities and we work on the upper extremities and ADLs.*
Client: *What are ADLs?*
OT: *That means I am here to help you do things like eat, bathe, and get dressed.*
Client: *Oh, can you fix my TV?*
OT: *No, I don't fix TVs. Can we begin the evaluation now sweetie?*

Suggestions to improve this interaction:

1.

2.

3.

4.

5.

6.

7.

8.

9.

10.

Learning Activity 1-1: Communication Basics

Over the course of your professional career as an OT, you will have the opportunity to meet and work with a variety of clients. When communicating with a client (or caregiver/significant others), make an effort not to talk from the doorway or across a room; try to move closer instead (Drench, Noonan, Sharby, & Ventura, 2012). If the client is seated in a chair or wheelchair, it is preferable for the therapist to be seated nearby at the client's level rather than standing and towering over him. Also, it is important that the therapist have an understanding of the client's literacy level, such as primary language spoken and level of education completed. If the therapist is unable to communicate effectively because the client is deaf or only speaks, reads, or understands a different language, the therapist should arrange for a qualified interpreter according to established standards for that setting.

It is useful to practice some standard opening lines ahead of time to help you display confidence and make a positive first impression. In the space provided, write several sentences you might use initially when introducing yourself to a new client, such as Susan Smythe, a 70-year-old woman who had total hip replacement surgery 2 days ago.

OT introduction:

Now check your introductory statement against the following suggestions in this chapter to determine whether all the necessary elements are present.

For an initial encounter with an adult client, it is more respectful for an OT to use an appropriate title such as "Mr." or "Mrs." and the client's last name. Ensure you are pronouncing the person's name correctly. For the client described earlier, Susan Smythe, her last name could be pronounced with either a short or long "i" sound in the middle. It is courteous to ascertain which pronunciation is correct. Next, tell the client your name and discipline. Make sure to also acknowledge your working relationship with the client's physician who referred the client to occupational therapy and other team members as appropriate, such as the PT and/or your fieldwork educator. The OT might also determine whether the client has an understanding of occupational therapy and/or ask how the client is feeling. Of course, each client encounter will be a little different depending on the circumstances. Here are some examples of introductory statements that an OT or student might use with a client recovering from hip surgery:

- *Hello, Mrs. Smythe, I am Valerie Veracity, an occupational therapy student. Am I saying your last name correctly? It is very nice to meet you. I have been working with your OT, Kevin, and he asked me to see you today to review your hip precautions and teach you how to manage putting on your socks and shoes. How are you feeling today?*

- *Good morning, Mrs. Smythe. My name is Valerie Veracity, and I am from the occupational therapy department. Dr. Smart ordered OT to help you recover from your hip surgery. I am an occupational therapy student working with Kevin Karing, the therapist who evaluated you yesterday. Do you have any questions about occupational therapy before we start?*

Learning Activity 1-1: Communication Basics (continued)

- *Hello, Mrs. Smythe. My name is Valerie Veracity. I am an occupational therapy student and this person next to me is Kevin Karing, my supervisor. Dr. Smart ordered occupational therapy to help you recover from your hip surgery so we are here to evaluate you. Before we begin, would you like me to explain what occupational therapy is?*

- *Good morning, Mrs. Smythe. I am Sally Smiley, an occupational therapist. Am I pronouncing your last name correctly? Your surgeon, Dr. Smart, asked me to teach you how to manage your daily activities without bending your hip too much. I would like to ask you about the kinds of things you need to be able to do for you to return home. First of all, how does your hip feel today?*

- *Hello, Mrs. Smythe. I am Sally Smiley, an occupational therapist. Am I saying your last name correctly? Your surgeon referred you to occupational therapy so that I can teach you how to manage safely at home with your hip precautions. I also work closely with Patty Patience, your physical therapist, whom you met earlier. Do you have any questions before we start the evaluation?*

- *Good morning, Mrs. Smythe. It is nice to meet you. I am Sally Smiley, your occupational therapist for today. Kevin, the OT whom you have been working with this week, has the day off. He asked me to teach you how to get dressed safely with your hip precautions. Do you remember what equipment Kevin gave you yesterday to help you dress?*

Now write an introduction you might use for John Valorie, whom you are meeting for the first time for the initial evaluation. He underwent surgery for a below knee amputation (BKA) 5 days ago.

OT introduction:

Learning Activity 1-2: What Is Occupational Therapy?

Clients, other professionals, and members of the public are not always aware of occupational therapy or may not fully understand the profession. The distinct value of occupational therapy should always be explained during the initial client contact or evaluation. Occupational therapy practitioners must provide a clear and simple definition of occupational therapy appropriate to the client's situation and explain briefly how that client will benefit from occupational therapy services. The AOTA website (www.aota.org) and official documents, such as *The Philosophical Base of Occupational Therapy* (AOTA, 2011) and *Occupational Therapy Practice Framework: Domain and Process* (AOTA, 2014b), are useful resources to help you define occupational therapy for different audiences. Also, Table 1-1 presents practical suggestions for communicating with clients and others effectively.

Create a brief definition of occupational therapy that you might use with clients or family/caregivers.

Occupational therapy is ...

Now develop a brief definition that you might use to explain occupational therapy to other professionals or service providers (i.e., medical interns, teachers, school administrators, optometrists, etc.).

Occupational therapy is ...

Table 1-1

Suggestions for Initial Client Encounters and Occupational Therapy Definition

Do

- Make a sincere effort to have eye contact with the person you are addressing, particularly if you must review paperwork, jot down notations, or enter information on the computer during the encounter
- Pay close attention to what the person is saying or doing
- Use simple, easy-to-understand language
- Make your definition brief and uncomplicated
- Explain what *occupation* means
- Relate to the individual client's condition, situation, or problem
- Discuss how occupational therapy can help
- Differentiate occupational therapy from other disciplines
- Consider what is appropriate for that practice setting, time frames, and reasonable for the client's circumstances
- Clarify the focus of your intervention *for that particular client* relating to occupation, such as enabling independence, remediating particular client factors to improve function, facilitating skills or occupational adaptations, assessing safety, providing caregiver education, modifying the environment, improving comfort or quality of life
- Provide examples or describe briefly the use of preparatory tasks and methods, therapeutic activities and occupations, adaptive equipment, or other specialized interventions indicated for this client

Don't

- Do not appear preoccupied with other matters, such as personal problems, casual conversations with staff, or paperwork
- Do not use technical jargon or abbreviations (unless you explain them). Clients may not know what ADL, COTA, OTR, CVA, etc., stand for or the meaning of terms such as *activities of daily living*, *dysphagia*, *sensory integration*, or *myocardial infarction*
- Do not talk down to the client or act as if the client is unintelligent
- Do not refer to an adult client with nicknames such as "honey" or "sweetie"
- Do not refer to an OTA as a "therapist"
- Do not use an identical explanation for each client. Not all clients will achieve complete independence or improved functional abilities as some conditions are irreversible or terminal. However, occupational therapy can help clients maintain function and manage chronic conditions for improved quality of life. The focus of OT interventions may be different according to various circumstances, but will contribute to occupational performance in some way
- Do not guarantee results but, instead, explain areas that will be addressed or may realistically improve based on sound clinical knowledge
- Do not overwhelm the client with too much information
- Do not ask the client a question you really do not want an answer to. For example, if you say, "Do you want to come to therapy today?" that sets up the client to refuse treatment. It would be better to say, "It is time for your occupational therapy session now." If you ask the client, "How was your day today?" be prepared to hear about bland hospital food, a noisy roommate, or how the television or phone did not work properly. You might decide it is better to target a question toward the client's condition, such as, "How does your hip feel today?"
- Do not lie or create false hope or unrealistic expectations. However, how you temper the truth can have a significant effect in helping to prevent client hopelessness and despair

Reprinted with permission from Morreale, M. J. (2015). *Developing clinical competence: A workbook for the OTA*. Thorofare, NJ: SLACK Incorporated.

Worksheet 1-2

It Looks Like You Play All Day

A group of physicians are taking a tour of the rehabilitation department. When they arrive at the occupational therapy clinic, the physicians observe the following client interventions happening:

- A 70-year-old female client baking cookies
- A 65-year-old male client navigating his power wheelchair around an obstacle course
- A 52-year-old male client standing while sanding a wood birdhouse
- A 50-year-old female client using a button hook on a button board
- A 48-year-old female client standing and using a reacher to place cereal boxes in an upper cabinet
- A 22-year-old male client playing checkers with an OTA

One of the physicians comments, "It looks like you must play with toys all day in here." How might an OT respond to this?

Learning Activity 1-3: Explaining Occupational Therapy's Distinct Value

For each of the following situations, role-play with a partner or write a few sentences below. Introduce yourself as an OT or student and explain the distinct value of occupational therapy for that client and general desired, realistic outcomes. For this exercise, assume each client has been referred to occupational therapy and that this is your initial contact with the client.

1. **Early Intervention:** Mary Mackie is a single parent of 20-month-old Alexis. Alexis was recently diagnosed with a developmental disability; she is nonverbal; has poor eye contact, oral-motor sensitivity, and tactile defensiveness; and does not walk yet.

2. **Outpatient clinic:** Jane Doe is a 40-year-old married bookkeeper with children aged 2 and 5 years. Jane sustained a Colle's fracture in her dominant upper extremity 6 weeks ago. The cast was removed last week, and she has not returned to work. Her hand is swollen, painful, and stiff, causing difficulty with activities of daily living (ADLs) and instrumental ADLs (IADLs).

3. **School Setting:** Jack Springer is the parent of Steven, a second-grade student with a learning disability. Steven demonstrates poor handwriting, difficulty using scissors, poor time management, and decreased organizational skills. Steven's delayed skills acquisition creates difficulty with completing class assignments and managing clothing for gym and recess.

4. **Skilled Nursing Facility:** Karen Kairgiver is the adult child and health care agent of Ruth Rezzydent, a client with moderate dementia. Ruth has lived in a long-term care facility for the past year but fell out of bed last week, breaking her hip. She is 1 week status post total hip replacement surgery.

5. **Acute Care Hospital:** Mike O'Malley, a 75-year-old retired plumber, had a heart attack 5 days ago. He lives with his wife in a private house and was independent before his hospitalization.

6. **Rehabilitation Hospital:** Marvin Billings is an 18-year-old male client who sustained a C-6 spinal cord injury in a diving accident in his backyard pool.

7. **Inpatient Behavioral Health Setting:** Judy Jones is a 21-year-old female diagnosed with a cocaine addiction. She lives at home with her parents, recently dropped out of college, and was arrested for drug possession a few days ago. She was admitted to an inpatient drug rehabilitation program in lieu of going to jail.

Worksheet 1-3

Delegating Clients to an OTA

OTs delegate aspects of the occupational therapy process to OTAs. Consider the following interaction between an OT and a client at the end of the initial evaluation session. Provide suggestions to improve this interaction.

OT: *Mr. Gonzalez, now that I have all your information and we have agreed on your goals for therapy, your treatment will begin tomorrow afternoon. The OTA, Joe, will be working with you for the next few weeks.*
Client: *Oh, will I see you again?*
OT: *Well, I'm sure you will see me running around the clinic or working with other clients. I will be re-evaluating you again in a few weeks to check on your progress. However, Joe, the OTA, will be providing your day-to-day treatment.*
Client: *What's an OTA?*
OT: *That stands for "occupational therapy assistant."*
Client: *If you don't mind, I would rather have a real therapist like you, not an aide.*
OT: *Don't worry, Joe is a great therapist. He has worked here for 10 years and is familiar with your diagnosis. All the clients really like him a lot.*
Client: *Will this Joe guy be asking me all these questions again?*
OT: *That should not be necessary. It was very nice to meet you, and I am sure you will do well here. I will call for someone to bring you back to your room now. Good-bye.*

Suggestions to improve this interaction:

1.

2.

3.

4.

5.

6.

7.

8.

9.

10.

Learning Activity 1-4: Occupational Therapy vs Physical Therapy

Indicate how an OT might respond to each of the following situations.

1. You are an OT working in a long-term care setting and attending the weekly team meeting today for one of the units. During the meeting, the head nurse states, *"Ellen Elderlee in room 468 hasn't had any rehab in awhile. She is developing some tightness in her right shoulder and elbow, which is making it hard to dress and bathe her. I think we should get PT involved."*

2. You are an OT working in an acute care setting. Your client, Helen, had shoulder surgery 2 days ago, and you completed the occupational therapy evaluation yesterday. You enter Helen's room and see that she has several visitors. Helen announces to her visitors, *"Oh, here's my physical therapist. I guess it is time for my arm exercises now. I hope the PT won't make you all leave."*

3. You are an OT working in an inpatient rehabilitation facility. Today you are in the occupational therapy room working with Mr. Getbetta. Your session entails having Mr. Getbetta work on preparatory interventions to improve sitting balance, range of motion, and fine motor skills needed for managing utensils and feeding. As the client is working on preparatory tasks, such as tossing beanbags and using a Velcro checkerboard, a PT comes to get the client and asks, *"Are you finished playing with Mr. Getbetta? It is time for me to walk him now so I will have to pull him away from fun and games."*

4. You are an occupational therapist working in a school setting. As you are walking down the hallway, a teacher asks to speak with you and says, *"See that student Marilyn over there?* [Teacher points to a student in classroom.] *She always fidgets like that, and she can't seem to sit up straight or focus on copying notes from the blackboard. Her desk is always a mess too. Should we have her evaluated by OT or would PT be better? Do you think it would even help?"*

Therapeutic Relationships

According to the *Occupational Therapy Practice Framework* (AOTA, 2014b), *therapeutic use of self* is an integral part of the occupational therapy process and is used in all client interactions. *The Intentional Relationship: Occupational Therapy and Use of Self* (Taylor, 2008) is a useful resource that discusses the occupational therapy historical perspective regarding the therapeutic use of self. This book also describes the Intentional Relationship Model, which Taylor (2008) developed to define the interpersonal dynamic between the occupational therapist and client. Taylor (2008) delineates, at length, six therapeutic communication modes that occupational therapy practitioners use most frequently in therapeutic relationships. These six ways of relating to clients include advocating, collaborating, empathizing, encouraging, instructing, and problem solving (Taylor, 2008). The occupational therapy "toolbox" used in professional practice consists of many therapeutic qualities and methods to foster appropriate and helpful client relationships. Some therapeutic qualities and practical tips are described below. Additional information about occupational therapy interventions used in mental health practice can be found in Chapter 8.

Therapeutic Qualities and Tips

Attending: Actively centering on the client allows the therapist to make astute observations and develop impressions to begin the professional reasoning process. Cole describes this as "the attentive physical presence the therapist focuses on the client.... Taking note of appearance, body language, posture, seating position, eye contact and facial expression are all part of attending" (2012, p. 72).

Active listening: This is the ability of the occupational therapy practitioner to show genuine interest in the client and demonstrate a caring approach, which can be conveyed by eye contact, facial expression, not interrupting, and nonverbal communication such as an appropriately relaxed posture, not fidgeting, and nodding to various client statements (Froehlich, Roy, Augustoni, Arsenault, & Eldredge, 2014a). The therapist should also occasionally pause and allow for silences that enable the person talking to "fill the space with what weighs heavily on them... If the speaker is struggling with what else to say, a simple '*Tell me more*' or '*What else*' may be all the speaker needs to hear in order to continue talking about what is on his or her mind" (Froehlich et al., 2014a, p. 92).

Genuine caring approach: Nonverbal communication, tone of voice, and the choice of words the therapist uses to speak to the client can either convey genuineness or give the impression that the therapist is disinterested or just going through the motions. Thus, it is important to spend enough time with the client, show active listening, follow through with promises, and provide competent, effective care. Demonstrating kindness and paying attention to detail might include taking the time to obtain a blanket or snack for the client as needed, neatly folding the client's clothing during a dressing intervention, and carefully adjusting the bed covers, for example. Also, the therapist making an effort to point out the "little things" can help clients to feel special and cared for (e.g., noticing that the nursing home client has a new manicure, commenting on the family photo on a nightstand, or praising incremental progress or client effort during a particular therapy task).

Respect and cultural sensitivity: Be cognizant and respectful of the client's cultural background and possible implications for emotional expression. For some clients, cultural factors may include a more stoic nature, limited eye contact, avoidance of touch, or special rituals, for example. Always demonstrate cultural sensitivity, and avoid personal bias or judgment regarding a client's gender, age, race, sexual orientation, socioeconomic status, level of education, appearance, diagnosis, among other characteristics (Froehlich et al., 2014a). Strive to believe in the dignity and worth of each individual despite his or her problems or challenging situations (Froehlich, Roy, Augustoni, Eldredge, & Arsenault, 2014b).

Empowerment: Believe in the client's potential for change. Foster a client-centered atmosphere that gives the client hope and empowers him or her to overcome obstacles and be an active part of his or her own solution (Froehlich et al., 2014b). This might also include teaching the client assertiveness and self-advocacy skills.

Empathy: Use primary accurate empathy, which is recognizing the feelings of the client. A helpful way to convey empathy is by using the statement, "You feel ________________ because ________________" (Cole, 2012, p. 74). Realize that different kinds of emotions (e.g., bad, glad, sad, mad) all have different levels of intensity (mild, moderate, high), so it is important that the therapist identify the accurate emotion (Cole, 2012). For example, Cole (2012, p. 74) describes the emotion of anger as a spectrum "from low intensity, like annoyed or perturbed, to very high intensity, like rage" and the emotion of "fearful" as levels going from mild (worried) to severe (petrified). Reflective listening and advanced accurate empathy enable the therapist to form an educated guess or hypothesis about the underlying feelings, topics, or concerns that the client is hinting about (Cole, 2012; Froehlich et al., 2014a).

Therapeutic Relationships (continued)

Restatement: This technique uses the form of a question to rephrase what the speaker said to reflect that the client was heard (Froehlich et al., 2014a).

Humor: In addition to the physiological benefits of true laughter, humor can be an effective tool in select situations to motivate clients, manage difficult situations, "break the ice," reduce client anxiety, or make the therapist seem more approachable.

Redirection: The therapist must recognize when the session is veering off in an unintended direction, such as if the client is being inattentive, asking personal questions, being too verbose, going off on another topic, not answering a question directly, or lacking focus for the conversation or task at hand. The therapist must tactfully and respectfully manage the behavior by directing the client's attention to the desired intervention activity/topic or close the session as appropriate.

Therapeutic self-disclosure: Indirect self-disclosure conveys to the client a sense of the therapist's approval or disapproval of the client's statements or behavior through nonverbal communication such as nodding "yes" or "no", smiling or frowning, or exhibiting tension or laughter, for example (Cole, 2012). Direct self-disclosure involves the therapist relating a personal vignette with a similar theme and describing how it was resolved or the coping mechanisms used to help the client with a challenging situation (Cole, 2012). This technique must be used judiciously, not just as an opportunity for the therapist to vent (Cole, 2012).

Maintain professional boundaries: Unlike personal relationships that involve reciprocal give-and-take, professional relationships should never make the client feel the need to provide any type of support to the therapist (Drench et al., 2012). In addition to limiting the disclosure of personal information, occupational therapy practitioners must also limit the extent of emotional involvement to maintain professional judgment and objectivity (Drench et al., 2012). Any use of comforting or therapeutic touch must be in accordance with facility policy and be culturally sensitive; it is critical that it not be misinterpreted as inappropriate personal touch (Drench et al., 2012). It is respectful to ask the client's permission before any essential physical procedures are performed such as range of motion, retrograde massage, or assessment of areas covered by clothing. Gifts from clients should not be expected, and many facilities have policies in place that clearly prohibit acceptance of client gifts or, perhaps, only allow nominal gifts such as candy, cookies, or flowers.

Worksheet 1-4

Do You Know What You Are Doing?

Your client, realizing you are a student or new practitioner, may express concern about your knowledge base or ability to handle his or her situation. The client may ask, *"Have you ever worked with someone like me before?"* or *"Do you know what you are doing?"*

How can you respond appropriately while being truthful about your limited experience?

Worksheet 1-5

Are You Really Sure You Can Do This?

Clients often experience anxiety and uncertainty regarding their health condition or circumstances. They may express various concerns regarding occupational therapy, other health team members, care received, or upcoming events. It is important that you follow protocols in place to ensure safety and respond appropriately to help put the client's mind at ease. Consider how you might respond to the following client scenarios, assuming that you are competent in the particular task at hand:

1. Your client is concerned about your ability to transfer him safely and states, *"I am a big guy and you are so tiny. I really don't think you can get me into that wheelchair."*

2. While performing a cooking task in occupational therapy, your client expresses fear regarding functional ambulation and states, *"I am afraid my weak leg will buckle and I will fall."*

3. As you are about to transfer a client from wheelchair to bed, your client states, *"I don't want you to get hurt moving me."*

Worksheet 1-6

I Want to Walk

Consider the therapeutic communication techniques you might use as an OT when responding to the following situations.

1. Your client, Hector, is a 22-year-old carpenter who recently sustained a C-6 spinal cord injury due to a fall from a roof. As you complete the initial evaluation and are discussing his occupational therapy goals for the next few weeks, Hector tells you the doctors are wrong and his main goal is to walk again. You know this is unrealistic based on the medical reports. What would you say to him?

2. Your client, Melvin, is a 68-year-old male with a total hip replacement. He has non-weight-bearing status for his affected lower extremity and is presently using a walker with moderate assistance. Today you are trying to teach Melvin how to don his socks and shoes using adaptive equipment. He tells you that the equipment is "silly," that his wife can help him dress, and that his only goal is to walk again. What would you say to him?

Worksheet 1-7

This Feels Like Kindergarten

Your client, Keith, is a 62-year-old defense attorney whose hobbies include gardening and woodworking. Keith has undergone surgery to repair a lacerated median nerve and is now at the strengthening phase in therapy. He has not returned to work yet due to hypersensitivity in his hand and difficulty grasping and manipulating objects. To implement the occupational therapy intervention plan, you place the client's affected hand in a plastic shoebox filled with uncooked rice and ask him to locate and remove small objects (e.g., blocks, beads) with the affected hand. The client seems offended and states, *"I feel like I am in kindergarten with my grandkids! My children would really laugh if they saw me, a pit bull defense lawyer, doing this."* How would you respond to those statements?

To address this client's specific deficits and likely goals, what activities and occupations could you choose that might be more meaningful for this client?

Learning Activity 1-5: I Don't Want Therapy

Consider the therapeutic communication techniques you might use as an OT when responding to the following situations.

1. A client was admitted to an acute care hospital with an exacerbation of chronic obstructive pulmonary disease, and her anticipated discharge is in 3 days. The OT evaluation was completed yesterday. Today, you enter the client's hospital room in the morning and tell her it is time for occupational therapy. The client states, *"Please go away. I just did a lot of leg exercises and walking in PT. I am too tired for any more therapy."* What would you say to her?
2. Your client is 80 years old and diagnosed with rheumatoid arthritis. He has pain and stiffness in both upper extremities, causing difficulties with ADLs. Today he arrives at the outpatient clinic for his OT initial evaluation. He is accompanied by his wife who states, *"My husband doesn't need all this. He had therapy before and it did not help. I don't know why the doctor made us come here."* What would you say to them?
3. Your client in home care is a 67-year-old male who has terminal pancreatic cancer. During his occupational therapy session he states, *"What's the use of all this therapy? The doctor told me I only have 6 months to live. This is a complete waste of time."* What would you say to him?
4. Your client was recently admitted to an acute behavioral health unit following a suicide attempt. You go to the client's room to take her to a scheduled occupational therapy activity group and the client states, *"Just leave me alone. I do not want to see anyone and I am not good with crafts. There is no point in me going."* What would you say to her?

Learning Activity 1-6: I Don't Need a Job

Clients who are unfamiliar with occupational therapy often take the word *occupation* literally, erroneously believing the profession entails finding jobs for people. Consider how an OT might respond to the following situations.

1. A 22-year-old college student was admitted to the hospital 2 days ago with bilateral leg fractures and internal injuries sustained from a motor vehicle accident. Today, you enter the client's hospital room to perform the OT evaluation. You tell the client your name and indicate that you are from the occupational therapy department. The client states, *"I don't need a job now. What I need is to get out of here to finish up my bachelor's degree and go to law school in the fall."* How would you respond to those statements?
2. Your client is 78 years old and diagnosed with Parkinson's disease. He has decreased bilateral upper extremity range of motion and strength, along with a history of falling. Today, he arrives at the outpatient clinic for his OT evaluation. He is accompanied by his wife, who states, *"My husband certainly doesn't need a job at his age. He hasn't worked in years! I don't know why the doctor made us come here."* How would you respond to those statements?
3. A toddler diagnosed with a developmental delay recently started receiving early intervention services. Today, the child's father took the day off from work to observe his daughter's OT evaluation. During the occupational therapy session the parent states, *"Do you always start training disabled kids this early for a job? My daughter is only 2! How do you know what she is going to want to be?"* How would you respond to those statements?
4. Your client is a 55-year-old plumber who recently had cardiac bypass surgery. During his occupational therapy session he states, *"What's the use of this job therapy? Forget about me getting a job. The doctor told me I won't be able to go back to work. This is all a waste of time."* How would you respond to those statements?
5. Your client, a 40-year-old woman diagnosed with substance use disorder, was admitted to an inpatient behavioral health unit yesterday. During your initial encounter with the client she states, *"I haven't worked since my kids were born. They are only 8 and 10 now so I am not planning to go back to work any time soon. It is ridiculous that the doctor is making me attend occupational groups here."* How would you respond to those statements?

Worksheet 1-8

Open-Ended and Closed-Ended Questions

When working with a client, you will often find it important to gather information to enhance your knowledge of the client for intervention planning. Open-ended questions that require full responses can elicit more information than closed-ended questions, which may only elicit single-word responses (Davis, 2011; Rollnick, Miller, & Butler, 2008).

Indicate whether the following questions and comments are open-ended (O), closed-ended (C), or neither (N):

1. _______ What flavor of yogurt did you eat?
2. _______ I respect your decision to do that.
3. _______ Please explain the reason for making that choice.
4. _______ How do you feel about that situation?
5. _______ Did you like the book?
6. _______ Would you be willing to tell me your life story?
7. _______ How old are you?
8. _______ What events were going on in the world the year you were born?
9. _______ I guess that is a pretty tough situation.
10. _______ What is your address?
11. _______ Tell me from the beginning how your pain developed.
12. _______ Have you been taking your medication?
13. _______ How do you fit exercise into your daily routine?
14. _______ How many hours per day do you study?
15. _______ How long have you been feeling dizzy?
16. _______ I see that you have been very busy knitting.
17. _______ What happened to make you feel that way?
18. _______ Did you fall in your house?
19. _______ You drew a very interesting picture.
20. _______ Tell me how you are feeling today.

Worksheet 1-9

Asking Open-Ended Questions

Clients may express vague, disingenuous, or limited statements about their condition, circumstances, or emotional status. Occupational therapy practitioners use professional reasoning to formulate targeted, thoughtful questions that elicit necessary, desired client information. Closed-ended questions are appropriate for situations that require only a very specific short response or "yes" or "no" answer, such as asking whether a sensory stimulus can be felt, determining a client's age, confirming that a medical test or procedure was completed, or inquiring if the person is tired or hungry. Open-ended questions help the occupational therapy practitioner gather further information to clarify the client's situation, perception, or emotions (Cole, 2012). Cole (2012, p. 74) suggests that to prevent a simple "yes" or "no" response, the occupational therapy practitioner should use words such as *what* and *how* as sentence starters and avoid the following: *do you, can you, would you, are you, have you*. You might also use words such as *tell me, explain,* or *describe* when asking pertinent open-ended questions. Use caution with the word *why* as it puts the client in a position of having to explain or defend a situation, possibly creating the perception of judgment on the part of the therapist (Cole, 2012). For each of the following client statements, develop several open-ended questions to obtain pertinent information from the client.

1. My shoulder hurts.

2. I can't do anything right.

3. I fell in my apartment.

4. My life is a charade.

5. I never thought I would turn out like this.

6. My hand is useless.

7. I'm so confused.

8. I lost my job.

9. I hate school.

10. I am no good in gym class.

Adapted from Cole, M. (2012). *Group dynamics in occupational therapy: The theoretical basis and practice application of group intervention* (4th ed.). Thorofare, NJ: SLACK Incorporated.

Worksheet 1-10

Eliciting Information Efficiently

Jean Jones is a 60-year-old female who was recently hospitalized for onset of Guillain-Barré syndrome. Yesterday, Jean was transferred from an acute care facility to a rehabilitation hospital. An OT, Nick, is covering for an OT colleague who evaluated Jean yesterday, but who has the day off today. Consider Nick and Jean's initial conversation, which follows. What suggestions would you make regarding the OT's interaction with the client?

OT: *Hello, Jean, I am Nick, an occupational therapist. Karen, your regular occupational therapist, has the day off and asked me to work with you today. It is very nice to meet you. Are you feeling better today?*
Client: *No.*
OT: *Why do you say that?*
Client: *I'm terrible. Don't you know how weak I am? I can't do anything!*
OT: *That's not true. When I came in I saw that you were doing a pretty good job feeding yourself with that device Karen gave you.*
Client: *Well, I spilled half of my food.*
OT: *The nurses will be in soon to get you cleaned up. Anyway, can I ask you some questions?*
Client: *I would rather be left alone.*
OT: *This won't take too long. Where do you reside?*
Client: *1374 East Main Street—just a few blocks from here.*
OT: *I mean, do you live in a house?*
Client: *No.*
OT: *An apartment?*
Client: *No, a condo.*
OT: *Do you have any stairs?*
Client: *Yes.*
OT: *How many stairs?*
Client: *Do you mean inside or outside?*
OT: *Both.*
Client: *Three steps outside and about 10 steps to the second floor.*
OT: *OK, now tell me about your bathroom situation.*
Client: *Well, I occasionally get constipated so I have to drink a lot of prune juice.*

Suggestions to improve this therapist's interaction with the client:

1.

2.

3.

4.

5.

Revise the interaction to incorporate more useful questions from the therapist.

Worksheet 1-11

Interaction Between an OT and an Elementary School Student

Marisol is an entry-level OT who works at an elementary school. Her client, Chrystal, is a second-grade student with a developmental delay. Marisol and Chrystal had the following conversation during an intervention session. Clearly, the OT's interaction with the student is inappropriate, unethical, and could result in disciplinary action and possibly being fired. What suggestions would you make that would create an appropriate and more productive exchange with the student?

OT: *OK, Chrystal, we are going to work some more on your handwriting today. Let's start with this worksheet.*
Student: *Do we have to?*
OT: *Yes. You know your parents and teacher would like your work to be much neater. It will only get better if you practice.*
Student: *Writing is boring. Can't we do something else?*
OT: *Not today. Would you like to choose a colored pencil from the box?*
Student: *No.*
OT: *Chrystal, pick up a pencil. Any color you would like.*
Student: *Nope.*
OT: *Don't be difficult. Please grab one of the pencils.*
Student: *What if I don't?*
OT: *Well, you'll be sorry.*
Student: *What does that mean?*
OT: *Do you want to see your parents again?*
Student: *Yes.*
OT: *Well, you can't go home until you pick up a pencil and finish this worksheet.*
Student: *You can't make me stay here.*
OT: *Oh yeah, missy? I will tie you to the chair if I need to. Now pick up a pencil. Why are you crying now?*
Student: *You are yelling at me. I don't like that.*
OT: *I am not yelling. I am just talking in a loud voice because you are being a bad girl. Come on, now, start this worksheet. I will give you a pretty sticker when you are finished.*

Suggestions to improve this interaction:

1.

2.

3.

4.

5.

6.

7.

8.

Learning Activity 1-7: Nonverbal Communication

With a partner, choose a contemporary TV talk show (e.g., *The View*, *The Talk*, *The Five*) that has a panel of diverse hosts who discuss current events or controversial subjects. Watch the opening segment of the show with the sound off and observe how the talk show hosts interact with each other. Jot down the nonverbal behaviors you observed during the exchange and determine if you can ascertain the overall tone of the conversation. Can you tell which panelists seem to agree or disagree with the others? Did you and your partner interpret what you saw in the same way? What are the specific behaviors you and your partner each observed to reach your conclusions? After you complete this worksheet, watch the segment again, but with the sound on, so you can determine whether your interpretation of nonverbal behaviors was correct.

Positive Nonverbal Behaviors Observed	***Negative Nonverbal Behaviors Observed***

- If you felt the panel's tone was congenial, did you observe any panelists smiling, nodding, hugging, lightly touching each other affectionately, or waiting to speak one's turn?
- If you felt the tone was aggressive or argumentative, did you observe panelists standing up, pointing, or exhibiting "in-your-face" behavior? Were people speaking over one another at the same time? What facial expressions did you observe? What behaviors indicated that people may have been shouting?
- Did any of the panelists "tune out" by looking away or moving elsewhere, crossing arms, sighing, or not actively participating?

Learning Activity 1-8: Communication Styles

Watch a one-on-one TV interview performed by a celebrity interviewer perceived as having a more gentle or empathetic approach (such as Barbara Walters or Oprah Winfrey). Also watch an episode of a show where real people are interrogated by someone with a more direct style or tougher reputation (such as Dr. Phil or Judge Judy). Compare and contrast the two styles of questioning and the nonverbal behavior of the interviewers. Consider the following as you are watching the two interviews:

- What did the interviewers do or say to elicit the information they were trying to obtain?
- What specific open-ended or closed-ended questions did they ask?
- What tone of voice did the interviewers use?
- Were the styles of both interviewers equally effective?
- How did the persons being questioned respond verbally and nonverbally? Did they appear comfortable or uncomfortable?
- Was information freely shared or were responses vague and resistant?
- Do you feel any of the interviewer's questions or behaviors were inappropriate? Why or why not?
- Which interviewer appeared more sympathetic to an individual's situation and why?
- Did an interviewer specifically acknowledge or guess at what the person was feeling? If so, was the interviewer's interpretation correct?
- What judgmental or empathetic words did the interviewers use?
- How was active listening evident?
- Was either of the interviewer's approaches too soft or too tough?
- Which approach do you like better and why?

Reprinted with permission from Morreale, M. J. (2015). *Developing clinical competence: A workbook for the OTA*. Thorofare, NJ: SLACK Incorporated.

Worksheet 1-12

People-First Language and Term Usage

People-first language and the appropriate use of diagnostic terms makes a profound difference on the focus and perception that others have on the individual with a disabling condition. In the list that follows, indicate whether the phrase is an appropriate (A) or inappropriate (I) use of descriptive language:

1. ______ the blind people
2. ______ the athetoid child
3. ______ crazy person
4. ______ individual who has served in combat
5. ______ person who has a disability
6. ______ victim of depression
7. ______ person who is crippled
8. ______ the child with leukemia is a heroic boy
9. ______ wheelchair user
10. ______ the epileptic
11. ______ Downs kid
12. ______ the schiz I am working with today
13. ______ the borderline
14. ______ the person with cancer
15. ______ the older man who is mentally retarded
16. ______ suffers from Alzheimer's
17. ______ wheelchair-bound
18. ______ senior who lives in an active adult community
19. ______ group of old people
20. ______ client is max assist

Worksheet 1-13

Better Communication

For each of the following scenarios, choose which of the two statements would likely be the better response from an occupational therapy practitioner. Write one or two sentences to explain your rationale for choosing each answer.

1. You go to a client's hospital room with the intent to transport the client to the OT room for therapy.
   ___ Would you like to come to therapy now?
   ___ It is time for occupational therapy now.
2. You are beginning an intervention session with a client who had hip replacement surgery.
   ___ Do you have hip pain today?
   ___ How are you today?
3. During an OT session, a client diagnosed with a cerebrovascular accident is having difficulty transferring to a commode and begins to cry.
   ___ What is making you cry?
   ___ Why are you so upset?
4. A child who is overweight is holding back tears and mentions the other students call him "fatty."
   ___ Just try to ignore them.
   ___ You feel sad because the other children are calling you names.
5. A 22-year-old female client with conservative religious beliefs mentions she is engaged and is looking forward to kissing her fiancé for the first time on her wedding day.
   ___ It is nice you have something special to look forward to.
   ___ How do you know you and your fiancé will be compatible?
6. An elderly client was admitted due to injuries sustained in a fall at home.
   ___ Tell me what happened to cause you to fall.
   ___ Did you fall because you were not using your walker?
7. An outpatient client with three young children mentions that her family does not celebrate Halloween because of their religious beliefs.
   ___ Do your kids feel like they are missing out?
   ___ I understand that many people prefer not to celebrate certain holidays.
8. An outpatient client states that she experienced pain while performing the new exercise program at home that the OTA told her to do.
   ___ Don't worry—no pain, no gain.
   ___ Show me how you are doing your exercises.
9. An OT working with a 3-year-old child in a preschool program would like the child to work on fine motor activities to improve play skills.
   ___ If you are a good girl today, you can pick a prize from the prize box.
   ___ If you complete these activities, I will give you a prize.
10. A client who sustained third-degree burns and has severe facial scars was admitted to a behavioral health program due to depression over his appearance. He is being evaluated by the OT.
    ___ I am sorry your scars make you feel depressed.
    ___ How have your injuries affected you?

Answers to Chapter 1 Worksheets

Worksheet 1-1: Initial Client Encounter

1. It is more respectful to call the elderly client "Mrs. Payshent" rather than by her first name.
2. *"Hey"* in the opening statement is not very professional. "Hello" or "Good morning" are more appropriate in this situation. Always use appropriate language for the particular context and geographical area.
3. *"How are things today?"* is vague, so the client responds about issues unrelated to her diagnosis.
4. The OT does not acknowledge the client's complaints.
5. The OT does not initially explain the purpose of the session, which is the initial evaluation.
6. The OT does not acknowledge her working relationship with the physician or PT and does not clearly explain the reason for the referral.
7. The OT uses unfamiliar abbreviations such as "OT" and "ADLs" with which the client is not familiar.
8. The explanation, *"help you do things like eat, bathe, and get dressed,"* does not reflect skilled occupational therapy. An aide or family member could simply help the client complete these tasks.
9. The OT does not adequately explain what occupational therapy is, such as the meaning of *occupation* or goals of improving the client's function. There also needs to be a better distinction between the disciplines of OT and PT.
10. Calling an adult client *"sweetie"* is disrespectful.
11. The OT is not using effective or efficient communication skills, which wastes time and does not convey professionalism.

Worksheet 1-2: It Looks Like You Play All Day

It is important to convey the distinct value of occupational therapy. You might discuss how real-life activities (such as cooking, carpentry, crafts, and wheelchair mobility) and the use of adaptive devices and techniques contribute to a client's occupational performance and goal attainment. You could also explain how occupational therapy practitioners use everyday objects to work on remediating different client factors and skills to improve a client's performance in daily living skills (occupations). For example, without breaching client confidentiality, you might relate how baking and playing checkers address specific cognitive/perceptual functions, such as sequencing, problem solving, or spatial relations. Performing activities while standing also help to restore balance, strength, and endurance, which are all necessary for ADL performance. You might also relate the use of preparatory media, such as therapy putty, cones, and pegs, to improve specific motor functions (e.g., elbow range of motion, grasp and release, or tip pinch) or relate them to other essential skills needed for daily activities, such as crossing midline. The OT department might also internally use this experience to reflect on whether enough occupation-based interventions are being regularly implemented.

Worksheet 1-3: Delegating Clients to an OTA

1. The OT uses an unfamiliar acronym "OTA" that requires clarification.
2. It is important to realize that an OTA should be referred to as an "occupational therapy practitioner" or "occupational therapy assistant" and *not* as a "therapist" (AOTA, 2010, 2014a; Centers for Medicare & Medicaid Services, 2008, 2012). The OT is considered a "therapist."
3. The OT does not explain role delineation regarding an OT and OTA.
4. The OT does not acknowledge her close working relationship with the OTA, Joe.
5. The OT does not acknowledge the ongoing supervisory process.

6. The client may perceive being "handed off" to an OTA as an insult. The OT indicates the client will see her working with other clients in the clinic instead.
7. The OT does not indicate that an OTA does have professional education, certification, and licensure.
8. It would be helpful to actually introduce the OTA in person to the client.
9. Although the OT indicates the OTA has "experience with this diagnosis," it is not clear whether this means personal experience (e.g., a family member or the OTA has had this diagnosis) or whether the OTA has actually worked with other clients who had this diagnosis.
10. The OT has not indicated that she will discuss the evaluation results and intervention plan with the OTA.
11. The OT does not ask whether the client has further questions.
12. The OT does not ask if the client is comfortable or needs anything while the client waits for the transporter.

Worksheet 1-4: Do You Know What You Are Doing?

In clinical practice, if you are expected to do a task you are very unsure of, you should discuss this with your supervisor (AOTA, 2014a). It is unethical to perform interventions for which you are not competent (AOTA, 2010, 2015). Assuming you are competent with a particular client task, your communicative style should convey confidence in your abilities and professionalism. However, an occupational therapy student or practitioner should never exaggerate or fabricate information about one's credentials or experience (AOTA, 2015). As an occupational therapy student, you might explain to the client that you have professional education in this area, are closely supervised, and would not do anything that would knowingly put the client in danger. As a new occupational therapist, you might add that you have fieldwork experience, have passed a national certification examination, and are licensed. If the client still appears concerned, you might ask another colleague or your supervisor to oversee or assist with the task.

Worksheet 1-5: Are You Really Sure You Can Do This?

For these kinds of situations, it is imperative that the client feel safe and that you demonstrate understanding of the client's concerns such as fear of falling or getting hurt. Your demeanor and communication should convey confidence and professionalism but you have an ethical obligation to only attempt tasks that are you are competent to perform (AOTA, 2010, 2015). When clients express concern about your ability to implement an intervention such as a transfer, you might convey your professional education, practice, and experience. Reassure the client that you would not do anything that would be unsafe. *However, never put yourself or your client at risk if you are at all unsure of your ability to transfer a client safely.* If a client is much bigger than you are, you might consider the option of having someone to assist with the transfer or, perhaps, take this opportunity to perform a cotreatment with the PT. *Know your facility's policies and procedures regarding transfers.* To prevent risk of injury, the facility might also require that more than one person be present or the use of a mechanical lift for specific client assist levels. When transferring a client, be sure to explain the procedure and also address the client's specific concerns such as, *"I will support your knee with my leg so it can't buckle"* or *"I have transferred a lot of people much bigger than you and will not let you fall. This transfer belt will ensure that you are safe."* If the client still appears concerned or, if there is likely potential for injury, you can ask another colleague or your supervisor to stand by or assist with the task. Sometimes humor can even be an effective method with select clients: *"I am a lot stronger than I look—this lab coat is hiding my huge muscles!"*

Worksheet 1-6: I Want to Walk

1. Sometimes clients have great difficulty accepting the reality of a situation. They may be scared, confused, angry, or in denial. You might acknowledge and validate the client's feelings, but without giving false hope. It is important that the OT convey a sense of respect and genuineness and use therapeutic communication techniques, such as active listening, asking open-ended questions, and primary accurate empathy. The following useful formula is suggested for OT practitioners to show empathy and understand feelings: "You feel ________ because ________" (Cole, 2012). You might say, *"You feel angry and overwhelmed because this is a huge life-changing event and you don't know how you will be able to cope. Is that correct?"* However, it is a balancing act to gently acknowledge the truth while avoiding causing hopelessness and despair. During the exchange you might

say, *"You had a very, very serious injury. We need to first focus on achieving your other goals during the next few weeks, like being able to feed yourself and operating a wheelchair"* or *"I am so sorry that your injury is not likely to make walking a feasible goal. However, we are all here to help you become as independent as possible. I can tell that you are very determined and will be able to manage many things on your own."* Of course, you may encourage the client to continue to express his feelings and to attend support groups and counseling as appropriate.

2. The intervention plan should include client-centered goals that the OT can reinforce with the client. You can acknowledge the client's frustration, *"You feel frustrated because you have to go through all this effort when you just want to be up and about."* You might then go on to say, *"Tomorrow we will be working on arm exercises so you can have enough strength and endurance to achieve your goal of using your walker safely at home"* or *"The doctor said you are not allowed to bend for several months because of your surgery. This equipment will allow you to work toward your goal of being independent again at home, like you were before your surgery. I am sure your wife would appreciate that too."*

Worksheet 1-7: This Feels Like Kindergarten

Make a sincere effort to incorporate activities and occupations into the client's intervention program whenever possible. Rather than presenting this client with the aforementioned preparatory task that offended him, this client may have benefited more from a "real-life" task such as handling soil for a gardening activity, using a sanding block to sand wood, or using a built-up pen for writing. If a client seems offended performing a preparatory task that is otherwise not normally age-appropriate, you might say something such as, *"It sounds like you might be feeling a bit insulted doing this. I'm sorry—that is not my intent."* Acknowledge that although the activity might appear "juvenile" on the surface, there is, indeed, a specific therapeutic purpose. When implementing preparatory interventions, you should make it a point to relate the task to the particular client factors and performance skills you are remediating. Also explain how this relates to occupational performance. In this case, the task was chosen to help reduce hypersensitivity and improve manipulation skills of the affected hand to enable occupations such as writing, using a computer keyboard, and performing hobbies.

Worksheet 1-8: Open-Ended and Closed-Ended Questions

Resources: (Davis, 2011; Rollnick et al., 2008).

Indicate if the question is open-ended (O), closed-ended (C), or neither (N):

1. __C__ What flavor of yogurt did you eat?
2. __N__ I respect your decision to do that.
3. __O__ Please explain the reason for making that choice.
4. __O__ How do you feel about that situation?
5. __C__ Did you like the book?
6. __C__ Would you be willing to tell me your life story?
7. __C__ How old are you?
8. __O__ What events were going on in the world the year you were born?
9. __N__ I guess that is a pretty tough situation.
10. __O__ What is your address?
11. __O__ Tell me from the beginning how your pain developed.
12. __C__ Have you been taking your medication?
13. __O__ How do you fit exercise into your daily routine?
14. __C__ How many hours per day do you study?
15. __C__ How long have you been feeling dizzy?
16. __N__ I see that you have been very busy knitting.
17. __O__ What happened to make you feel that way?

18. __C__ Did you fall in your house?
19. __N__ You drew a very interesting picture.
20. __O__ Tell me how you are feeling today.

Worksheet 1-9: Asking Open-Ended Questions

Here are some suggestions, although you may come up with other questions.

1. My shoulder hurts.
   Describe your shoulder pain or *What does your shoulder pain feel like?*
   What makes your shoulder pain better or worse?
   How does the pain affect your daily activities?
   When does the pain occur?
2. I can't do anything right.
   What do you mean by that?
   How long have you felt this way?
   Describe a situation that causes you to feel that way.
   What would you like to change?
3. I fell in my apartment.
   How long ago did you fall in your apartment?
   What happened after you fell?
   When did you fall in your apartment?
   What might you have done differently to prevent falling?
4. My life is a charade.
   What do you mean by that statement?
   How is your life a charade?
   What are your plans for the future?
   What are some things you wish you had done differently?
5. I never thought I would turn out like this.
   How do you see yourself?
   How would you describe the way that other people see you?
   How do you feel about ... (e.g., your arrest, addiction to cocaine, homelessness).
   How do you think you could turn things around?
   What are your goals?
   What would you like to change?
6. My hand is useless.
   What specific problems are you having with your hand?
   When did you start having difficulty with your hand?
   How does your hand condition affect your daily activities?
   What types of things are hard to do with your hand?
7. I'm so confused.
   What things are confusing you?
   What else are you feeling?
   What would help you to understand?
   How can you get more information?

8. I lost my job.
   What are your plans?
   How does that affect you and your family?
   Why do you think you lost your job?
   What happened that caused you to lose your job?
   What might have happened differently to avoid getting fired?
9. I hate school.
   What do you hate about school?
   What would you like to change about school?
   Describe what makes you feel that way about school.
   How long have you felt this way?
10. I am no good in gym class.
   What specific things in gym class are hard for you?
   Tell me how that makes you feel.
   What would you like to be better at?
   What are some things you feel you are good at in school?

Worksheet 1-10: Eliciting Information Efficiently

Clearly, in this scenario, the OT is not using appropriate open-ended questions to elicit the desired information in a timely manner. Cole (2012, p. 74) suggests that to prevent a simple yes or no response, the OT practitioner should avoid the following as question starters: *do you*, *can you*, *would you*, *are you*, or *have you*. Here are some additional suggestions for improving this client interaction:

1. It is more respectful to call the client "Mrs. Jones" rather than "Jean."
2. The OT should explain the purpose of the session.
3. The OT should demonstrate empathy and address Mrs. Jones's concerns when the client reports feeling "terrible" or when the client expresses frustration regarding spilling her food.
4. The OT should acknowledge that the client has particular feelings, but, instead, the OT insinuates that Mrs. Jones should not feel that way.
5. The OT should use open-ended rather than closed-ended questions.
6. The OT needs to phrase questions more clearly to target the desired information in a concise manner.

Here is the same exchange in a more useful format:

OT: *Hello, Mrs. Jones, I am Nick, an occupational therapist. Your regular occupational therapist, Karen, has the day off. Karen asked me to work with you today to discuss your living situation so we can start planning how you will manage at home. It is very nice to meet you. How are you today?*
Client: *Terrible.*
OT: *What is making you feel terrible?*
Client: *Don't you know how weak I am? I can't do anything!*
OT: *You are feeling very frustrated because your illness is making everything more difficult for you. Is that correct?* [Client nods her head "yes".] *However, I can tell by the way you were just feeding yourself that you are a very determined person. I am sure you will make a lot of progress here.*
Client: *Do you really think so?*
OT: *Absolutely. Now please tell me about your living situation—what type of place do you live in, and who might be around to help?*

(continued on next page)

Client: *I live with my husband in a condo. My daughter lives a few miles away, and I have a good friend who lives next door to me.*

OT: *That's great. I would like to know more about the physical layout of your condo, such as the number of steps and how the bathroom is situated.*

Client: *I have 3 steps outside and about 10 steps to the second floor. There is a powder room on the first level and a full bathroom on the second level, next to my bedroom.*

The OT would continue interviewing the client in this manner until all the desired information is obtained.

Worksheet 1-11: Interaction Between an OT and an Elementary School Student

1. Schools strive to create a welcoming and safe environment for students. Policies are created to prevent harassment, intimidation, and bullying (HIB) of students, and a variety of resources are available (New Jersey Department of Education, 2010; Ohio Department of Education, 2014). This OT is intimidating the student with language that is unacceptable. Scaring the student by threatening, *"I will tie you to the chair"* and *"I will not let you see your parents"* may cause emotional harm to the student. The OT's behavior is clearly unprofessional, unethical, and may result in severe disciplinary action or firing.
2. The OT is not maintaining professional composure as she is yelling at the student.
3. Do not ask a client if he or she "wants" to do a task if the answer "no" would be unacceptable.
4. It may be better to offer a specific choice to the student, such as: *"What color pencil do you want to use today, the red or green one?"* or *"Choose one of these two worksheets to work on today."*
5. It might be better for the OT to present the activity more positively, such as: *"Let's show your parents how much better you are doing with your handwriting"* or *"We are going to do this worksheet in pretty rainbow colors. You can use a different colored pencil for each line."*
6. By using appropriate verbal and nonverbal communication, the OT must "set the tone" that he or she is an authority figure that deserves respect. However, it is not productive or professional to lose one's temper, yell, or get into an argument with a student.
7. Do not call a student "bad." It is the child's specific behavior and language that are unacceptable. The OT might say, *"You are talking back to me and not following directions. That is not acceptable."*
8. Incorporate therapeutic use of self and techniques, such as behavior modification or making the activity into a "game." Here are some examples:

   "If you form all the letters correctly now, I will give you a special prize today."

   or

   "If you can finish this worksheet before the timer goes off, I will give you an extra sticker."

   or

   "After you finish this worksheet, I will put it on my bulletin board because I am proud of how hard you have been working on your handwriting this month."

   or

   "You feel writing is boring because it is not easy for you and you don't like to practice—is that right? I understand. Let's just work on this for 10 minutes and then we will do something fun."

Worksheet 1-12: People-First Language and Term Usage

People-first language and appropriate use of diagnostic terms make a profound difference on the focus and perception that others have on the individual with a disabling condition. In the list that follows, indicate if the phrase is an appropriate (A) or inappropriate (I) use of descriptive language:

1. _I_ the blind people—*This should read "The persons who have blindness"*
2. _I_ the athetoid child—*This should read "The child who has athetoid cerebral palsy"*

3. __I__ crazy person—*This should read "The person who has serious mental illness"*
4. __A__ individual who has served in combat
5. __A__ person who has a disability
6. __I__ victim of depression—*People should not be referred to as victims of a disease. A more empowering statement would be "the person who has depression"*
7. __I__ person who is crippled—*The word* crippled *is no longer appropriate for use in conversation. More appropriate terms are "The person who has a disability" or "The client who is unable to ambulate."*
8. __I__ the child with leukemia is a heroic boy—*People facing a disease process do not typically describe themselves as heroes; they are simply dealing with a disease.*
9. __A__ wheelchair user
10. __I__ the epileptic—*People should not be referred to as a diagnosis. It would be better to say, "The client who has epilepsy."*
11. __I__ Downs kid—*This is not people-first language. It would be better to say "The child who has Down syndrome."*
12. __I__ the schiz I am working with today—*This is not people-first and also is a derogatory way to say "schizophrenia."*
13. __I__ the borderline—*This is not people-first and dehumanizes individuals with the diagnosis of borderline personality disorder.*
14. __A__ the person with cancer
15. __I__ the older man who is mentally retarded—*Although this is people-first language, the term* intellectual disability *is preferred* (American Psychiatric Association, 2013; Harris, 2013).
16. __I__ suffers from Alzheimer's—*It is more appropriate to say the "person who is diagnosed with Alzheimer disease."*
17. __I__ wheelchair bound—*The correct term is* wheelchair user.
18. __A__ senior who lives in an active adult community
19. __I__ group of old people—*Terms such as* seniors, mature adults, *and* elderly clients *are more respectful.*
20. __I__ client is max assist—*The client is not an assist level. It is better to say "Client requires max assist for ..."* (Morreale & Borcherding, 2013).

Worksheet 1-13: Better Communication

For each of the following scenarios, choose which of the two statements would likely be the better response from an OT.

1. You go to a client's hospital room with the intent to transport the client to the OT room for therapy.

   ___ Would you like to come to therapy now?

   __*__ It is time for occupational therapy now.

   Do not ask a question for which the answer "no" would be unacceptable. However, clients do have the right to refuse therapy.

2. You are beginning an intervention session with a client who had hip replacement surgery.

   ___ Do you have hip pain today?

   __*__ How are you today?

   An open-ended question would elicit more information rather than just a simple "yes" or "no" response.

3. During an OT session, a client diagnosed with a cerebrovascular accident is having difficulty transferring to a commode and begins to cry.

   __*__ What is making you cry?

   ___ Why are you so upset?

   The word why may sound judgmental and give the impression the therapist is insinuating the client should not be feeling the way he or she is feeling (Cole, 2012).

4. A child who is overweight is holding back tears and mentions the other students call him "fatty."

   ____ Just try to ignore them.

   _*_ You feel sad because the other children are calling you names.

   An empathic response acknowledges the child's feelings. The OT must also adhere to facility policies and procedures regarding reporting of the bullying.

5. A 22-year-old female client with conservative religious beliefs mentions she is engaged and is looking forward to kissing her fiancé for the first time on her wedding day.

   _*_ It is nice you have something special to look forward to.

   ____ How do you know you and your fiancé will be compatible?

   It is important to respect this client's moral and religious beliefs and not inject personal bias.

6. An elderly client was admitted due to injuries sustained in a fall at home.

   _*_ Tell me what happened to cause you to fall.

   ____ Did you fall because you were not using your walker?

   In this scenario, an open question would sound less judgmental and elicit more information rather than just a yes or no response.

7. An outpatient client with three young children mentions that her family does not celebrate Halloween because of their religious beliefs.

   ____ Do your kids feel like they are missing out?

   _*_ I understand that many people prefer not to celebrate certain holidays.

   It is important to respect this client's moral and/or religious beliefs and not express personal bias.

8. An outpatient client states that she experienced pain while performing the new exercise program at home that the OTA told her to do.

   ____ Don't worry—no pain, no gain.

   _*_ Show me how you are doing your exercises.

   It is important to ascertain whether the client is performing the exercises accurately and safely. The OT also needs to determine whether the pain is typical and expected or is a concern that needs to be addressed.

9. An OT working with a 3-year-old child in a preschool program would like the child to work on fine-motor activities to improve play skills.

   ____ If you are a good girl today, you can pick a prize from the prize box.

   _*_ If you complete these activities, I will give you a prize.

   Do not label a child as good or bad. Focus on the behavior instead.

10. A client who sustained third-degree burns and has severe facial scars was admitted to a behavioral health program due to depression over his appearance. He is being evaluated by the OT.

    ____ I am sorry your scars make you feel depressed.

    _*_ How have your injuries affected you?

    An open question will help elicit the client's feelings rather than reinforcing the negativity of the scars.

References

American Occupational Therapy Association. (2010). Standards of practice for occupational therapy. *American Journal of Occupational Therapy, 64*(Suppl. 6), S106–S111.

American Occupational Therapy Association. (2011). The philosophical base of occupational therapy. *American Journal of Occupational Therapy, 65*(Suppl. 6), S65.

American Occupational Therapy Association. (2014a). Guidelines for supervision, roles, and responsibilities during the delivery of occupational therapy services. *American Journal of Occupational Therapy, 68*(Suppl. 3), S16–S22.

American Occupational Therapy Association. (2014b). Occupational therapy practice framework: Domain and process (3rd ed.). *American Journal of Occupational Therapy, 68*(Suppl. 1), S1–S48.

American Occupational Therapy Association. (2015). Occupational therapy code of ethics (2015). *American Journal of Occupational Therapy, 69*(Suppl. 3), 6913410030. http://dx.doi.org/10.5014/ajot.2015.696S03

American Psychiatric Association. (2013). *Diagnostic and Statistical Manual of Mental Disorders Fifth Edition*. Arlington, VA: American Psychiatric Association.

Centers for Medicare & Medicaid Services. (2008). *Medicare Benefit Policy Manual* (Pub. 100-02: Ch. 15, Section 230.2). Baltimore: Centers for Medicare & Medicaid Services. Retrieved from http://www.cms.gov/Regulations-and-Guidance/Guidance/Manuals/Downloads/bp102c15.pdf

Centers for Medicare & Medicaid Services. (2012). *Medicare Benefit Policy Manual* (Pub. 100-02: Ch. 15, Section 220). Baltimore: Centers for Medicare & Medicaid Services. Retrieved from http://www.cms.gov/Regulations-and-Guidance/Guidance/Manuals/Downloads/bp102c15.pdf

Cole, M. (2012). *Group dynamics in occupational therapy: The theoretical basis and practice application of group intervention* (4th ed.). Thorofare, NJ: SLACK Incorporated.

Davis, C. (2011). *Patient practitioner interaction: An experiential manual for developing the art of heath care* (5th ed.). Thorofare, NJ: SLACK Incorporated.

Drench, M. E., Noonan, A.C., Sharby, N., & Ventura, S. H. (2012). *Psychosocial aspects of health care* (3rd ed.). Upper Saddle River, NJ: Pearson Education Incorporated.

Froehlich, J., Roy, M. C., Augustoni, B., Arsenault, A. K., & Eldredge, J. (2014a). Effective communication. In K. Jacobs, N. MacRae, & K. Sladyk (Eds.), *Occupational therapy essentials for clinical competence* (2nd ed., pp. 85–112) Thorofare, NJ: SLACK Incorporated.

Froehlich, J., Roy, M. C., Augustoni, B., Eldredge, J., & Arsenault, A. K. (2014b). Therapeutic use of self. In K. Jacobs, N. MacRae, & K. Sladyk (Eds.), *Occupational therapy essentials for clinical competence* (2nd ed., pp. 113–125). Thorofare, NJ: SLACK Incorporated.

Harris, J. C. (2013). New terminology for mental retardation in DSM-5 and ICD-11. *Current Opinion in Psychiatry, 26*, 260–262. Retrieved from http://www.medscape.com/viewarticle/782769

Morreale, M. J. (2015). *Developing clinical competence: A workbook for the OTA*. Thorofare, NJ: SLACK Incorporated.

Morreale, M. J., & Borcherding, S. (2013). *The OTA's guide to documentation: Writing SOAP notes* (3rd ed.). Thorofare, NJ: SLACK Incorporated.

New Jersey Department of Education. (2010). *Harassment, intimidation, & bullying (HIB)*. Retrieved from http://www.state.nj.us/education/students/safety/behavior/hib

Ohio Department of Education. (2014). *Anti-harassment, intimidation and bullying resources*. Retrieved from http://education.ohio.gov/Topics/Other-Resources/School-Safety/Safe-and-Supportive-Learning/Anti-Harassment-Intimidation-and-Bullying-Resource

Rollnick, S., Miller, W., & Butler, C. (2008). *Motivational interviewing in health care: Helping patients change behavior.* New York: Guilford Press.

Taylor, R. (2008). *The intentional relationship: Occupational therapy and use of self.* Philadelphia: F.A. Davis.

Chapter 2

Demonstrating Professionalism

Professional behaviors for occupational therapy practitioners include traits such as dependability, punctuality, a well-groomed appearance, and appropriate demeanor. Occupational therapists (OTs) and occupational therapy assistants (OTAs) must also meet professional standards for attire, workplace conduct, oral and written communication, and ethical behavior. In addition, occupational therapy practitioners must demonstrate good time management, organizational skills, and abide by the many standards in place to ensure safety. This chapter presents worksheets, and learning activities to help you identify and describe professional behaviors and skills necessary for fieldwork and clinical practice. Answers to worksheet exercises are provided at the end of the chapter.

Contents

Morreale, M. J., & Amini, D.
The Occupational Therapist's Workbook for Ensuring Clinical Competence (pp. 35-78).

Worksheet 2-1

Scheduling Fieldwork

Always follow your academic fieldwork coordinator's specific instructions regarding the scheduling of fieldwork—for example, whether you should contact your fieldwork educator by phone or e-mail.

For this exercise, consider the following information when answering the first two questions. *You have just been assigned Level I fieldwork for the spring semester. Your academic fieldwork coordinator provided the facility name and address, name of your fieldwork educator, a contact phone number, and e-mail address. The fieldwork consists of 3 full days that do not have to be consecutive, but must be completed by May 15. It is now February 1.*

1. You would really like to complete your fieldwork during spring break (the third week of April) when you do not have classes. When should you first attempt to contact the fieldwork site to set up your fieldwork dates?
   A. One week before you plan on completing the fieldwork
   B. One month before you plan on completing the fieldwork
   C. Beginning of February
   D. Beginning of March
   E. Beginning of April

2. You called your fieldwork site as directed, but your fieldwork educator was not available at that time. You left a message with the department secretary asking the fieldwork educator to call you back. It is 2 days later, and you have still not heard back. Which of the following is your best course of action?
   A. Contact your academic fieldwork coordinator
   B. Wait another day or two for the fieldwork educator to call back
   C. Wait another week for the fieldwork educator to call back
   D. Call again and leave another message if your fieldwork educator is again unavailable
   E. Call again and ask to speak with the rehabilitation director if your fieldwork educator is still unavailable

3. You contact your fieldwork educator by phone, who informs you that you have been assigned a different fieldwork educator at that site. Which of the following is your best course of action?
   A. Thank the person and state that you will need to cancel the fieldwork
   B. Thank the person but afterward ask your academic fieldwork coordinator for a new fieldwork site
   C. Ask to speak with that new fieldwork educator and notify your academic fieldwork coordinator of the change
   D. Tell the person on the phone that the change is not acceptable because you need to complete the fieldwork exactly as it was assigned to you
   E. Ask to speak with the rehabilitation director

4. You contacted your fieldwork educator several weeks ago to schedule your Level I fieldwork. The fieldwork is supposed to begin tomorrow, but you've just become ill with a bad stomach virus that is causing severe nausea and diarrhea. Which of the following is your best course of action?
   A. Contact the site immediately to inform your fieldwork educator that you are ill and must reschedule the fieldwork
   B. Take some medicine, get a good night's sleep, and attend fieldwork even if you are still having symptoms
   C. Request that your academic fieldwork coordinator notify the site about your pending absence tomorrow
   D. Ask a family member or friend to call the site and notify your fieldwork educator about your pending absence tomorrow
   E. Bring a doctor's note to fieldwork tomorrow to prove your illness and ask your fieldwork educator if you should stay or not

Worksheet 2-1 (continued)

Scheduling Fieldwork

5. A week before you are to begin Level II fieldwork, your fieldwork educator calls to inform you that, because several staff members are on sick leave, your fieldwork must be rescheduled to a month later than you were originally scheduled to begin. This will conflict with your next Level II fieldwork. Which of the following is your best course of action?
   A. Thank the person for calling, but state that you must cancel fieldwork at that site
   B. Thank the person for calling, but state you will need to discuss this with your academic fieldwork coordinator
   C. Let the fieldwork educator know this will inconvenience you greatly and indicate it is unfair this happened so close to your scheduled starting date
   D. Insist strongly that you must complete the fieldwork during the exact dates that were assigned to you.
   E. Ask to speak with the rehabilitation director

6. You contact your fieldwork educator, Carrie Capable, by e-mail. Carrie sends the following reply: "Dear Student, I am sorry, but the rehabilitation director has already assigned another fieldwork student to me at this time. However, I have forwarded your message to Ellen Ethical, OTR, who will be your supervisor instead. She will contact you by e-mail today or tomorrow." Which of the following is your best course of action?
   A. Send an e-mail to the rehabilitation director regarding this situation
   B. Reply by e-mail to thank Carrie Capable, but also state that you will need to cancel the fieldwork
   C. Reply by e-mail to thank Carrie Capable and then wait several days for the new fieldwork educator to contact you
   D. Call the fieldwork site and ask to speak with Ellen Ethical today as you do not have her e-mail address
   E. Reply by e-mail and ask Carrie Capable if it is possible for her to switch students

7. As directed, you send an e-mail to your fieldwork educator to set up your Level I fieldwork. It is a week later and you have not gotten any reply. Which of the following is your best course of action?
   A. Resend the original e-mail to your fieldwork educator at this time
   B. Wait several more days for the fieldwork educator to reply
   C. Send another e-mail to the fieldwork educator asking why that person has not replied and whether there is a problem with the fieldwork
   D. Send an e-mail to the rehabilitation director and copy it to the fieldwork educator and your academic fieldwork coordinator
   E. Send an e-mail to your academic fieldwork coordinator asking for assistance

8. You contacted your fieldwork educator several weeks ago to schedule your Level I fieldwork. The fieldwork is supposed to begin tomorrow, but the weather forecast calls for severe weather. You are nervous about driving in these weather conditions. Which of the following is your best course of action?
   A. Contact the site immediately to inform your fieldwork educator that you are not able to attend fieldwork tomorrow
   B. Get a good night's sleep and check the weather forecast in the morning to decide whether you will attend fieldwork
   C. Request that your academic fieldwork coordinator notify the site about your pending absence tomorrow.
   D. Follow your college's policy regarding fieldwork absences
   E. Have your parent or guardian call to inform the fieldwork educator that you are not allowed to drive in severe weather

Worksheet 2-1 (continued)

Scheduling Fieldwork

9. You are supposed to begin Level I fieldwork today at 8:30 a.m. However, you are stuck in traffic and will not be arriving until about 9:15 a.m. Which of the following is your best course of action?
   A. Once you arrive late, apologize profusely and promise it will not happen again
   B. Only when it is safe to do so, attempt to call, text, or e-mail your fieldwork educator to notify the person that you are delayed
   C. Turn around to return home and reschedule fieldwork for another day
   D. When you arrive at fieldwork, act as if nothing happened and hope that no one notices you were late
   E. Once you arrive, tell the fieldwork educator it really wasn't your fault that you were late and complain about all the traffic you encountered

10. Your Level I fieldwork is scheduled to begin tomorrow. However, your fieldwork educator contacts you today to inform you that he needs to take the day off and must reschedule fieldwork to the following week. This change will cause you to be late handing in your fieldwork paper and timesheet to the academic fieldwork coordinator. Which of the following is your best course of action?
    A. Tell the fieldwork educator that this is not fair because you scheduled the fieldwork way ahead of time and will now get a bad grade in class
    B. Firmly insist that you be assigned to another person tomorrow so you can complete the fieldwork on time.
    C. Once the conversation is completed, hang up and call your fieldwork educator's supervisor
    D. Reschedule fieldwork and contact your academic fieldwork coordinator to explain the situation
    E. Start crying and hope the fieldwork educator will do something to help you

Worksheet 2-2

Fieldwork Phone Interview

You must call your fieldwork educator as directed to set up your Level I fieldwork schedule. You have never been to this facility before and are not very familiar with the area. For each of the items below, indicate with a Y (yes) or N (no) if it is an appropriate topic for you to ask during the initial phone contact.

1. ___ Directions to the fieldwork site
2. ___ Start and end times for the day
3. ___ Where to meet in the facility
4. ___ If the facility is in a "bad" area
5. ___ Date(s) to complete fieldwork
6. ___ Amount of time for lunch
7. ___ Permission to come in late because you have to drive your kids to school
8. ___ Whether a lab coat is required
9. ___ Wearing of sneakers
10. ___ Availability of coffee or tea in the morning
11. ___ Permission to use your cell phone so you can monitor your children
12. ___ Permission to come in late or leave early to accommodate your bus or train schedule
13. ___ Permission to leave early to pick your children up from school
14. ___ Permission to leave early due to a dental appointment to get your teeth cleaned
15. ___ Permission to wear a head covering if required by your religion
16. ___ What paperwork to bring
17. ___ Whether it will be a particularly difficult fieldwork because a classmate failed fieldwork there last semester
18. ___ Reimbursement for gas and tolls
19. ___ If the fieldwork will require a lot of homework
20. ___ Types of diagnoses you will observe

Reprinted with permission from Morreale, M. J. (2015). *Developing clinical competence: A workbook for the OTA*. Thorofare, NJ: SLACK, Incorporated.

Worksheet 2-3

Stress Reduction for That First Day

Your fieldwork is scheduled to begin next week. List at least 10 things you can do ahead of time to help reduce your stress level and arrive on time your first day.

1.

2.

3.

4.

5.

6.

7.

8.

9.

10.

Worksheet 2-4

Fieldwork Attire

Imagine you have been assigned fieldwork at an inpatient medical setting. You have contacted your fieldwork educator, and this person indicated that your client interventions will primarily consist of self-care occupations, transfers, and therapeutic exercises. Your fieldwork educator also informed you that the dress code is "business casual with a lab coat." For each of the following items listed, indicate with a Y (yes) or N (no) whether it is an appropriate choice for a fieldwork student to wear at this site. Explain why you chose each of your answers.

1. ____ Scrubs ____________________
2. ____ Sneakers ____________________
3. ____ Flat, closed-toe shoes with rubber soles ____________________
4. ____ Dressy flip-flops ____________________
5. ____ Low-heeled leather sandals ____________________
6. ____ Heavy perfume/cologne/aftershave ____________________
7. ____ Stud earrings ____________________
8. ____ Eyebrow piercing ____________________
9. ____ Head covering ____________________
10. ____ Visible underwear above pants waistband ____________________
11. ____ Neatly pressed dark jeans ____________________
12. ____ Khaki pants and a polo shirt ____________________
13. ____ Plain black sweatpants ____________________

Worksheet 2-4 (continued)

Fieldwork Attire

14. ___ Sport T-shirt/jersey ___

15. ___ Button-down Oxford shirt ___

16. ___ Dress slacks ___

17. ___ Cargo pants ___

18. ___ Polo shirt with collar and small designer logo emblem ___

19. ___ 32-inch plain gold necklace ___

20. ___ Charm bracelet ___

21. ___ Well-groomed, long artificial nails without polish ___

22. ___ Dark gray suit ___

23. ___ Name tag ___

24. ___ Solid-color leggings ___

25. ___ Solid-color hoodie ___

Reprinted with permission from Morreale, M. J. (2015). *Developing clinical competence: A workbook for the OTA*. Thorofare, NJ: SLACK Incorporated.

Learning Activity 2-1: Presentation and Demeanor

Kaser and Clark (2000) developed this next exercise to help participants improve awareness of how one is perceived and how one judges others on the basis of appearance and behavior. This exercise is a useful tool to facilitate understanding of the direct effects of one's demeanor, language, posture, and presentation, and to explore how pre-existing attitudes and values affect professionalism (Kaser & Clark, 2000). The steps for completing the activity are as follows:

Process

1. The instructor distributes worksheets.
2. Participants instructed to look about the room, observe other participants. Participants may walk about but refrain from talking.
3. Participants encouraged to observe body language, clothing, hairstyles, or any feature that would form an opinion.
4. Participants encouraged to make note of a previous event in their life that caused them to formulate a certain opinion/judgment/belief about the participant they are observing.
5. After 30 minutes observing time, instructor begins to encourage participants to disclose their observations and the reasons for their observations/opinions.
6. The worksheets have been constructed to elicit positive characteristics. However, the instructor should be sensitive to certain observations that may emerge and be prepared to handle comments that some of the participants may find discouraging/offensive.

Judging a Book by the Cover

1. Find someone who looks like they enjoy children.
   A. Reason:

2. Find someone who looks like they play sports.
   A. Reason:

3. Find an animal lover. One who takes care of and raises animals.
   A. Reason:

4. Find a person who looks ambitious. One who gets the job done.
   A. Reason:

5. Find one who appreciates classical music.
   A. Reason:

6. Find the one who likes modern rock and roll music.
   A. Reason:

Learning Activity 2-1: Presentation and Demeanor (continued)

7. Find someone who looks daring and would appreciate exciting activities.
   A. Reason:

8. Find an interesting conversationalist. Someone you could listen to.
   A. Reason:

9. Find a gourmet cook or one who would enjoy gourmet cooking.
   A. Reason:

10. Find a sophisticated-looking person. Go for the refined look.
    A. Reason:

11. Who looks intelligent in this group (you cannot list yourself).
    A. Reason:

Reprinted with permission from Kaser, J., & Clark, E. N. (2000). *Developing professional behaviors*. Thorofare, NJ: SLACK Incorporated.

Worksheet 2-5

Professional Behaviors

For each of the following professional behaviors, list the professional characteristics or traits it represents (e.g., attention to detail, reliability, initiative, veracity, respect).

	Professional Behavior	***Professional Characteristic***
1.	Administering a standardized assessment accurately	*Example: Service competency Attention to detail*
2.	Offering to put your fieldwork educator's clinical notes back into the clients' charts without being asked	
3.	Admitting you did not complete your notes on time, apologizing, and offering to stay late or come in early to complete them	
4.	Arranging self-feeding interventions predawn or after dusk for an occupational therapy client who is fasting during Ramadan	
5.	Switching a client's treatment time so it does not conflict with physical therapy	
6.	Addressing an adult client by using "Mr." or "Mrs." and client's surname	
7.	Not refusing to work with a client who is positive for HIV or tuberculosis	
8.	Writing a thank-you note to your fieldwork educator after your interview	
9.	Arriving to your fieldwork interview 5 minutes early	
10.	Asking a senator to vote for a proposed law that improves access to mental health services	
11.	Cleaning up water that you notice on the floor near the hydrocollator	
12.	Preparing and assembling all the information packets in time for a workshop that the occupational therapy department is sponsoring	
13.	Not billing Medicare B for a session consisting only of skilled instruction lasting 7 minutes	
14.	Closing the computer screen after entering client information	
15.	Nodding and maintaining eye contact when a client is answering questions	
16.	Participating in an event to raise awareness of a specific disease	
17.	Being the "go-to" person for solving problems regarding manual wheelchairs	
18.	Not dating a cute client your age who asks you out	
19.	Ensuring that all the OTA's notes are cosigned when required by law or facility policy	
20.	Knocking on a closed door before entering the client's room or an examination room	
21.	Discussing a client's discharge plan with the PT and social worker	
22.	Acknowledging that the client feels disappointed when his or her son did not come for a visit	
23.	Not complaining when you have to stay late one day to order a client's durable medical equipment (DME) before the client is discharged home	

Worksheet 2-5 (continued)

Professional Behaviors

	Professional Behavior	Professional Characteristic
24.	Writing several drafts of a SOAP (subjective, objective, assessment plan) note to ensure an accurate, professional presentation before showing it to your fieldwork educator	
25.	Reporting suspected child or elder abuse to appropriate personnel/agencies to prevent further harm to the individual	
26.	Arranging for an interpreter when the client speaks a different language than you do	
27.	Ensuring that the OTAs you are supervising receive appropriate levels of supervision	
28.	Arranging for more copies when you take the last client handout from the file cabinet	

Worksheet 2-6

Ethics Sanctions

Occupational therapy practitioners who demonstrate unethical behavior may face disciplinary action at work and, possibly, legal consequences depending on the nature and severity of the behavior. In addition, unethical behavior may result in sanctions issued by state licensure boards, the National Board for Certification in Occupational Therapy ([NBCOT] 2009, 2011), and/or the American Occupational Therapy Association ([AOTA] 2015, 2014a). Define the following disciplinary action terms and put them in order from less severe to more severe.

A. Probation
B. Reprimand
C. Revocation
D. Suspension
E. Censure

1. ______________________________

2. ______________________________

3. ______________________________

4. ______________________________

5. ______________________________

Reprinted with permission from Morreale, M. J. (2015). *Developing clinical competence: A workbook for the OTA*. Thorofare, NJ: SLACK Incorporated.

Ethical Decision Making

Kornblau and Burkhardt (2012) developed a process for ethical decision making titled Clinical Ethics & Legal Issues Bait All Therapists Equally (CELIBATE) Method for Analyzing Ethical Dilemmas. This approach, summarized in Figure 2-1, helps health practitioners analyze ethical dilemmas by considering the legal aspects of the situation along with other factors. In addition to regulations regarding occupational therapy licensure and scope of practice, situations may be influenced by various laws addressing areas such as child/elder/spousal abuse, insurance fraud, sexual harassment, confidentiality, discrimination, theft, assault and/or battery, and malpractice (Kornblau & Burkhardt, 2012).

1. **What is the problem?**
2. **What are the facts of the situation?**
3. **Who are the interested parties?**
   - Facility
   - Patient
   - Other therapists
   - Observers
   - Payers
   - Others
4. **What is the nature of their interest? Why is this a problem?**
   - Professional
   - Personal
   - Business
   - Economic
   - Intellectual
   - Societal
5. **Is there an ethical issue?**
   - Does it violate a professional code of ethics? Which section(s)?
   - Does it violate moral, social, or religious values?
6. **Is there a legal issue?**
   - Practice act/licensure law and regulations? Which section(s)?
   - Check the CELIBATE Checklist for other possible legal issues.
7. **Do I need more information?**
   - What information do I need?
   - Is there a treatment, policy, procedure, law, regulation, or document that I do not know about?
   - Can I obtain a copy of the treatment, policy, procedure, law, regulation, or document in writing?
   - Do I need to research the issue further? What does the literature say?
   - Do I need to consult with a mentor, an expert in this area, and/or a lawyer?
8. **Brainstorm possible action steps.**
9. **Analyze action steps.**
   - Eliminate the obviously wrong or impossible choices.
   - How will each alternative affect my patients, other interested parties, and me?
   - Do my choices abide by the applicable code of ethics?
   - Do my choices abide by the applicable practice act and regulations?
   - Are my choices consistent with my moral, religious, and social beliefs?
10. **Choose a course of action (considering ethical principles and philosophies).**
    - The Rotary Four-Way Test:
      1. Is it the *truth*?
      2. Is is *fair* to all concerned?
      3. Will it build *goodwill* and *better friendships*?
      4. Will it be *beneficial* to all concerned?
    - Is it win-win?
    - How do I feel about my course of action?

Figure 2-1. CELIBATE method for analyzing ethical dilemmas. (Reprinted with permission from Kornblau, B. L., & Burkhardt, A. [2012]. *Ethics in rehabilitation: A clinical perspective* [2nd ed.]. Thorofare, NJ: SLACK Incorporated.)

Worksheet 2-7

Ethical Behavior

Determine whether the following statements are true (T) or false (F).

1. T___ F___ If an OT is found guilty of committing a severe unethical act, the AOTA can take away the OT's license to practice.
2. T___ F___ An occupational therapy volunteer can report an OT's unethical behavior to the NBCOT.
3. T___ F___ An occupational therapy student should begin following the Code of Ethics when Level II fieldwork commences.
4. T___ F___ An occupational therapy practitioner who commits an unethical act could have his or her name listed publicly as an ethics violator by the AOTA or NBCOT.
5. T___ F___ AOTA guidelines take precedence over state laws.
6. T___ F___ Committing a felony may limit a person's ability to practice occupational therapy.
7. T___ F___ If an occupational therapy practitioner did not know about a particular law, the OT or OTA cannot be sanctioned for an unethical act that violates that law.
8. T___ F___ An occupational therapy state license is only affected by occupational therapy ethical infractions and not other legal violations that an OT might have committed.
9. T___ F___ An occupational therapy practitioner has an obligation to report a colleague's unethical behavior only if it is occupational therapy related.
10. T___ F___ The NBCOT implements sanctions within 1 week when a very serious complaint is lodged against an occupational therapy practitioner.
11. T___ F___ A state can suspend an occupational therapy aide's license for unethical behavior in an occupational therapy clinic.
12. T___ F___ A person visiting a hospital patient can file a complaint with an occupational therapy state licensure board.
13. T___ F___ An OT accused of practicing under the influence of drugs automatically loses NBCOT certification if reported to NBCOT.
14. T___ F___ An OT receiving 6 months' probation from an OT state licensing board cannot practice occupational therapy for the entire 6 months.
15. T___ F___ An OT sanctioned by the NBCOT cannot appeal the decision.
16. T___ F___ Minimizing a client's progress when documenting is not considered unethical if it helps the person receive essential therapy services from the insurance company.
17. T___ F___ An occupational therapy practitioner cannot be disciplined by the AOTA, NBCOT, and an occupational therapy state licensure board all at the same time.
18. T___ F___ It is acceptable for an OT to refuse to treat a person with HIV if the therapist is concerned about catching the disease.
19. T___ F___ A therapist censured by an occupational therapy state licensure board cannot practice occupational therapy during the time of the censure.
20. T___ F___ When an occupational therapy licensure board's sanction is revocation, the therapist can only practice occupational therapy with daily, direct supervision.

Learning Activity 2-2: Unprofessional Conduct

For each of the following negative behaviors of an occupational therapy practitioner, list several possible consequences. Consider how the actions might create specific safety concerns or problems, affect relationships with client or colleagues, or merit disciplinary action by not complying with facility policy and procedures or professional standards, such as the AOTA's *Code of Ethics* (AOTA, 2015). Also, under each item, list the specific trait or type of conduct it represents (e.g., dishonesty, poor safety awareness, unreliability, discrimination, carelessness).

	Unprofessional Behavior	*Potential Safety Concerns or Problems*	*Possible Effect on Relationship With Clients or Colleagues*	*Possible Disciplinary Action That May Result*
1.	Cosigning an OTA's notes (when required by law or facility policy) without reading them Trait:			
2.	Badmouthing your boss or place of employment on a social media site Trait:			
3.	Realizing that a pair of scissors is missing after leading an occupational therapy crafts group in a mental health setting Trait:			
4.	Taking client paperwork home to complete it Trait:			
5.	Habitually arriving late to work Trait:			
6.	Not putting therapy equipment away when finished using it Trait:			
7.	Playing games on your work computer while waiting for your outpatients to arrive Trait:			
8.	Immediately providing an inpatient client with a copy of your documentation when he or she requests that information during an intervention session Trait:			
9.	During Level I fieldwork at a hospital, giving a client one's home phone number so that the client can call to ask questions or just to talk Trait:			

	Unprofessional Behavior	Potential Safety Concerns or Problems	Possible Effect on Relationship With Clients or Colleagues	Possible Disciplinary Action That May Result
10.	Accidentally sending an e-mail containing confidential client information to the wrong e-mail address or leaving a printed copy on the copying machine Trait:			
11.	Telling a client that he or she looks "hot and sexy" in an outfit Trait:			
12.	Talking to a colleague about a client while buying candy in the hospital gift shop Trait:			
13.	Calling in sick to go to a concert with a friend Trait:			
14.	Forgetting to fill out the purchase requisition for reachers, sock aids, and long shoehorns Trait:			
15.	Not washing hands after treating a client Trait:			
16.	Signing a note written by another OT because the other therapist forgot to sign it before going home Trait:			
17.	Looking at the medical records of a relative or friend who was admitted to your facility, but is not on your caseload Trait:			
18.	Jokingly telling a first-grader that he needs to complete therapy activities now or you will not let the student go home today Trait:			
19.	Forgetting to bring your professional name tag to work Trait:			
20.	Using a client in a clinical research study without informed consent Trait:			

Learning Activity 2-3: Unprofessional Conduct—More Examples

For each of the following negative behaviors of an occupational therapy practitioner, list several possible consequences. Consider how the actions might create specific safety concerns or problems, affect relationships with client or colleagues, or merit disciplinary action by not complying with facility policy and procedures or professional standards, such as the AOTA's *Code of Ethics* (AOTA, 2015). Also, under each item, list the specific trait or type of conduct it represents (e.g., dishonesty, poor safety awareness, unreliability, discrimination, carelessness).

	Unprofessional Behavior	*Potential Safety Concerns or Problems*	*Possible Effect on Relationship With Clients or Colleagues*	*Possible Disciplinary Action That May Result*
1.	Casually conversing with colleagues while a client is performing exercises or an activities of daily living (ADL) activity Trait:			
2.	At lunchtime with colleagues, making fun of clients who demonstrate peculiar behaviors or mannerisms Trait:			
3.	Trying a physical agent modality, for which you have no formal training, with a client because a sales representative tells you it is beneficial and teaches you how to use it Trait:			
4.	Billing Medicare for time spent reviewing a client's chart or writing a contact note Trait:			
5.	Giving a glass of water to an unfamiliar nursing home client when the client asks you for a drink Trait:			
6.	Asking an occupational therapy aide to perform a skilled occupational therapy intervention with a client because you are too busy to manage all the clients today Trait:			
7.	Losing occupational therapy paperwork that was previously entered in the client's chart Trait:			
8.	Not informing nursing staff that the occupational therapy client experienced an episode of incontinence and has soiled clothing Trait:			
9.	Throwing draft SOAP notes in the trash without shredding or removing identifying information Trait:			

Learning Activity 2-3: Unprofessional Conduct—More Examples (continued)

	Unprofessional Behavior	Potential Safety Concerns or Problems	Possible Effect on Relationship With Clients or Colleagues	Possible Disciplinary Action That May Result
10.	Leaving an 8-hour continuing education seminar after 6 hours but submitting the full course completion certificate for NBCOT recertification or occupational therapy license renewal Trait:			
11.	"Borrowing" adaptive equipment or an orthotic device from your facility so that a family member can use it at home Trait:			
12.	Minimizing a client's progress in a treatment note so the insurance company will approve additional sessions Trait:			
13.	Criticizing a colleague's skills in front of clients or staff Trait:			
14.	When supervising a fieldwork student, changing scores to a passing grade because you "think" the student will gain those skills on the job Trait:			
15.	Forgetting to lock wheelchair brakes during a client transfer Trait:			
16.	Telling a postsurgical client with poor recovery that his surgeon is a "quack" with a reputation for botching surgery Trait:			
17.	Accepting cash gifts from your client in home care Trait:			
18.	Keeping a client with Medicare on your caseload and billing for provision of routine maintenance therapy when skilled care is not necessary Trait:			
19.	Forgetting to set a timer when placing a hot or cold pack on a client Trait:			
20.	Before trying other alternatives, applying a vest restraint to a client who is at risk for falling out of the wheelchair Trait:			

Worksheet 2-8

Student and Client Interaction

Laura is an occupational therapy student completing Level II fieldwork at a skilled nursing facility. Her client, Peggy, is 75 years old and has a diagnosis of chronic obstructive pulmonary disease. Laura and Peggy had the following conversation at the end of an intervention session. What suggestions would you make regarding the OT student's interaction with the client?

OT student: *Peggy, as you know, I have to say goodbye to you today as I am finished with my 12-week fieldwork at the nursing home. However, I am sure you are looking forward to going back home next week.*
Client: *To tell you the truth, I am a bit nervous about it.*
OT student: *Why?*
Client: *As you know, I live alone, and my children live across the country. My sister hasn't been well lately, and the neighbor who used to help me once in awhile just got a new job and is moving away.*
OT student: *Honey, don't worry. Everything will be fine. We would not be discharging you unless you were ready.*
Client: *Yes, but I do not really know anyone else in my apartment building.*
OT student: *Now you have an excuse to make some new friends then.*
Client: *That is not so easy at my age.*
OT student: *Well, you have a nice personality. I certainly enjoyed talking with you, and I will miss you. You remind me of my grandma.*
Client: *I like talking to you too. Maybe we can talk once in awhile after I go home, or you can come visit me. Can I have your cell phone number? I won't be able to call you at this place anymore.*
OT student: *Sure, let me write it down for you.* [Student writes phone number on a piece of paper and hands it to Peggy.]
Client: *Also, I have a something for you to show my appreciation. Let me get it out of my pocket.* [Peggy removes a $50 bill and hands it to the student.]
OT student: *Peggy, that really isn't necessary.*
Client: *I insist. Put it toward your certification exam. You have been so nice to me the whole time I have been here.*
OT student: *Wow, thank you so much Peggy. That is very kind of you.* [She gives Peggy a hug]. *Unfortunately, I do have to go now and finish up my paperwork. Good luck to you. Bye.*

Suggestions to improve this interaction:

1.

2.

3.

4.

5.

6.

7.

8.

Worksheet 2-9

Written Communication

Critique the following e-mail that an occupational therapy student wrote to her professor. List 10 suggestions to improve this note.

Hey Prof Jones,

> *I don't think it is fare that u failed me on my research paper. ☹ I SPEND A LOT OF TIME AND WORKED REALLY HARD ON IT! I wanna meat with u ASAP to discuss. Thx.*
>
> *Mary Smith*

Suggestions to improve this note:

1.

2.

3.

4.

5.

6.

7.

8.

9.

10.

Learning Activity 2-4: Professional Communication

Imagine you just had a 1-hour interview with your fieldwork educator, Nick Knack, regarding your upcoming Level II fieldwork experience. You learned you will be working primarily on the spinal cord and traumatic brain injury units. During the interview, it was confirmed that you are scheduled to begin fieldwork on the first Monday of next month. Your fieldwork educator requested that, on your first day, you meet him in the Human Resources office at 8:00 a.m. to fill out required paperwork. In the box below (or using a computer), write a sample e-mail to the fieldwork educator as a follow-up to your recent interview. Switch notes with a partner and critique each other's note.

Considering the note created for this exercise, does it thank the fieldwork educator for his time, demonstrate enthusiasm for the upcoming experience, and confirm the meeting place and time? Is the note free from slang and errors in spelling and grammar? Does the note convey a professional image and include a respectful greeting and an appropriate closing?

Reprinted with permission from Morreale, M. J. (2015). *Developing clinical competence: A workbook for the OTA*. Thorofare, NJ: SLACK Incorporated.

Worksheet 2-10

Medical Terminology and Abbreviations

Using a medical terminology book or an approved abbreviations list from your program or facility, translate the following abbreviations, diagnoses, and doctor's orders into full English phrases or sentences.

1. Client Ⓘ w/c ↔ toilet but exhibits SOB
2. Client O × 3 but requires SBA when performing functional mobility using NBQC
3. The student's limited Ⓡ shoulder ER/IR was noted in IEP.
4. Pt. mod Ⓐ EOB → commode c̄ walker
5. Resident's LUE strength WFL but demonstrates ↓ FM skills 2° tremors
6. Child c/o discomfort LLE when AMB due to AFO
7. CXR – for TB, VS stable, NKA
8. EMG + Ⓛ CTS
9. Dx: Ⓡ AKA 2° MVA, HTN, UTI
10. Dx: PTSD, OCD. PMH: Fx Ⓡ DRUJ 2° GSW while serving in Iraq
11. Dx: Fx Ⓡ index PIP c̄ ORIF, CRPS
12. Dx: PDD-NOS, ADHD
13. Client s/p Ⓡ THR 2° DJD, TTWB RLE, OOB c̄ walker
14. OT 3 × wk × 1 mo. for P/AROM RUE, ADL retraining, PAMs PRN
15. OT 2/wk × 6 wks: eval & tx, ADL/IADLs, TENS, US, HEP

Adapted from Morreale, M., & Borcherding, S. (2013). *The OTA's guide to documentation: Writing SOAP notes* (3rd ed.). Thorofare, NJ: SLACK Incorporated.

Worksheet 2-11

Avoiding Documentation Errors

Rewrite the following sentences to make them more professional by correcting errors in spelling, abbreviations, grammar, and fundamentals of documentation.

1. The client was able to preform wheelchair mobility independently to go from his hospital room to the dinning room.

2. The students musical instruments were stored in the band teacher's office.

3. The COPD client stated she becomes OBS when performing heavy activities for more then a few minutes.

4. The Occupational Therapy Assistant instructed the client on therapy puddy exercises.

5. The PT. was seen for 30 minutes bedside to help her eat breakfast.

6. The client's dysphasia contributed to his inspiration pnumonia.

7. The child needed modified assistance to donn his orthosis.

8. The client stated "he cannot wait to go home."

9. The client used his bad hand to grasp the bed rail when rolling to the left.

10. The TBI worked on ↓ safety and ↑ left neglect to improve IADL performance.

Worksheet 2-12

Avoiding Documentation Errors—More Practice

Rewrite the following sentences to make them more professional by correcting errors in spelling, abbreviations, grammar, and fundamentals of documentation.

1. The student asked if the OTA could help her write her name?

2. The resident exhibited urinary incontinents and stated "I have a urinary track infection".

3. The client was instructed in arom exercises so that her bad arm does not get stiff.

4. The home health aid was adapt at transfering clients.

5. The client's throat was sore because the speech pathologist made the client speak two long in therapy.

6. The pt.'s torn rotary cuff required surgery and afterwards his deltoid was painful when palpitated.

7. The two OTA's treated the OT's to lunch when they got a promotion.

8. The child griped the toy steering wheel with her dominate right hand and used her left hand to press the horn.

9. The clients' tremers made it unsafe for her to use the parrafin machine.

10. The toddler with Autism exhibited a positive babinski sign.

Reprinted with permission from Morreale, M. J. (2015). *Developing clinical competence: A workbook for the OTA*. Thorofare, NJ: SLACK Incorporated.

Worksheet 2-13

Documentation Fundamentals

An OT wrote the following note after contact with a client. Use AOTA's *Guidelines for Documentation of Occupational Therapy* (AOTA, 2013) or other documentation resources to help determine which fundamental elements are incorrect or missing in the OT's note that follows.

Really Good Rehabilitation Center
Restful Springs, Florida

Name: Rhezzydent, R. *Date of Birth: 4/1/1932*

Dx: Right mastectomy 2° Breast Cancer *Physician: Dr. Seth Oscope*

11:30 *Client in bed and refusing therapy this morning due to side eff. from chemotherapy. Client stated she vomited ~~two~~ three times this morning and is tired from not sleeping well last night. Plan: attempt therapy again this aft. and instruct client on right upper extremity AROM exercises.*

J.W.

1.

2.

3.

4.

5.

6.

7.

8.

9.

10.

Adapted from Morreale, M. J., & Borcherding, S. (2013). *The OTA's guide to documentation: Writing SOAP notes* (3rd ed.). Thorofare, NJ: SLACK Incorporated.

Worksheet 2-14

Managing a Schedule

Imagine you are an OT working at an inpatient facility and are responsible for supervising an OTA. The work hours for the OT department are from 8:30 a.m. to 4:30 p.m., and the staff is allowed a 30-minute lunch break and two 15-minute breaks (one in the morning and one in the afternoon). Your caseload consists of 10 clients, described below, and you have a mandatory 30-minute staff meeting today at 11:00 a.m. In addition, you must also set aside time to supervise and collaborate with the OTA and complete all of your daily paperwork and departmental tasks. Fill in your schedule below, including the best time frames for treating your clients.

Time	***Client***
8:30	
9:00	
9:30	
10:00	
10:30	
11:00	
11:30	
12:00	
12:30	

Time	***Client***
1:00	
1:30	
2:00	
2:30	
3:00	
3:30	
4:00	
4:30	

Client Caseload (Approximately 30 minutes each session)

1. Mary sustained a stroke and requires instruction in self-feeding. Her schedule includes physical therapy (PT) at 9:00 a.m. and speech therapy (ST) at 3:00 p.m.
2. Tim has colon cancer and requires instruction in energy conservation. He receives chemotherapy at 1:00 p.m.
3. Mabel sustained a stroke and requires instruction in grooming. She receives PT daily at 10:30 a.m. and ST at 2:00 p.m.
4. Leroy has undergone rotator cuff surgery and requires instruction in postsurgical care of the involved extremity before his discharge at noon.
5. Jim has Parkinson's disease and requires instruction in safe transfers. He is scheduled for PT at 3:00 p.m.
6. Leila sustained a left femur fracture and now must use a walker. She needs recommendations for durable medical equipment (DME)/adaptive equipment before her discharge home at noon. She is scheduled for PT at 8:30 a.m.
7. Natasha has undergone surgery for a right below-knee amputation (BKA) and needs exercises to increase her upper body strength and endurance for functional ambulation with a walker. She receives PT daily at 11:00 a.m.
8. Ellen recently sustained multiple trauma from a motor vehicle accident. She needs a right resting hand orthosis today. PT is scheduled for 2:00 p.m.
9. Mario sustained a stroke and needs activities to decrease his left neglect and improve cognition for activities of daily living (ADL) performance. He is scheduled for an MRI at 3:00 p.m.
10. Harvey is recovering from pneumonia and is being discharged tomorrow. He needs a home exercise program to increase activity tolerance for ADLs. He is scheduled for PT at 12:30 p.m.

Learning Activity 2-5: Gathering and Organizing Therapy Items

Because occupational therapy practitioners are often pressed for time in a working day, it is important to perform tasks efficiently. To avoid wasted time, gather and organize therapy materials ahead of time whenever possible, such as when planning to implement a home health or school-based intervention, work with a client bedside, or assess client factors.

Consider the following clients on your caseload. Make a list of all the items you will need to gather and bring with you to implement each client intervention. Be sure to consider any paperwork or documentation materials you may also need.

1. **Home Health:** Stanley is a 75-year-old male diagnosed with Parkinson's disease. He was recently discharged from an acute care hospital to his assisted living residence, but never received occupational therapy while in the hospital. The occupational therapy evaluation in home health determined that Stanley has fair plus muscle strength in both upper extremities and fair activity tolerance, which limit functional ambulation with a walker. Stanley also demonstrates decreased dynamic sitting balance and reports dizziness when bending over. The plan for today's session is to initiate upper extremity strengthening and to teach Stanley lower body dressing using adaptive equipment.

   ____

   ____

   ____

   ____

2. **School Setting:** Tamika is an 8-year-old student diagnosed with a developmental delay. She has decreased muscle tone, resulting in poor posture while sitting at her desk. Tamika also demonstrates difficulty holding a pencil properly, maintaining wrist extension, and staying within the lines when writing. The plan for today's session is to work with Tamika in the classroom and provide some adaptations for her challenges.

   ____

   ____

   ____

   ____

3. **Acute Care Hospital:** Brad was involved in a motor vehicle accident and sustained multiple trauma, including bilateral femur fractures, internal injuries, and a wrist sprain. He is currently on bed rest, but is conscious and awake. The doctor has ordered an ulnar gutter orthosis for Brad's wrist. Because the rehabilitation department does not have this type of orthotic device as a prefabricated option, Brad's orthosis will need to be custom fabricated at bedside. A rolling cart is available to transport items.

   ____

   ____

   ____

   ____

4. **Outpatient clinic:** Margaret is 50 years old and has carpometacarpal osteoarthritis in her right, nondominant thumb. The plan for today is to reassess Margaret's affected hand to determine progress in thumb AROM, grip and pinch strength, and work on fine motor skills to improve ADL and instrumental ADL (IADL) performance.

   ____

   ____

   ____

   ____

Worksheet 2-15

Infection Control

Worker and client safety are of great concern in the health care environment of today. Infections by multidrug-resistant organisms (MDROs) are increasing throughout the world. Limiting the spread of and controlling MDROs is urgent as the current number of antibiotics able to treat these infections is limited and new drugs are not yet available (World Health Organization [WHO], 2014). This worksheet reviews infectious diseases and the precautions put into place by the Centers for Disease Control and Prevention (CDC) and WHO (CDC, 2014; WHO, 2014). For the health and well being of occupational therapy clients and personnel, it is essential that managers and practitioners understand the importance of infection control and abide by the many standards in place to ensure safety.

For each of the numbered items, match the aspect of infection control with the description that follows. Answers may be used more than once.

Personal Protective Equipment (PPE)	Safe Injection Practices	Respiratory Hygiene/ Cough Etiquette	Environmental Cleaning
Hand hygiene	Standard precautions	MDROs	Education and training
Methicillin-resistant *Staphylococcus aureus* (MRSA)	Vancomycin-resistant *Enterococci* (VRE)	PPE doffing	Alcohol-based hand rub

1. The term used by the CDC and WHO that identifies the minimal set of precautions that must be employed in health care settings.
____

2. Considered by the CDC and WHO to be the most critical activity to reduce the risk of spreading infections in health care settings.
____

3. Wearable equipment designed to safeguard health care workers from exposure to or contact with infectious agents.
____

4. Ensuring that transmission of diseases from one client to another via needles and syringes is minimized. A new syringe and needle must be used for each person, syringes and medication must be kept away from contaminated equipment, and used syringes and needles cannot be inserted or reinserted into a vial of medication.
____

5. Cleaning equipment and treatment surfaces with appropriate detergent and water using friction, or cleaning with an electronic tool, such as an ultrasonic cleaning device and chemical agents.
____

6. Preventing the spread of respiratory infection by limiting contamination from secretions of individuals who have signs and symptoms of a respiratory infection. Examples include posting signs with instructions to cover mouths and noses when coughing or sneezing, providing tissues, and encouraging hand hygiene.
____

7. The action that should be completed first if an OT is accidently cut with a tool being used to debride a partial-thickness wound.
____

Worksheet 2-15 (continued)

Infection Control

8. Used syringes and needles must be disposed of, at the point of use, in a closed, puncture-resistant, and leak-proof sharps container.

 ____

9. Two of the most common bacteria causing health care–associated infections (HAIs).

 ____

10. Use of alcohol-based rub as the primary mode in health care settings, unless visible soil is present (blood, fecal matter), which requires soap-and-water cleansing.

 ____

11. A critical element of standard precautions that facilitates appropriate decision making and promotes adherence.

 ____

12. The method an OT completing feeding activities with a drooling child should use to minimize potential infection from infected saliva.

 ____

13. Recommended for use on a regular basis in health care settings because of its activity against a broad spectrum of epidemiologically important pathogens.

 ____

14. Ensuring that the outside of contaminated PPE does not come in contact with skin of the user; remove items while turning the outside in and grasping the clean inside surface to place into appropriate laundry container.

 ____

15. The generic term for organisms that are resistant to treatment and are associated with increases in morbidity, length of stay, increased costs, and mortality in health care settings.

 ____

Answers to Chapter 2 Worksheets

Worksheet 2-1: Scheduling Fieldwork

1. C. Attempts to schedule fieldwork should be made as soon as possible because it may take several weeks just to connect with your fieldwork educator. Also, although you may want to complete fieldwork during a particular time frame, this may not fit with your supervisor's schedule. Your fieldwork educator may be on vacation, or there may be other students scheduled at that time. If you wait until only a short time frame before your desired time frame and cannot be accommodated, then it may be too late to complete fieldwork by your program deadline. Contacting your fieldwork educator as soon as possible after fieldwork has been assigned should give you enough time to schedule a mutually agreeable time frame.
2. D. Occupational therapy practitioners are very busy at clinical sites and may not be able to return your call immediately. Also, that person may not have received the message or may forget to call you back. You should call again. If you cannot contact your fieldwork educator after three or four attempts over several weeks, then you should discuss this with your academic fieldwork coordinator. It would not be appropriate to ask for the rehabilitation director at this time.
3. C. Because of staffing changes, scheduled vacations, and other factors, the facility may assign a different fieldwork educator to you. You should schedule your fieldwork with this new supervisor, but also immediately inform your academic fieldwork coordinator regarding this change.
4. A. A student should not attend fieldwork with an illness that could be contagious to clients or staff or significantly affect job performance. People understand that emergencies and illnesses occur, but expect that situations be handled appropriately. The professional action to take is for you to immediately notify your fieldwork educator that you will be absent, humbly apologize for the inconvenience your illness causes, and ask politely to reschedule. Realize the site may not agree to reschedule, and, if this is the case, do not get upset or argue with the site. You should also notify your academic fieldwork coordinator about your illness and absence and determine whether the site is able to reschedule your fieldwork. If you are planning to see a health professional for treatment of your illness, it is helpful to offer your fieldwork educator and academic fieldwork coordinator medical documentation to verify that you have a valid reason to be absent.
5. B. First of all, do not panic! Fieldwork schedules can change for a variety of reasons, so this is not an uncommon situation. It would not be productive to argue with the fieldwork educator. Your first course of action would be to immediately contact your academic fieldwork coordinator, who can discuss your situation with the two sites and help you find a workable solution. Perhaps the second site can be rescheduled, or your fieldwork coordinator may be able to substitute a different site for your first or second fieldwork, although you may need to be flexible with time frames.
6. C. This is not an uncommon situation. Thank the person for contacting you, notify your academic fieldwork coordinator of the change, and wait a day or two for the new person to contact you as directed. If you do not hear from the new person in several days, be sure to follow up. It would be inappropriate to speak to the rehabilitation director or ask the person to switch students.
7. A. A week is more than adequate time to wait for a reply, so you should follow up immediately and resend your e-mail. The fieldwork educator may have overlooked the e-mail or deleted it accidentally, so do not be defensive or accusatory. There is no need to contact the rehabilitation director. You should make further attempts to contact the fieldwork educator before asking your academic fieldwork coordinator to intervene.
8. D. Follow your college's policy regarding fieldwork absences for inclement weather, emergencies, or other situations. You should also understand the consequences for unexcused absences. Health facilities count on staff being present to provide essential client care, but do realize that it may be unsafe or impossible for some staff to get to work in very severe weather conditions, such as a hurricane, tornado, or blizzard. Of course, differences exist between such weather conditions as snow flurries vs an active blizzard; or between a thunderstorm vs a hurricane evacuation. Another option is to consider other means of getting to fieldwork, such as public transportation or, perhaps, spending the night at a hotel (or a friend/relative's house) within walking distance of the facility. The weather forecast may change by the next morning and may not even be an issue. It would be unprofessional to have a parent or guardian call.

9. B. As soon as you realize you are going to be late, the professional action to take is to attempt to notify your fieldwork educator. However, if you are doing the driving, be sure to follow the rules of the road and only text, e-mail, or call when it is safe and legal to do so, such as after having pulled over into a parking space. Then, once you arrive late, accept responsibility, apologize profusely, and promise it will not happen again. Do not lie or make excuses. Lateness, particularly on the first day, gives a negative impression. It is prudent to plan properly to allow enough travel time for unexpected situations or traffic.
10. D. Emergencies and other situations happen occasionally, so you might find that your fieldwork schedule changes. You should remain patient, understanding, and flexible. It would be unprofessional to cry, whine, or to contact the supervisor. Reschedule the fieldwork and contact your academic fieldwork coordinator to discuss the situation. It is best to not wait until the last minute to complete fieldwork to allow for unexpected changes.

Worksheet 2-2: Fieldwork Phone Interview

1. N Directions to the fieldwork site

   Working occupational therapy practitioners are very busy. It may be perceived as unprofessional to ask for non-clinical information you can easily obtain on your own. It is better to obtain directions by other means, such as the Internet or by using a navigation system.

2. Y Start and end times for the day
3. Y Where to meet in the facility
4. N If the facility is in a "bad" area

   This type of question is not professional and might be perceived as discriminatory.

5. Y Date(s) to complete fieldwork
6. N Amount of time for lunch

   This type of question may be perceived as unprofessional because it implies you are more interested in breaks that your fieldwork. You might ask, "Can you tell me about a typical day's schedule?"

   It may be prudent to pack a lunch to bring with you the first day because there may not be enough time to purchase lunch offsite or wait in line in the cafeteria.

7. N Permission to come in late because you have to drive your kids to school

   You are expected to be at the site during typical working hours. You should try to make other arrangements for your children.

8. Y Whether a lab coat is required
9. N Wearing of sneakers

   Sneakers are not considered professional attire, so it is best not to initiate asking about them. Plan to wear comfortable, low-heeled shoes, preferably with rubber soles. If your supervisor happens to indicate that sneakers may be worn, realize the sneakers must be clean (no scuff marks or dirt), low-profile, and tasteful (e.g., no blinking lights, sparkles, or bright colors).

10. N Availability of coffee or tea in the morning

    Your focus should be on the clinical experience. Plan to have your breakfast or beverage before coming to the fieldwork site.

11. N Permission to use your cell phone so you can monitor your children

    Your entire focus should be on the clinical experience while you are at the site. Although a brief call at lunchtime should be acceptable, it is best to make alternate arrangements for your children for the rest of the workday.

12. N Permission to come in late or leave early to accommodate your bus or train schedule

    You are expected to be at the site during typical working hours even if it is not the most convenient for you. Plan to take an earlier or later bus/train, or make other arrangements, such as taking a taxi or asking a friend or family member to drive you.

13. __N__ Permission to leave early to pick your children up from school

    You are expected to be at the site during typical working hours. You should try to make other arrangements for your children.

14. __N__ Permission to leave early due to a dental appointment to get your teeth cleaned

    You are expected to be at the site during typical working hours. It is not appropriate to leave early for a routine appointment that can be rescheduled.

15. __Y__ Permission to wear a head covering if required by your religion

    Head coverings are normally not allowed except for those required for religious reasons. It is prudent to discuss any religious accommodations you might need.

16. __Y__ What paperwork to bring

17. __N__ Whether it will be a particularly difficult fieldwork because a classmate failed fieldwork there last semester

    It is not appropriate to discuss another student's experience and could also be perceived as a negative attitude.

18. __N__ Reimbursement for gas and tolls

    Commuting costs are typically the student's responsibility.

19. __N__ If the fieldwork will require a lot of homework

    A question phrased that way could be perceived as a negative attitude. It would be better to ask whether there will be any assignments that you might start preparing for now.

20. __Y__ The types of diagnoses you will observe

Worksheet 2-3: Stress Reduction for That First Day

Your fieldwork is scheduled to begin next week. Box 2-1 provides practical suggestions of what you can do ahead of time to help reduce your stress level and to arrive on time your first day.

Box 2-1.

Stress Reduction for That First Day

- Obtain clear and correct directions to the fieldwork site ahead of time and determine availability of parking.
- Perform at least one "dry run" ahead of time to determine how long it will take to get to your fieldwork site and also to ensure you will not get lost your first day. Ideally, your practice run should be during the same time frame that you will need to travel for fieldwork.
- On your fieldwork day, allow more time than you deem necessary to travel to your site. This will give you an extra "cushion" of time if you have several red lights, experience road construction, or get stuck in extra traffic.
- Set an alarm clock or timer the evening before your fieldwork and get a good night's sleep.
- A day or two ahead of time, make sure you will have enough gas in the car if you are driving.
- Check the weather report to determine if the weather may affect driving conditions.
- A day or two ahead of time, make sure you have enough cash for parking, tolls, lunch, and other necessities so you do not have to go to an ATM right before fieldwork.
- A day or two ahead of time, confirm any essential plans such as a babysitter, car availability, and train or bus schedule.
- Select and prepare your clothes and accessories the night before fieldwork, making sure they are clean and neatly pressed.
- Pack your lunch the evening before fieldwork.
- Gather necessary items such as your name tag, any required documentation, car keys, and wallet the night before so you are not searching for them in the morning.
- If a lab coat is required, make sure it fits and is clean and neatly pressed ahead of time.

(continued)

Box 2-1 (continued)

Stress Reduction for That First Day

- Review information about the fieldwork site. Study up on the diagnoses you are likely to see at that site and take steps to become culturally competent regarding typical clients who receive services there.
- Take steps to prepare yourself for various situations at that site (such as seeing open wounds, blood transfusions, or severe burns) that you fear will make you feel "woozy."
- Eat a healthy breakfast to help ensure you will not get lightheaded or faint at the site.
- Remember that fieldwork educators realize that you are a student and do not expect that you will know everything. However, initiative, a positive attitude, thoughtful questions, and appropriate communication with clients will go a long way in helping to make a good impression.

Worksheet 2-4: Fieldwork Attire

Always check with your facility regarding the required dress code. Although some settings are more formal or casual than others, attire must meet standards for client care and safety. Realize that in many practice settings, such as physical rehabilitation and schools, an occupational therapy practitioner might be standing and walking a lot, going up and down flights of stairs, bending, transferring clients, for example. Attire should be comfortable, clean, neat, and modest and allow for safe client care. "Business casual" means clothing that gives a professional appearance, but is not overly dressy or formal. Here are some typical guidelines based on the inpatient scenario presented.

1. __N__ Scrubs: *In this situation, scrubs would not be appropriate because they do not conform to the designated dress code. However, in some settings, scrubs might be the required dress code for rehabilitation staff.*
2. __N__ Sneakers: *Sneakers are not considered business casual attire. However, some settings may allow rehabilitation staff to wear clean, low-profile sneakers.*
3. __Y__ Flat, closed-toe shoes with rubber soles: *Professional and safer for client care.*
4. __N__ Dressy flip-flops: *Unacceptable for inpatient client care as they can be a safety hazard during transfers or exposure to body fluids. Hosiery and closed toe shoes are often mandatory.*
5. __N__ Low-heeled leather sandals: *Hosiery and closed toe shoes are often mandatory for direct care. Exposed feet can be a safety hazard during transfers or exposure to bodily fluids.*
6. __N__ Heavy perfume/cologne/after shave: *Clients may be allergic or sensitive to smell.*
7. __Y__ Stud earrings: *One or two small, tasteful earrings are usually acceptable.*
8. __N__ Eyebrow piercing: *This does not give a professional appearance. It is best to remove visible facial piercings.*
9. __N__ Head covering: *Typically, only head coverings for religious requirements are allowed. Baseball hats, fedoras, bonnets, and other headwear are not appropriate.*
10. __N__ Visible underwear above pants waistband: *This looks sloppy and is unprofessional.*
11. __N__ Neatly pressed dark jeans: *Jeans are not professional attire, although some settings may allow them.*
12. __Y__ Khaki pants and a polo shirt: *These are standard types of garments that occupational therapy practitioners may wear.*
13. __N__ Plain black sweatpants: *These are not professional attire and are better suited for a gym or leisure activities.*
14. __N__ Sport T-shirt/jersey: *These are not professional attire and are better suited for a gym or leisure activities.*
15. __Y__ Button-down oxford shirt: *Standard type of garment that occupational therapy practitioners may wear.*
16. __Y__ Dress slacks: *Acceptable as long as they are tasteful and not extremely fancy or garish.*
17. __N__ Cargo pants: *These generally do not give a professional appearance.*
18. __Y__ Polo shirt with collar and small designer logo emblem: *Standard type of garment that occupational therapy practitioners may wear.*

19. __N__ 32-inch plain gold necklace: *Although necklaces may not be prohibited, long chains could be an infection control or safety hazard during transfers or bed mobility (such as hitting the client in the face or getting caught on something), or clients may pull on it, potentially hurting the health practitioner.*
20. __N__ Charm bracelet: *Although bracelets may not be prohibited, dangling charms could be an infection control or safety hazard when handling clients because they may injure skin or catch on client's clothing.*
21. __N__ Well-groomed, long artificial nails without polish: *Long nails, particularly artificial nails (of any length), can harbor bacteria* (CDC, 2011). *Long nails may also rupture gloves or injure clients.*
22. __N__ Dark gray suit: *This would generally be considered overdressed.*
23. __Y__ Name tag: *An identification badge is usually required in health care settings per facility policy and/or state regulation.*
24. __N__ Solid-color leggings: *These are unprofessional as the only lower body covering. Might be acceptable worn under a dress or skirt.*
25. __N__ Solid-color hoodie: *This is not professional attire and is better suited for a gym, school, or leisure activities.*

Worksheet 2-5: Professional Behaviors

Resources: AOTA, 2014b, 2015; Jacobs, MacRae, & Sladyk, 2014.
You may identify additional pertinent traits/characteristics.

	Professional Behavior	***Professional Characteristic***
1.	Administering a standardized assessment accurately	*Example: Service competency* *Attention to detail*
2.	Offering to put your fieldwork educator's clinical notes back into the clients' charts without being asked	*Initiative*
3.	Admitting you did not complete your notes on time, apologizing, and offering to stay late or come in early to complete them	*Accepts responsibility*
4.	Arranging self-feeding interventions predawn or after dusk for an occupational therapy client who is fasting during Ramadan	*Cultural sensitivity* *Flexibility*
5.	Switching a client's treatment time so it does not conflict with physical therapy	*Flexibility* *Cooperation*
6.	Addressing an adult client by using "Mr." or "Mrs." and client's surname	*Respect* *Courtesy*
7.	Not refusing to work with a client who is positive for HIV or tuberculosis	*Unbiased* *Nondiscrimination* *Inclusion*
8.	Writing a thank you note to your fieldwork educator after your interview	*Courtesy*
9.	Arriving to your fieldwork interview 5 minutes early	*Punctuality* *Dependability*
10.	Asking a senator to vote for a proposed law that improves access to mental health services	*Social justice* *Advocacy*
11.	Cleaning up water that you notice on the floor near the hydrocollator	*Initiative* *Safety awareness*
12.	Preparing and assembling all the information packets in time for a workshop that the occupational therapy department is sponsoring	*Time management* *Organizational skills* *Reliability*

	Professional Behavior	**Professional Characteristic**
13.	Not billing Medicare B for a session consisting only of skilled instruction lasting 7 minutes [*Billable units are 8 minutes or more*]	*Honesty* *Veracity*
14.	Closing the computer screen after entering client information	*Confidentiality*
15.	Nodding and maintaining eye contact when a client is answering questions	*Active listening*
16.	Participating in an event to raise awareness of a specific disease	*Social justice* *Altruism*
17.	Being the "go-to" person for solving problems regarding manual wheelchairs	*Dependability* *Service competency*
18.	Not dating a cute client your age who asks you out	*Professional boundaries*
19.	Ensuring that all the OTA's notes are cosigned when required by law or facility policy	*Attention to detail* *Conscientiousness* *Reliability*
20.	Knocking on a closed door before entering the client's room or an examination room	*Respect* *Courtesy*
21.	Discussing a client's discharge plan with the PT and social worker	*Interprofessional collaboration* *Teamwork* *Cooperation*
22.	Acknowledging that the client feels disappointed when his or her son did not come for a visit	*Empathy*
23.	Not complaining when you have to stay late one day to order a client's durable medical equipment (DME) before the client is discharged home today	*Good attitude* *Flexibility*
24.	Writing several drafts of a SOAP note to ensure an accurate, professional presentation before showing it to your fieldwork educator	*Conscientiousness* *Attention to detail*
25.	Reporting suspected child or elder abuse to appropriate personnel/agencies to prevent further harm to the individual	*Beneficence*
26.	Arranging for an interpreter when the client speaks a different language than you do	*Autonomy*
27.	Ensuring that the OTAs you are supervising receive appropriate levels of supervision	*Conscientiousness* *Intraprofessional collaboration*
28.	Arranging for more copies when you take the last client education handout from the file cabinet.	*Courtesy* *Initiative*

Worksheet 2-6: Ethics Sanctions

The order of sanctions from less severe to more severe is as follows (AOTA, 2014a; NBCOT, 2011):

- Reprimand
- Censure
- Probation
- Suspension
- Revocation

Worksheet 2-7: Ethical Behavior

Resources: AOTA, 2014a, 2014b, 2015; NBCOT, 2009, 2011. Also refer to any federal guidelines affecting occupational therapy practice and the state agency that regulates occupational therapy in the state in which you are working.

1. T ___ F _*_ If an OT is found guilty of committing a severe unethical act, the AOTA can take away the OT's license to practice *(The AOTA cannot issue state regulatory sanctions, but can report the individual's behavior to the appropriate state regulatory agency and take action regarding his or her AOTA membership.)*
2. T _*_ F ___ An occupational therapy volunteer can report an OT's unethical behavior to the NBCOT *(Anyone can formally report unethical behavior. However, the volunteer should use judgment to consider the nature of behavior that would warrant a complaint to the NBCOT vs simply reporting unprofessional conduct to a supervisor or administrator at that facility.)*
3. T ___ F _*_ An occupational therapy student should begin following the Code of Ethics when Level II fieldwork commences *(Professional conduct should be exhibited throughout an occupational therapy educational program, including Level I and Level II fieldwork.)*
4. T _*_ F ___ An occupational therapy practitioner who commits an unethical act could have his or her name listed publicly as an ethics violator by the AOTA or NBCOT *(This is the disciplinary action of censure.)*
5. T ___ F _*_ AOTA guidelines take precedence over state laws *(State and federal laws take precedence.)*
6. T _*_ F ___ Committing a felony may limit a person's ability to practice occupational therapy *(Refer to the NBCOT website* (www.nbcot.org) *and the state agency that regulates OT.)*
7. T ___ F _*_ If an occupational therapy practitioner did not know about a particular law, the OT or OTA cannot be sanctioned for an unethical act that violates that law *(An OT practitioner is expected to be knowledgeable about applicable laws affecting occupational therapy practice.)*
8. T ___ F _*_ An occupational therapy state license is only affected by occupational therapy ethical infractions and not other legal violations that an OT might have committed (*Committing a felony may limit a person's ability to practice occupational therapy. Refer to the NBCOT website* [www.nbcot.org] *and the state agency that regulates occupational therapy.)*
9. T ___ F _*_ An occupational therapy practitioner has an obligation to report a colleague's unethical behavior only if it is related to occupational therapy *(For example, an OT may report a PT or nurse's unethical conduct.)*
10. T ___ F _*_ The NBCOT implements sanctions within 1 week when a very serious complaint is lodged against an occupational therapy practitioner *(The process of information gathering and appeals require a longer time frame.)*
11. T ___ F _*_ A state can suspend an occupational therapy aide's license for unethical behavior in an occupational therapy clinic *(occupational therapy aides are not typically licensed professionals.)*
12. T _*_ F ___ A person visiting a hospital patient can file a complaint with an occupational therapy state licensure board (*Any member of the public may file a complaint.)*
13. T ___ F _*_ An OT accused of practicing under the influence of drugs automatically loses his or her NBCOT certification if reported to the NBCOT *(Any complaint must be substantiated, and there is a formal disciplinary process.)*
14. T ___ F _*_ An OT receiving 6 months' probation from an occupational therapy state licensing board cannot practice occupational therapy for the entire 6 months *(That is not the definition of probation.)*
15. T ___ F _*_ An OT sanctioned by the NBCOT cannot appeal the decision (The *NBCOT has a formal appeals process.)*
16. T ___ F _*_ Minimizing a client's progress when documenting is not considered unethical if it helps the person receive essential therapy services from the insurance company *(It is unethical to falsify or "fudge" client information.)*
17. T ___ F _*_ An occupational therapy practitioner cannot be disciplined by the AOTA, NBCOT, and an occupational therapy state licensure board all at the same time (*Each organization has different functions.)*

18. T ___ F _*_ It is acceptable for an OT to refuse to treat a person with HIV if the OT is concerned about catching the disease *(Communicable diseases always pose a concern for health providers whether it is HIV, hepatitis B, tuberculosis, or any other communicable condition. However, it is unethical to discriminate on the basis of a person's diagnosis, and clients must always be treated with dignity and respect. Because health practitioners may not even know a person has a communicable disease, the health worker must always incorporate standard precautions as appropriate.)*
19. T ___ F _*_ An OT censured by an occupational therapy state licensure board cannot practice occupational therapy during the time of the censure. (*A public disapproval statement does not prevent the practice of occupational therapy.)*
20. T ___ F _*_ When an occupational therapy licensure board's sanction is revocation, the therapist can only practice occupational therapy with daily, direct supervision. (*The license has been taken away.)*

Worksheet 2-8: Student-Client Interaction

1. It is condescending to call an adult client such nicknames as "honey" or "sweetie."
2. The student does not use primary accurate empathy to acknowledge the client's feelings about going home and being alone. It might be better to say, "*You feel worried about being home alone because you do not have a support system nearby. Is that correct?*" or "*You feel like you will be lonely at home because your sister and neighbor are not able to visit. Is that correct?*"
3. The student does not discuss any available community supports.
4. The student does not indicate any follow-up by the OT before the client's discharge.
5. It is unprofessional to state that the client reminds the student of her grandmother. A client may also perceive this statement as an insult.
6. It is not appropriate for the student to give the client her personal phone number or to imply that she will visit the client at home. The student must maintain professional boundaries.
7. *Students and employees must always adhere to the facility's policies and procedures regarding any gifts from clients.* Usually, there are rules in place against accepting "tips" or gifts worth more than a nominal amount. In this scenario, the student should not be accepting this monetary gift. Facilities often only allow acceptance of small items, such as flowers or food that can be shared with the department (such as a box of doughnuts, cookies, or candy). If the client would like to express appreciation with a larger gift, the facility might allow a monetary donation to the rehabilitation department (e.g., to purchase a piece of equipment) or the facility's charitable foundation.
8. Do not make guarantees such as, "*Everything will be fine*" or "*You will make a complete recovery.*" In this situation, it might be better to say something like, "*The health team will try to make your transition home as smooth as possible. We will do our best to address your concerns before you are discharged.*"

Worksheet 2-9: Written Communication

Resource: Braveman, 2011.

1. Proofread written communication. This note contains misspelled words (e.g., correct words are *fair* and *meet* rather than *fare* and *meat*) and poor grammar (e.g., correct verb is *spent* rather than *spend*).
2. Do not use slang such as "hey" and "wanna."
3. Do not use unprofessional abbreviations such as "u" or "thx."
4. Use a greeting or salutation such as "Dear."
5. Use the person's full, appropriate title (e.g., Professor Jones, Mrs. Jones). *Ensure you have spelled the person's name correctly.* Both authors of this book have often experienced students spelling the authors' surnames incorrectly on homework assignments and e-mails (e.g., Morreal or Morales rather than the proper spelling of Morreale, and Armini or Ameene instead of the correct spelling of Amini).
6. Do not use all capitals in a sentence because this denotes shouting.
7. The use of emoticons or emojis do not give a professional appearance.

8. Consider the tone of what is written and how it may be perceived. This note conveys an angry and accusatory tone.
9. It is better to spell out such standard abbreviations as *as soon as possible*.
10. Use a closing, such as *Sincerely*.

Here is the same note written in a more useful format:

Dear Professor Jones,

I would like to meet with you to discuss my research paper grade. Please let me know a time that would be convenient for you. Thank you.

Sincerely,
Mary Smith

Worksheet 2-10: Medical Terminology and Abbreviations

Suggested resources: Gateley & Borcherding, 2012; Morreale & Borcherding, 2013; Sames, 2015.

1. Client Ⓘ w/c ⟷ toilet but exhibits SOB.
   Client is independent transferring wheelchair to toilet and back to wheelchair, but exhibits shortness of breath.
2. Client O × 3 but requires SBA when performing functional mobility using NBQC
   Client is alert and oriented to person, place, and time but requires standby assistance when performing functional mobility using a narrow-base quad cane.
3. The student's limited Ⓡ shoulder ER/IR was noted in IEP
   The student's limited right shoulder external and internal rotation was noted in the Individualized Education Program.
4. Pt. mod Ⓐ EOB → commode c̄ walker
   Patient requires moderate assistance to transfer from the edge of bed to commode with use of a walker.
5. Resident's LUE strength WFL but demonstrates ↓ FM skills 2° tremors
   Resident's left upper extremity strength is within functional limits, but resident demonstrates decreased fine motor skills secondary to tremors.
6. Child c/o discomfort LLE when AMB due to AFO
   Child complains of discomfort in left lower extremity when ambulating due to ankle-foot orthosis.
7. CXR – for TB, VS stable, NKA
   Chest x-ray is negative for tuberculosis, vital signs are stable, and client has no known allergies.
8. EMG + Ⓛ CTS
   Electromyogram test is positive for diagnosis of left carpal tunnel syndrome.
9. Dx: Ⓡ AKA 2° MVA, HTN, UTI
   Diagnoses are right above-knee amputation secondary to a motor vehicle accident, hypertension, and urinary tract infection.
10. Dx: PTSD, OCD. PMH: Fx Ⓡ DRUJ 2° GSW while serving in Iraq
    Diagnoses are posttraumatic stress disorder and obsessive-compulsive disorder. Past medical history: sustained fracture to right distal radioulnar joint due to a gunshot wound while serving in Iraq.
11. Dx: Fx Ⓡ index PIP c̄ ORIF, CRPS
    Diagnoses are fracture of the right index finger proximal interphalangeal joint with open reduction and internal fixation and complex regional pain syndrome.
12. Dx: PDD-NOS, ADHD
    Diagnoses are pervasive developmental disorder not otherwise specified and attention-deficit/hyperactivity disorder.

13. Client s/p Ⓡ THR 2° DJD, TTWB RLE, OOB c̄ walker

    Client is status post right total hip replacement secondary to degenerative joint disease. Client has toe-touch weight-bearing status right lower extremity and is allowed to get out of bed using a walker.

14. OT 3 × wk × 1 mo. for P/AROM RUE, ADL retraining, PAMs PRN

    Occupational therapy ordered three times weekly for 1 month for passive and active range of motion to the right upper extremity, activities of daily living retraining, and physical agent modalities as needed.

15. OT 2/wk × 6 wks: eval & tx, ADL/IADLs, TENS, US, HEP

    Occupational therapy ordered two times weekly for 6 weeks for evaluation and intervention, basic and instrumental activities of daily living, transcutaneous electrical nerve stimulation, ultrasound, and instruction in a home exercise program.

Worksheet 2-11: Avoiding Documentation Errors

Here are some corrections and suggestions for professional documentation (Gateley & Borcherding, 2012; Merriam-Webster, 2001; Morreale & Borcherding, 2013; Sames, 2015).

1. The client was able to <u>preform</u> wheelchair mobility independently to go from his hospital room to the <u>dinning</u> room.

   The client was able to perform wheelchair mobility independently to go from his hospital room to the dining room.

2. The <u>students</u> musical instruments were stored in the band teacher's office.

   This sentence does not indicate whether only one student had multiple instruments stored (i.e., The student's musical instruments were stored in the band teacher's office) or multiple students had their instruments stored (i.e., The students' musical instruments were stored in the band teacher's office).

3. The <u>COPD client</u> stated she becomes <u>OBS</u> when performing heavy activities for more <u>then</u> a few minutes.

   The client with COPD stated she becomes SOB when performing heavy activities for more than a few minutes.

4. The <u>Occupational Therapy Assistant</u> instructed the client on therapy <u>puddy</u> exercises.

   The sentence may vary depending on the intended purpose or audience of the notation:

   The OTA instructed the client on therapy putty exercises.

   The client was instructed on therapy putty exercises.

   The client was instructed on therapy putty exercises by the OTA.

5. The <u>PT. was seen</u> for 30 minutes bedside <u>to help</u> her eat breakfast.

   The pt. participated in therapy 30 minutes bedside for skilled feeding instruction during breakfast. ("PT" stands for physical therapist or physical therapy whereas "pt." stands for patient.)

   "Help" does not denote a skilled intervention.

6. The client's <u>dysphasia</u> contributed to his <u>inspiration pnumonia</u>.

   The client's dysphagia contributed to his aspiration pneumonia.

7. The child needed <u>modified assistance</u> to <u>donn</u> his orthosis.

   This sentence needs a standard term for assist level:

   The child needed moderate assistance to don his orthosis.

   or

   The child donned his orthosis with modified independence.

8. The client <u>stated "he cannot wait to go home."</u>

   The client stated he could not wait to go home.

   The client stated that he "cannot wait" to go home.

   The client stated, "I cannot wait to go home."

9. The client used his <u>bad</u> hand to grasp the bed rail when rolling to the left.

   The client used his affected hand to grasp the bed rail when rolling to the left.

   The client used his weak hand to grasp the bed rail when rolling to the left.

10. The TBI worked on ↓ safety and ↑ left neglect to improve IADL performance.

    The client with traumatic brain injury worked on increasing safety and decreasing left neglect to improve IADL performance.

    Use people-first language.

Worksheet 2-12: Avoiding Documentation Errors—More Practice

Here are some corrections and suggestions for professional documentation (Gateley & Borcherding, 2012; Merriam-Webster, 2001; Morreale & Borcherding; 2013; Sames, 2015.

1. The student asked if the OTA could help her write her name?

   The student asked if the OTA could help her write the student's name.

2. The resident exhibited urinary incontinents and stated "I have a urinary track infection".

   The resident exhibited urinary incontinence and stated, "I have a urinary tract infection."

3. The client was instructed in arom exercises so that her bad arm does not get stiff.

   The client was instructed in AROM exercises to prevent stiffness of her affected arm.

   The client was instructed in AROM exercises to prevent stiffness of her weak upper extremity.

4. The home health aid was adapt at transfering clients.

   The home health aide was adept at transferring clients.

5. The client's throat was sore because the speech pathologist made the client speak two long in therapy.

   It is best to write objectively and avoid criticizing or blaming another professional, student, or colleague in a therapy note (Kettenbach, 2009; Scott, 2013). Also, "two" should be "too."

   The client reported throat soreness following his speech therapy session.

   The client reported that his sore throat started around 3:00 p.m.

6. The pt.'s torn rotary cuff required surgery and afterwards his deltoid was painful when palpitated.

   The pt.'s torn rotator cuff needed surgical repair, after which the client reported pain in deltoid upon palpation.

7. The two OTA's treated the OT's to lunch when they got a promotion.

   In the above sentence it is not clear who got the promotion:

   The two OTAs treated the OTs to lunch when the OTs got a promotion.

   The two OTAs treated the OTs to lunch when the OTAs got a promotion.

8. The child griped the toy steering wheel with her dominate right hand and used her left hand to press the horn.

   The child gripped the toy steering wheel with her dominant right hand and used her left hand to press the horn.

9. The clients' tremers made it unsafe for her to use the parrafin machine.

   The client's tremors made it unsafe for her to use the paraffin machine.

10. The toddler with Autism exhibited a positive babinski sign.

    The toddler with autism exhibited a positive Babinski sign.

Worksheet 2-13: Documentation Fundamentals

Resource: AOTA, 2013. Additional resources: Gateley & Borcherding, 2012; Morreale & Borcherding, 2013; Sames, 2015.

1. No case number present
2. Client's full name not delineated
3. Date of client contact not indicated
4. Time does not indicate if it is a.m. or p.m.
5. Department of occupational therapy not indicated
6. Type of note not delineated (contact note)
7. Initials are not acceptable for OT's signature

8. Occupational therapy credentials not indicated with signature
9. Error not corrected properly (not initialed or dated)
10. Blank space exists between end of note and signature
11. Nonstandard abbreviations used (eff. and aft.)
12. Note does not relate AROM to occupational performance

Worksheet 2-14: Managing a Schedule

Daily schedules will vary based on factors such as actual number of clients, length of intervention sessions, unexpected circumstances, and actual time spent for chart review, supervision, staff communication, client transport, and documentation, for example. In the examples that follow, the two blank time frames mid-morning and mid-afternoon allow for breaks and "catching up" if needed. Although there are a number of time frames that would work for the caseload presented, the following are two suggested schedules:

Time	*Sample Schedule A*	*Sample Schedule B*
8:30	Organize workday/collaborate with OTA	Organize workday/collaborate with OTA
9:00	Mabel	Mabel
9:30	Leroy	Leila
10:00	Leila	Leroy
10:30		Tim
11:00	Meeting	Meeting
11:30	Tim	
12:00	Lunch	Mary
12:30	Mary	Lunch
1:00	Ellen	Jim
1:30	Jim	Mario
2:00	Mario	Natasha
2:30	Harvey	
3:00		Ellen
3:30	Natasha	Harvey
4:00	Complete paperwork/collaborate with OTA	Complete paperwork/collaborate with OTA
4:30	Workday ends	Workday ends

1. Mary sustained a stroke and requires instruction in self-feeding. Her schedule includes PT at 9:00 a.m. and ST at 3:00 p.m. *It is preferable to do a feeding session at mealtime. Scheduling Mary at lunchtime today should be appropriate.*
2. Tim has colon cancer and requires instruction in energy conservation. He receives chemotherapy at 1:00 p.m. *Tim may feel ill after his chemotherapy, so OT should be implemented before that time.*
3. Mabel sustained a stroke and requires instruction in grooming. She receives PT daily at 10:30 a.m. and ST at 2:00 p.m. *A good time would be during normal morning self-care. The suggested schedule allows for Mabel to have a rest period before PT.*
4. Leroy has undergone rotator cuff surgery and requires instruction in postsurgical care of the involved extremity before his discharge at noon. *Leroy must be seen in the morning.*
5. Jim has Parkinson's disease and requires instruction in safe transfers. He is scheduled for PT at 3:00 p.m. *He should be allowed time for a rest period before or after PT. After PT would probably be too late in the day.*

6. Leila sustained a left femur fracture and now must use a walker. She needs recommendations for durable medical equipment (DME)/adaptive equipment before her discharge at noon. She is scheduled for PT at 8:30 a.m. *Therapy must begin after 9 a.m. (after PT session) and by 11:30 (before noon discharge).*
7. Natasha has undergone surgery for a right below-knee amputation (BKA) and needs exercises to increase her upper body strength and endurance for functional ambulation with a walker. She receives PT daily at 11:00 a.m. *Natasha's time frame is flexible, but occupational therapy cannot conflict with PT.*
8. Ellen sustained multiple trauma from a motor vehicle accident. She needs a right resting hand orthosis today. PT is scheduled for 2:00 p.m. *Ellen's time frame is flexible but cannot conflict with PT.*
9. Mario sustained a stroke and needs activities to decrease his left neglect and improve cognition for activities of daily living (ADL) performance. He is scheduled for an MRI at 3:00 p.m. *It is prudent to schedule Mario at least 1 hour before his MRI to complete his session.*
10. Harvey is recovering from pneumonia and is being discharged tomorrow. He needs a home exercise program to increase activity tolerance for ADLs. He is scheduled for PT at 12:30 p.m. *Harvey will require a rest period between therapy sessions.*

Worksheet 2-15: Infection Control

Resources: CDC, 2014; WHO, 2014.

1. The term used by the CDC and WHO that identifies the minimal set of precautions that must be employed in health care settings. *Standard precautions*
2. Considered by the CDC and WHO to be the most critical activity to reduce the risk of spreading infections in health care settings. *Hand hygiene*
3. Wearable equipment designed to safeguard health care workers from exposure to or contact with infectious agents. *Personal protective equipment (PPE)*
4. Ensuring that transmission of diseases from one client to another via needles and syringes is minimized. A new syringe and needle must be used for each person, syringes and medication must be kept away from contaminated equipment, and used syringes and needles cannot be inserted or reinserted into a vial of medication. *Safe injection practices*
5. Cleaning equipment and treatment surfaces with appropriate detergent and water using friction. Also, cleaning with an electronic tool such as an ultrasonic cleaning device and chemical agents. *Environmental cleaning*
6. Preventing the spread of respiratory infection by limiting contamination from secretions of individuals who have signs and symptoms of a respiratory infection. Examples include posting signs with instructions to cover mouths and noses when coughing or sneezing, providing tissues, and encouraging hand hygiene. *Respiratory hygiene/cough etiquette*
7. The action that should be completed first if an OT is accidently cut with a tool being used to debride a partial-thickness wound. *Hand hygiene*
8. Used syringes and needles must be disposed of, at the point of use, in a closed, puncture-resistant, and leak-proof sharps container. *Safe injection practices*
9. Two of the most common bacteria causing health care–associated infections (HAIs). *Methicillon-resistant* Staphylococcus aureus *(MRSA), vancomycin-resistant* enterococci *(VRE)*
10. Use of alcohol-based rub as the primary mode in health care settings, unless visible soil is present (blood, fecal matter), which requires soap and water cleansing. *Hand hygiene*
11. A critical element of standard precautions that facilitates appropriate decision making and promotes adherence. *Education and training*
12. The method an OT completing feeding activities with a drooling child should use to minimize potential infection from infected saliva. *Personal protective equipment (gloves)*
13. Recommended for use on regular basis in health care settings because of its activity against a broad spectrum of epidemiologically important pathogens. *Alcohol-based hand rub*

14. Ensuring that the outside of contaminated PPE does not come in contact with skin of the user; remove items while turning the outside in and grasping the clean inside surface to place into appropriate laundry container. PPE Doffing
15. The generic term for organisms that are resistant to treatment and are associated with increases in morbidity, length of stay, increased costs, and mortality in health care settings. MDROs

Chapter 2 References

American Occupational Therapy Association. (2013). Guidelines for documentation of occupational therapy. *American Journal of Occupational Therapy, 67*(Suppl. 6), S32–S38.

American Occupational Therapy Association. (2014a). Enforcement procedures for the Occupational Therapy Code of Ethics and Ethics Standards. *American Journal of Occupational Therapy, 68*(Suppl. 3), S3–S15.

American Occupational Therapy Association. (2014b). Occupational therapy's commitment to nondiscrimination and inclusion. *American Journal of Occupational Therapy, 68*(Suppl. 3), S23–S24.

American Occupational Therapy Association. (2015). Occupational therapy code of ethics (2015). *American Journal of Occupational Therapy*, 69 (Suppl. 3), 6913410030. http://dx.doi.org/10.5014/ajot.2015.696S03

Braveman, B. (2011). Communication in the workplace. In K. Jacobs & G. L. McCormack (Eds.), *The occupational therapy manager* (5th ed., pp. 195–208). Bethesda, MD: American Occupational Therapy Association.

Centers for Disease Control and Prevention. (2011). Hand hygiene in health care settings guidelines. Atlanta: Author. Retrieved from http://www.cdc.gov/handhygiene/guidelines.html

Centers for Disease Control and Prevention. (2014). Guide to infection prevention for outpatient settings: Minimum Expectations for Safe Care. Retrieved from http://www.cdc.gov/HAI/settings/outpatient/outpatient-care-gl-standared-precautions.html#asp

Gateley, C. A., & Borcherding, S. (2012). *Documentation manual for occupational therapy: Writing SOAP notes* (3rd ed.). Thorofare, NJ: SLACK Incorporated.

Jacobs, K., MacRae, N., & Sladyk, K. (2014). *Occupational therapy essentials for clinical competence* (2nd ed.). Thorofare, NJ: SLACK Incorporated.

Kaser, J., & Clark, E. N. (2000). *Developing professional behaviors*. Thorofare, NJ: SLACK Incorporated.

Kettenbach, G. (2009). *Writing patient/client notes: Ensuring accuracy in documentation* (4th ed.). Philadelphia: F.A. Davis.

Kornblau, B. L., & Burkhardt, A. (2012). *Ethics in rehabilitation: A clinical perspective* (2nd ed.). Thorofare, NJ: SLACK Incorporated.

Merriam-Webster (2001). *Merriam-Webster's guide to punctuation and style* (2nd ed.). Springfield, MA: Merriam-Webster.

Morreale, M. J. (2015). *Developing clinical competence: A workbook for the OTA*. Thorofare, NJ: SLACK Incorporated.

Morreale, M. J., & Borcherding, S. (2013). *The OTA's guide to documentation: Writing SOAP notes* (3rd ed.). Thorofare, NJ: SLACK Incorporated.

National Board for Certification in Occupational Therapy. (2009). *Professional conduct*. Retrieved from http://nbcot.org/index.php?option=com_content&view=article&id=126&Itemid=119

National Board for Certification in Occupational Therapy. (2011). Procedures for the enforcement of the NBCOT Candidate/Certificant Code of Conduct. Retrieved from http://nbcot.org/pdf/Enforcement_Procedures.pdf?phpMyAdmin=3710605fd34365e380b9ab41a5078545

Sames, K. M. (2015). *Documenting occupational therapy practice* (3rd ed.). Upper Saddle River, NJ: Pearson Education.

Scott, R. W. (2013). *Legal, ethical, and practical aspects of patient care documentation: A guide for rehabilitation professionals* (4th ed.). Burlington, MA: Jones & Bartlett Learning.

World Health Organization. (2014). Evidence of hand hygiene to reduce transmissions and infections by multi drug resistant organisms in health care settings. Retrieved from http://www.who.int/gpsc/5may/MDRO_literature-review.pdf?ua=1

Chapter 3

Understanding Professional Roles and Responsibilities

Professional roles and responsibilities in occupational therapy include such factors as maintaining professional credentials, ensuring appropriate supervision, demonstrating cultural sensitivity, and performing services competently (American Occupational Therapy Association [AOTA], 2010a, 2010b, 2014b, 2014c, 2015). Occupational therapy practitioners also have a professional duty to behave ethically, attain ongoing professional development, advocate for the profession, and collaborate intraprofessionally and interprofessionally (AOTA, 2010a, 2010b, 2014a, 2015). This chapter presents worksheets and learning activities to help you understand professional roles, responsibilities, service delivery methods and settings, and various expectations for fieldwork and clinical practice. Answers to worksheet exercises are provided at the end of the chapter.

Contents

Morreale, M. J., & Amini, D.
The Occupational Therapist's Workbook for Ensuring Clinical Competence (pp. 79-120).

Worksheet 3-1

Roles and Responsibilities

For each of the tasks below, indicate whether it is generally a skilled role/responsibility of an OT and/or OTA. Realize this will often depend on the state's occupational therapy practice act. For this exercise, assume the occupational therapy practitioner is competent in the designated tasks.

	Task	*OT*	*OTA*
1.	Instruct client in a home exercise program		
2.	Develop the occupational therapy intervention plan		
3.	Determine whether a client performs a cooking task safely		
4.	Gait training		
5.	Teach positioning techniques to a parent of a child with cerebral palsy		
6.	Upgrade an exercise program		
7.	Determine discharge from occupational therapy		
8.	Respond to a referral to occupational therapy		
9.	Implement occupational therapy interventions		
10.	Teach one-handed shoe-tying		
11.	Complete the occupational therapy initial evaluation report independently		
12.	Administer a standardized assessment		
13.	Interpret initial evaluation results		
14.	Fabricate an orthotic device		
15.	Customize a resident's wheelchair with specialized inserts		
16.	Administer superficial thermal modalities as the sole client intervention during a session		
17.	Document occupational therapy intervention		
18.	Provide intervention to a home care client		
19.	Instruct client in workplace ergonomics		
20.	Provide specialized instruction in self-care		
21.	Help a student put on boots for recess		
22.	Develop goals for an Individualized Education Program (IEP)		
23.	Assess transfer skills		
24.	Provide occupational therapy in a neonatal intensive care unit		
25.	Attain certification in hand therapy		
26.	Attain AOTA board certification in pediatrics		
27.	Attain AOTA specialty certification in low vision		
28.	Make recommendations to a teacher regarding compensatory techniques for a student receiving occupational therapy services		
29.	Delegate aspects of an occupational therapy initial evaluation		
30.	Write short-term goals in a treatment note as a substep toward implementing an established intervention plan		
31.	Update a client's intervention plan		
32.	Write a discharge report independently		

Worksheet 3-1 (continued)

Roles and Responsibilities

	Task	***OT***	***OTA***
33.	Adapt an activities of daily living (ADL) device to improve a client's self-care performance		
34.	Assess range of motion using a goniometer		
35.	Teach nursing staff how to apply a client's orthotic device		
36.	Provide a handout on cardiac precautions		
37.	Supervise a rehabilitation aide		
38.	Supervise a volunteer in the OT department		
39.	Supervise a Level I OTA student		
40.	Supervise a Level II OTA student		
41.	Supervise a Level I OT student		
42.	Supervise a Level II OT student		
43.	Lead an occupational therapy group in a behavioral health setting		
44.	Observe a child coloring a picture		
45.	Recommend durable medical equipment upon client's discharge home		
46.	Assess a client's orientation to person, place, and time		
47.	Inform nursing staff about a client's report of pain		
48.	Provide an inservice to the rehabilitation staff about an evidence-based practice article		
49.	Assess vital signs		
50.	Attend a team meeting to discuss a client's care and progress		

Adapted from Morreale, M. J. (2015). *Developing clinical competence: A workbook for the OTA*. Thorofare, NJ: SLACK Incorporated.

Learning Activity 3-1: State Regulation

Each state has its own requirements regarding occupational therapy practice. Information on credentialing and links to individual state regulatory boards can be found on the AOTA website (www.aota.org), the National Board for Certification in Occupational Therapy (NBCOT) website (www.nbcot.org), or by using an Internet search engine. Consider the state in which you plan to work as an OT and answer the following questions.

State in which you plan to work as an OT ____________________

1. **Licensure:**
   a. How does that state regulate occupational therapy practice for OTs?
   ___ Licensure ___ Authorization ___ State certification ___ Not regulated
   b. What department in that state has jurisdiction over occupational therapy? In New York, for example, occupational therapy is regulated by the New York State Education Department, Office of the Professions. Occupational therapy in the state you wish to work in is regulated by:
   ____
   ____
   ____
   c. What is the contact information for occupational therapy regulatory information for the state in which you want to work?
      a. Website address: ____________________
      b. Phone number: ____________________
   d. Does that state require *passing* the NBCOT examination to practice as an OT in that state? ___ Yes ___ No
   e. Does that state require *maintaining* NBCOT certification to renew licensure and continue practicing as an OT in that state? ___ Yes ___ No
   f. Does that state offer an option of a temporary license or limited permit allowing occupational therapy practice before the NBCOT examination is taken or passed? ___ Yes ___ No
   g. If applicable, what is the cost to apply for a temporary license or limited permit? ____________________
   h. If applicable, how long is a temporary license or limited permit good for? ____________________
   i. What is the cost to apply for licensure? ____________________
   j. In that state, licensure must be renewed every ____________________ years.
   k. What continuing education or other requirements are needed to maintain licensure in that state? ________
   ____
   ____
   ____

2. **Scope of Practice:**
   a. Does that state require a prescription in order for an occupational therapy evaluation to be performed?
   ___ Yes ___ No
   b. Does that state require a prescription for an occupational therapy intervention program to be implemented?
   ___ Yes ___ No
   c. What health professionals can legally write a prescription for occupational therapy in that state (e.g., physician, nurse practitioner, optometrist)?
   ____
   ____
   ____

Learning Activity 3-1: State Regulation (continued)

d. Can an OTA perform an evaluation in that state? ____ Yes ____ No
Explain briefly ____________________

e. What supervision requirements for an OTA are specified in that state?

f. What types of interventions are specified under the scope of occupational therapy practice in that state? ____

g. What occupational therapy practitioners are allowed to use superficial thermal modalities in that state (e.g., hot packs, paraffin, etc.)? ____ OT ____ OTA ____ None

h. What occupational therapy practitioners are allowed to use advanced physical agent modalities in that state (e.g., ultrasound, electrical stimulation, etc.)? ____ OT ____ OTA ____ None

i. What additional training, supervision, continuing education, or other criteria, if any, are required in that state for an occupational therapy practitioner to use physical agent modalities?

j. Describe other types of occupational therapy interventions in that state, if any, requiring additional training, supervision, continuing education, or other criteria (e.g., vision training, feeding and swallowing)?

Continuing Competency/Professional Development: As an OT, your professional responsibilities include competency in the aspects of client care that you plan/implement and ongoing professional development (AOTA, 2010a, 2010b, 2015). It is also essential that you understand and adhere to occupational therapy licensure requirements for the specific state in which you wish to work. Realize that individual states may mandate different or additional professional development requirements than what is needed to maintain NBCOT certification. To create a professional development plan, complete Learning Activity 3-3 in this chapter.

Learning Activity 3-2: National Certification

Information regarding national certification can be found at the NBCOT website (www.nbcot.org). Use that website to answer the questions below

1. How is NBCOT certification different than state regulation? ______
2. How does NBCOT certification help consumers of occupational therapy?
3. How many questions are on the certification exam? ______
4. What is the scoring scale for the certification exam? ______ to ______ and the passing score is ______
5. How much time is allotted for the certification exam? ______
6. What is the cost to take the exam?
7. What is the physical address of the testing site where you plan to take the certification exam (www.prometric.com)?
8. Of the acceptable forms of identification listed on the NBCOT website, which two will you use for entry to the exam?
   1. ______
   2. ______
9. Can a felony conviction prevent an OT from initial certification or OT practice? Explain briefly. ______
10. The initial certification period is good for how many years? ______
11. What professional development or continuing education requirements are needed to maintain national certification? ______
12. Review the Professional Development Units [PDU] Activities Chart on the NBCOT website. To remain certified, list several types of activities you might choose to participate in after successful completion of the exam.
    1
    2.
    3.
    4.
    5.
13. As an OT, your professional responsibilities include competency in the aspects of client care that you plan and implement and ongoing professional development (AOTA, 2010a, 2010b, 2015). Realize that an individual state's occupational therapy licensure law may mandate different or additional professional development requirements than what is needed to maintain NBCOT certification. To create a professional development plan, complete Learning Activity 3-3 in this chapter.

Learning Activity 3-3: Professional Development Plan

A professional development plan will help you to achieve personal career goals and meet professional requirements for credentialing. You might consider such professional opportunities as attaining an advanced academic degree; AOTA specialty or board certification in various practice areas; and credentialing by other professional organizations in areas such as hand therapy, driver rehabilitation, lymphedema management, and sensory integration. Perhaps you see yourself eventually switching to a completely different area of occupational therapy practice or aspire to a managerial role. You might even desire to give back to the profession of occupational therapy through volunteerism opportunities, such as supervising students, joining an AOTA committee, running for an elected occupational therapy office, providing some pro bono services, or participating in advocacy efforts for people with disabilities.

As an OT, your professional responsibilities include competency in the aspects of client care that you plan/implement and ongoing professional development (AOTA, 2010a, 2010b, 2015). It is also essential that you attain any mandated continuing education requirements related to occupational therapy licensure in the particular state in which you wish to work. Professional development requirements are also delineated for practitioners who wish to maintain NBCOT certification for personal/professional reasons or, in some instances, as mandated by state licensure laws. Realize that states may have different or additional professional development requirements than what is needed to maintain national certification.

To develop a professional development plan, reflect on your vision for where you would like to see yourself professionally a year from now, several years from now, and perhaps 5 or 10 years from now. Think about areas of knowledge or specific skills you would like to obtain or improve on that are relevant to your current or desired occupational therapy role(s). Also, consider your interest in possible volunteer opportunities (including special causes, pet projects, or humanitarian efforts) and other ways to promote or give back to the profession of occupational therapy. Fill in the blanks below with your professional goals and the activities that will help you to develop the desired knowledge or skills on your list and/or "give back" to the profession. Also, establish the specific sequence of steps and timeline as to how and when you plan to complete each of those goals and methods.

1. List a projected area of practice and the professional/career role(s) where you would like to see yourself working in for each of the following time frames:
   a. 1 year from now: ______________________________
   ____
   b. 2 to 3 years from now: ______________________________
   ____
   c. 5 years from now: ______________________________
   ____
   d. 10 years from now: ______________________________
   ____
2. List several areas of knowledge or specific skills you would like to obtain or improve on at this time.
   a. ______________________________
   b. ______________________________
   c. ______________________________
   d. ______________________________
   e. ______________________________
   f. ______________________________
3. List personal areas of interest for volunteerism, advocacy, or to promote the profession of occupational therapy (e.g., supervise a Level I fieldwork student, volunteer for an AOTA or state occupational therapy association committee, write an article about occupational therapy, advocate for people with mental illness).
   a. ______________________________
   b. ______________________________
   c. ______________________________
   d. ______________________________

Then, for each of the items you listed, use the following format to help you create a plan for professional development to meet your goals.

Personal Goal: Desired role, area of knowledge, or a specific skill you would like to obtain or improve on; area of interest for advocacy or promoting the profession	***Time frame to attain this goal***	***List the general methods you would choose for goal attainment (e.g., attend a workshop, participate in a journal club/study group, volunteer for a local Alzheimer's disease or multiple sclerosis organization, work with a mentor)***	***List the specific steps for how each of these methods will be accomplished (e.g., locate potential workshops within a 50-mile home radius, complete application for a doctorate program, contact 5 peers to form a journal club or study group, join a state's OT association)***	***Indicate a time frame in which each step/method will have been completed (e.g., by the end of this week, within 30 days, within 3 months, by end of this year, second year)***	***Date actually completed***

Worksheet 3-2

Supervision

1. Steve, an OTA, was recently hired to work at a facility that has two OTs and three other OTAs on staff. Steve feels he needs more supervision from his supervising therapist than he has been receiving since starting work 2 weeks ago. What primary action should Steve take?
   A. Ask coworkers how much supervision time they each receive
   B. Discuss concerns with the rehabilitation director
   C. Discuss concerns with his supervising OT
   D. Wait and see whether supervision improves over the next several weeks

2. Leila, an occupational therapy student, is performing Level II fieldwork in a school setting. During the first week, her fieldwork educator asked her to perform various standardized formal assessments on clients without direct supervision. Because Leila has never administered those particular assessments and did not learn about them in school, she informed her fieldwork educator about her inexperience. The fieldwork educator responded that the caseload is much busier than normal this week, she is confident in Leila's abilities, and that those assessments really need to be completed. The fieldwork educator also apologized for not having the time to watch Leila perform those assessments this week, but suggested that Leila take the assessments home to review them ahead of time. What should Leila's primary action be?
   A. Contact her academic fieldwork coordinator
   B. Take the assessments home to review them
   C. Quit fieldwork
   D. Speak to the rehabilitation director

3. An OT has delegated a particular client intervention to an OTA today. The OTA tells the OT that he feels this intervention is not in the best interest of the client and is uneasy about implementing it. What is the therapist's best course of action?
   A. Have a brief discussion to emphasize that the OT is his supervisor and the OTA must comply according to AOTA role delineation guidelines
   B. To avoid conflict, tell the OTA to do whatever he wants to do
   C. Tell the OTA not to treat the client and ask the rehabilitation director to fire the OTA
   D. Have an honest and open discussion with the OTA to explain why this treatment is appropriate and provide evidence-based resources

4. An entry-level OT was hired recently to work in an inpatient rehabilitation setting. The therapist is a bit overwhelmed and is running behind with today's schedule. The occupational therapy aide, who has worked there for 15 years and is very good with clients, offers to help out. Which of the following tasks is most appropriate for the therapist to delegate to the occupational therapy aide?
   A. Teaching a client with a recent heart attack how to use a sock assist
   B. Reviewing a client's home exercise program for accurate performance
   C. Asking a client to fill out a leisure inventory
   D. Determining whether the client requires any durable medical equipment (DME) for home

5. An OT is supervising a volunteer in the outpatient occupational therapy department. The volunteer is enrolled in college and studying to be an OT. As a result, the volunteer is familiar with how to use adaptive equipment. The volunteer is at the site because she wants to learn more about occupational therapy on her own. It is not a fieldwork experience. Which of the following is most appropriate for the OT to allow the volunteer to do?
   A. Cut out Velcro tabs for splint making
   B. Review charts to learn more about occupational therapy documentation
   C. Teach a client how to use a buttonhook
   D. Provide hand-over-hand assistance to help a client with decreased hand strength learn to use a reacher

Worksheet 3-3

Student Supervision

George is an OT working in a rehabilitation center. He is supervising Lauren, an occupational therapy Level II fieldwork student who began her fieldwork at that facility 5 days ago. Consider the following conversation that George and Lauren had about a client. What suggestions would you make regarding the interaction between the therapist and student?

OT: *Lauren, this morning I would like you to work on dressing with a new stroke patient. His name is Phil Betta, and he is in room 225. He has left hemiparesis and is mod assist for dressing and transfers. You can teach him how to use some adaptive equipment.*

OT student: *Will you be there with me?*

OT: *No. Unfortunately, I will be in a meeting all morning to prepare for our upcoming reaccreditation site visit. Don't worry. Mr. Betta is a very nice man. He isn't very large so he shouldn't be too difficult to transfer into a chair.*

OT student: *Oh. I have never transferred a "real" patient before. Do I have to get him out of bed?*

OT: *Well, he has some decreased trunk control, so it will be easier for him to perform dressing seated in a chair rather than sitting on the edge of the bed.*

OT student: *To be honest, I am a bit nervous. I don't think I am capable of transferring him by myself. Can someone else treat him this morning?*

OT: *Lauren, you will have to learn sometime. Now is a good time as any. Didn't you practice transfers in school?*

OT student: *Yes, but only with my classmates.*

OT: *It will be OK. Just make sure you block his affected knee so it does not buckle. Also, use a transfer belt so you can control him better.*

OT student: *I really think it will be better for me to just work with him sitting in bed. What adaptive equipment does he need?*

OT: *I already told you he should perform dressing while seated in a chair. You need to figure out what equipment CVA patients like him should use for dressing. Just review his chart, take your time with him, and you should be fine. I really have to go to my meeting now. I will see you later at lunchtime.*

Suggestions to improve this interaction:

1.

2.

3.

4.

5.

6.

7.

8.

Learning Activity 3-4: Supervision and Leadership Skills

Imagine you graduated recently and began your first job as the sole OT at a nursing home. The rehabilitation director at that facility, whom you report to, is a physical therapist (PT). Your job responsibilities include client care and supervising an OTA employed by the nursing home. The OTA is 20 years older than you and has worked there full time for 15 years. Reflect on the scenarios that follow, considering these two different employment situations.

Employment Situation 1: You are a full-time employee hired by the nursing home.

Employment Situation 2: You work for an agency that contracts you to be at the nursing home three mornings a week, primarily for evaluations and supervision. (Assume this meets that state's licensure requirements regarding OTA supervision.)

As you complete the questions, determine whether the actions you would take would be the same or different if working at either of the two jobs.

1. Upon meeting the OTA for the first time to discuss a supervision schedule and expectations, what might you say to set the tone for a positive collaborative working relationship?
2. What are some things you could learn from the OTA?
3. You would like to implement some new evidence-based procedures for occupational therapy client interventions that you learned in school, but the OTA tells you, "We have never done that this way here." How might you respond?
4. The facility has not yet switched to an electronic documentation system. You notice that the two staff PTs and the speech therapist all document using a Subjective, Objective, Assessment, and Plan (SOAP) note format but the OTA uses a narrative format. You feel it would be beneficial for all the rehabilitation disciplines to be consistent, but the OTA tells you she does not like writing SOAP notes. What would you do?
5. The OTA you are supervising is competent in the use of electrotherapeutic agents. She asks you whether she can try using neuromuscular electrical stimulation (NMES) on a current client who has shoulder subluxation resulting from a stroke. You did not learn about this particular modality in school and did not see it used during your fieldwork. What would you do if the client could potentially benefit from this specialized intervention?
6. You observe that the OTA is much better at making orthotic devices than you because you have not had much experience in this area. What are your thoughts about this?
7. You notice that some equipment shared with the PT department is showing signs of wear and tear, such as several of the hot packs and terry cloth covers. You also would like to get some new adaptive equipment for occupational therapy meal preparation training (e.g., cutting board, angled knife, jar opener) and would like the facility to purchase a washer and dryer for the occupational therapy room to work on instrumental activities of daily living (IADLs; laundry) with clients. What actions would you take, if any?
8. When you are being introduced to the nursing staff by the rehabilitation secretary, several of the nurses refer to the OTA as "the other occupational therapist." What would you do or say?
9. The OTA has arrived 30 minutes late to work 3 days this week, but no one has said anything about this. This has limited your supervision time. How would you handle this situation?
10. Although you feel the OTA is competent and a nice person, you do not have much in common with her due to the large age gap and your different political and/or religious views. What are some things you could do to promote a congenial working environment?

Worksheet 3-4

Cultural Competence

1. Carl, a 45-year-old man, has multiple sclerosis and has been referred to outpatient occupational therapy. Today the OT, Cindy, is meeting and working with him for the first time. Carl was accompanied by another man, whom he introduced as his husband. Cindy has deep religious beliefs that oppose gay marriage, causing personal uneasiness. What should the therapist do?
   A. Explain to the client her discomfort with his lifestyle but that she will try to do her best to help him
   B. Immediately speak to the rehabilitation director and refuse to treat the client
   C. Educate the client regarding the OT's religious beliefs and offer to pray for him
   D. Ignore personal feelings and treat client and his partner with respect

2. Ali sustained a myocardial infarction and was admitted to an acute care hospital. Sarah, an OT, is scheduled to teach him skilled bathing techniques today. When she gets to Ali's room, he tells her it is against his religion to have a female other than his wife help him with bathing. There are no male occupational therapy practitioners on staff. Which of the following is the best course of action for the therapist?
   A. Reassure Ali that she is a trained health professional and tell him not to worry
   B. Work on pertinent client factors necessary for bathing
   C. Ask a male nurse to teach Ali bathing techniques
   D. Document that the client refused occupational therapy today

3. Chava, a 65-year-old woman and homemaker, devoutly follows the Orthodox sect of Judaism. She is in a rehabilitation hospital following an exacerbation of chronic obstructive pulmonary disease (COPD). Her occupational therapy goals include increasing activity tolerance for home management. To enhance participation in meal preparation, the plan for today's occupational therapy session is for Chava to prepare her own lunch and incorporate energy conservation techniques. To obtain the proper ingredients from the food service department for the session, which of the following items are the most culturally sensitive for an OT to offer Chava as a possible lunch choice, assuming there are no medical dietary restrictions?
   A. Cheeseburger
   B. Scrambled eggs and bacon
   C. Turkey and cheese sandwich
   D. Fresh fruit salad with cottage cheese

4. Parita is 78 years old and recently emigrated from India to the United States. Parita sustained a cardiovascular accident that resulted in left hemiparesis. She is currently in a rehabilitation hospital where the clients are expected to wear regular clothes during the day. The occupational therapy intervention plan includes goals for independent transfers and safe functional ambulation for home management tasks. Parita is able to use a hemi-walker with minimal assistance, but the OT notes the hemi-walker keeps getting caught in Parita's sari, her traditional clothing. The OT discusses this safety hazard with her and suggests alternate garments, but Parita refuses to wear clothing other than her traditional saris. Besides planning to try pinning or modifying the garments (if the client will agree to this) and also discussing the situation with the PT, which of the following should the OT document?
   A. Document that Parita has poor safety awareness
   B. Document that Parita needs to use a narrow-based quad cane
   C. Document the safety hazard and client education
   D. Recommend discharge from occupational therapy

Worksheet 3-4 (continued)

Cultural Competence

5. Martin is a 60-year-old man who recently had surgery for a rotator cuff repair. As part of the postsurgical protocol, the OT is instructing Martin on a home program of range of motion (ROM) exercises that the physician wants Martin to perform several times daily. Martin informs the therapist he cannot perform the exercises during a 24-hour period each weekend because his faith requires rest on the Sabbath. Which of the following is the best course of action for the therapist?
   A. Educate Martin regarding the medical necessity of the exercises and insist that Martin perform his exercises daily over the weekend
   B. Educate Martin regarding the medical necessity of the exercises and suggest Martin discuss this with his religious leader
   C. Tell Martin not to perform the exercises on the Sabbath
   D. Document that Martin is noncompliant

6. Howard, a 38-year-old devout follower of the Orthodox sect of Judaism, is receiving outpatient occupational therapy after a flexor tendon repair to his dominant right hand. Which of the following goals would most likely be inappropriate for Howard?
   A. Ability to hold a prayer book
   B. Ability to don a prayer shawl
   C. Ability to manipulate rosary beads during prayer ritual
   D. Ability to use tefillin during prayer ritual

7. Olivia is a 25-year-old Christian woman who follows a vegan lifestyle. She was admitted to an inpatient behavioral health unit with a diagnosis of depression. The occupational therapy intervention plan includes having Olivia complete a project in crafts group to improve her self-esteem. The OT determines that to promote decision-making skills for today's session, Olivia should be given a choice of only two craft projects. Which of the following would likely be the most culturally sensitive to present as one of her choices?
   A. A basket-weaving project using bamboo reeds
   B. Egg decorating for upcoming Easter holiday
   C. A dream-catcher project using branches and wool yarn
   D. A coin purse leather-lacing project with a cross design

8. Eva is a 65-year-old woman of Haitian descent. She has been receiving outpatient occupational therapy for several weeks to address her severe, chronic shoulder pain. Today when Eva arrives, she informs the OT that her pain has recently subsided due to a healing service she attended in her community 2 days ago. What should the therapist's primary response be?
   A. Express happiness that the client's pain is better
   B. Ignore what the client said. Given the client's condition, this sudden recovery defies logic, and the OT does not want to offend the client by telling her that
   C. Tell the client that that this seems very unlikely and that her improvement is really from the therapy she has received
   D. Inform the client that she should have a psychological evaluation

Worksheet 3-4 (continued)

Cultural Competence

9. Claire, a 56-year-old devout Catholic, is in a rehabilitation hospital following surgery for removal of a brain tumor. Today happens to be Good Friday. As Claire will be discharged to home next week, the plan is for her to prepare her own lunch today so that the OT can evaluate Claire's safety for meal preparation tasks. To obtain the requisite ingredients from the food service department for the session, which of the following items is the most culturally sensitive for a therapist to offer Claire as a possible lunch choice, assuming there are no dietary medical restrictions?
   A. Turkey sandwich
   B. Grilled cheese sandwich
   C. Canned chicken noodle soup
   D. Microwavable pepperoni pizza

10. Lin is a 30-year-old Asian man who immigrated to the United States 8 months ago. After back surgery, he unknowingly became addicted to prescription painkillers when following the recommended dosage and was recently admitted to an inpatient chemical dependency program. Lin tends to be quiet during group and does not make eye contact with the OT. He barely interacts with the other clients and does not openly express his feelings. What should the therapist document?
    A. That the client is depressed
    B. That the client's interpersonal behaviors may be influenced by his culture
    C. That the client is noncompliant with group process
    D. That the client has a poor prognosis

Worksheet 3-5

Cultural Competence—More Practice

1. Tamara is an 18-year-old single mother of two toddlers aged 2 and 3. Her 2-year-old is diagnosed with a developmental delay and is receiving early intervention services at home. Tamara is 5' 4" and weighs 220 pounds. Her two children are at the top end of normal developmental ranges for weight. Which of the following is most appropriate for the OT to express to Tamara during the initial evaluation?
   A. "You should go on a diet."
   B. "It concerns me that your children are overweight."
   C. "Do you understand that your obesity will prevent you from taking care of your kids properly?"
   D. "Would you be open to having a dietician come talk to you about strategies for purchasing a variety of snacks and meals for the children?"

2. Priya is a 22-year-old premed student from India who has been attending college in the United States. She has been referred to outpatient occupational therapy because of a hand injury resulting from a fall. During the initial evaluation, Priya mentions that her fiancé will be arriving in the United States soon. The OT asks how long they have been dating, and Priya replies, "Oh, I haven't met him yet, but we have been texting and e-mailing each other for the past 2 months. Our families think we are a good match and have arranged for us to marry soon." This arouses the therapist's curiosity. Which of the following choices should be the therapist's primary response?
   A. "I did not know arranged marriages still happen in this day and age."
   B. "That seems like a very old-fashioned concept."
   C. "Sounds like you have something great to look forward to."
   D. "What if you do not like him—do you have any choice about getting married?"

3. Antonio and his family emigrated from Italy 6 months ago to become U.S. citizens. His 9-month-old son is diagnosed with cerebral palsy and recently started receiving early intervention services. To improve motor development to enhance ADLs and play, the OT is teaching Antonio and his wife how to position the infant properly. As the therapist asks Antonio to demonstrate holding the infant for the tasks of diapering and bathing, Antonio refuses and states, "It is the women's job to change the baby's diaper and bathe him. My wife always does that. You can't expect a man to do those things." Which of the following is the OT's best course of action?
   A. Insist that Antonio participate in diapering and bathing tasks as they are part of the child's intervention plan.
   B. Tell Antonio that fathers in the United States actively participate in diapering and bathing tasks so he should also.
   C. Work with Antonio on other aspects of the child's care that he feels are acceptable for him to participate in.
   D. Tell Antonio and his wife that he is sexist and that Antonio's help is needed with the baby.

Worksheet 3-5 (continued)

Cultural Competence—More Practice

4. Huan is a 91-year-old Chinese male living in the home of his adult son and daughter-in-law, as is traditional for their culture. Huan is diagnosed with end-stage dementia and is frail, bedridden, and dependent in ADLs. The family expresses that they desire to keep their beloved elder in their home. Huan is beginning to develop Stage 1 pressure areas on his ankle and sacrum. In addition to skilled nursing to address skin integrity, the physician-ordered home care occupational therapy to educate the family on bed mobility and positioning. As the OT completes the evaluation, which of the following is the therapist's best course of action?
   - A. Provide the family education as ordered while communicating respect for their interest in keeping Huan at home.
   - B. Insist that the family place the client in a nursing home to care for him better.
   - C. Recommend that Huan participate in an adult day care program.
   - D. Recommend PT to improve Huan's mobility using a walker.

5. Abraham, a 65-year-old male diagnosed with COPD, has been referred to outpatient OT after a short stay in a rehabilitation hospital. Abraham devoutly follows an ultra Orthodox sect of Judaism and owns a small retail business. His OT, Sarah, recognizes him from shopping at his store. Which of the following is most appropriate for Sarah to do when first greeting Abraham?
   - A. Shake hands and introduce herself as his OT.
   - B. Lightly touch his arm or back and introduce herself as his OT.
   - C. Give him a slight side hug and introduce herself as his OT.
   - D. Avoid physical contact and introduce herself as his OT.

Learning Activity 3-5: Improving Cultural Awareness

Interview someone who has different religious beliefs than you do or has a different cultural or ethnic affiliation. Choose one or more of the categories in the following table and compare and contrast them for the two of you. Some suggested topics are presented. Can you think of other questions you might ask to further improve cultural awareness? Each person should volunteer information based on their personal level of comfort for disclosure.

Category	*Topics You Might Explore*	*My Religion, Culture, or Ethnicity Is:*	*Other Person's Religion, Culture, or Ethnicity Is:*
Appearance and Attire	Are there specific requirements or special types of clothing? What types of religious garments/accessories are worn (e.g., shawl, fringes, cross, turban)? Is modesty important? Are head coverings important? What are the attitudes toward body size, tattoos piercings, makeup, hairstyles? Are there gender differences?		
More-Valued/ Less-Valued Professions	What professions are revered in that culture (e.g., rabbi, doctor, teacher, master craftsman)? What professions are considered least desirable?		
Dating Rituals/ Courtship	How do people typically meet (e.g., arranged marriage, matchmaker, bars or clubs)? What is the length of a courtship/engagement? What is the level of physical contact allowed? Is family approval needed?		
Marriage Rituals	Is ceremony inside a house of worship? What is the type of ceremony? What is the attire/adornment worn by bride/groom (e.g., color of dress, henna designs, headwear, tuxedo)? Besides the couple, who else is involved in ceremony? What type of celebration follows the ceremony?		
Rites of Passage	Is there a special ceremony/celebration for transition to adulthood (e.g., bar mitzvah, quinceañera, debutante ball)?		

Learning Activity 3-5: Improving Cultural Awareness (continued)

Category	*Topics You Might Explore*	*My Religion, Culture, or Ethnicity Is:*	*Other Person's Religion, Culture, or Ethnicity Is:*
Special Holidays	What cultural, secular, or religious holidays are celebrated? Why and how are each of those holidays celebrated?		
Death Rituals	Is there a specific time frame for burial? What type of services (e.g., wake, Shiva, church service)? Is there a special gathering following the burial or wake? What is the disposition of the body (mausoleum, burial, scattering of ashes)? What type of clothing is worn by the deceased? What type of clothing is worn by persons mourning/paying respect? What type of burial container is used (e.g., pine box, ornate casket, urn)? Is there belief in an afterlife? Is there ongoing visiting of the deceased's final resting place by survivors?		
Family Roles	Who provides care for elderly relatives? Are parents expected to live with married children? Are there gender/family member roles and responsibilities (e.g., matriarch, patriarch, do the women work outside of home, do fathers change diapers?) What are the styles of parenting (e.g., authoritarian, permissive, coparenting)?		
Lifestyle and Behaviors	What are the attitudes toward smoking, alcoholic beverages, and caffeine? Are there dancing restrictions? What are the attitudes toward TV, the Internet, movies, newspapers?		

Learning Activity 3-5: Improving Cultural Awareness (continued)

Category	*Topics You Might Explore*	*My Religion, Culture, or Ethnicity Is:*	*Other Person's Religion, Culture, or Ethnicity Is:*
Lifestyles, Health, and Sickness	What are the attitudes toward sickness or disability (e.g., punishment from God, stoic nature)? Is there belief in natural, holistic, or alternative treatments? Is there belief in cures from spiritual or healing rituals?		
Foods	Are there special foods for meals, holidays, and celebrations? Are there dietary considerations (e.g., kosher diet, specific meat products prohibited)? Are there religious rituals or special methods involving food?		
Religious Beliefs and Rituals	Is there belief in a higher power or deity? Are there specific rituals within a house of worship (e.g., kneeling, receiving Holy Communion)? Are there specific rituals outside of a house of worship (e.g., observing the Sabbath, lighting candles, saying the rosary)? Is there a sense of community? What are the types of sacraments?		

Reprinted with permission from Morreale, M. J. (2015). *Developing clinical competence: A workbook for the OTA*. Thorofare, NJ: SLACK Incorporated.

Worksheet 3-6

Attaining Service Competency

1. At her new job, an entry-level OT is expected to perform transfer training with a particular client who requires maximum assistance. The therapist is unsure that she knows how to do this safely by herself. Which primary course of action should the therapist take?

   A. Ask the PT or nursing staff to transfer the client instead.

   B. Ask for instruction in use of a lift device and for another professional to be present when the OT first uses it.

   C. Obtain more information on transfer techniques from textbooks and the Internet.

   D. Perform a different intervention.

2. Today an entry-level OT was delegated an outpatient client who had hand surgery 4 weeks ago. The surgical site is healed, and there are no surgical precautions at this time. The doctor's orders and supervising OT's intervention plan indicate that the client needs to work on increasing grip strength and fine motor skills to better manage ADLs and return to work. The therapist did not learn about that particular surgical procedure in school. Which of the following is the best course of action for the entry-level therapist before the client arrives several hours from now?

   A. Ask another occupational therapy practitioner to treat the client.

   B. Tell the occupational therapy supervisor it is unethical for the entry-level therapist to treat the client at this time.

   C. Review the client's chart and use resources to obtain more information regarding the client's diagnosis.

   D. Reschedule the client for another day when the OT's supervisor can be in the room at the same time to supervise.

3. An occupational therapy student is performing Level II fieldwork in an outpatient setting. The fieldwork educator informs the student that students at that site are expected to fabricate orthotic devices for clients. The student has not made an orthotic device since taking her skills class in school 6 months ago. One of the fieldwork educator's clients coming to therapy tomorrow needs a wrist extension orthosis. Which of the following is the best course of action for the student?

   A. Make the orthotic device on the client with the occupational therapist supervising.

   B. Review an orthotics textbook and videos.

   C. Ask the OT to fabricate the client's orthosis because students are not allowed to fabricate orthotic devices.

   D. Ask permission to make an orthotic device on an occupational therapy practitioner today.

4. An OT would like to learn more about techniques to address sensory functioning for children with autism. Which of the following is the best method that the therapist should implement?

   A. Read evidence-based professional literature

   B. Attend professional seminars

   C. Ask a more experienced occupational therapy practitioner to mentor the therapist

   D. All of the above

Worksheet 3-6 (continued)

Attaining Service Competency

5. An entry-level OT just started a job in a school setting. When would it be most appropriate for the therapist to stop participating in professional development activities?
   A. When the OT is fully competent in the current job
   B. When the OT is no longer working as a therapist
   C. When the OT has 10 years of clinical experience
   D. When the OT has 5 years of clinical experience

6. After attending 25 hours' worth of occupational therapy seminars during a current NBCOT recertification cycle, a hospital-based OT is on a tight budget and cannot afford any more professional seminars this year. To help accrue remaining professional development hours needed for NBCOT recertification, the therapist can do all of the following except:
   A. Develop a client satisfaction survey for the hospital's occupational therapy department
   B. Supervise Level I fieldwork students
   C. Publish an article in a local newsletter regarding the hospital's occupational therapy low-vision program
   D. Publish an article in an occupational therapy magazine that is not peer-reviewed

Learning Activity 3-6: Developing Professional Reasoning

During your fieldwork experience, you are expected to teach energy conservation techniques for home management to a group of clients with COPD. Your supervisor tells you that an essential component of the client instruction is teaching them how to incorporate proper breathing techniques as the IADLs are performed. You have never worked with anyone with COPD and are not sure how to implement the task properly. The group is scheduled for 2 days from now. Consider how you will approach this dilemma and the possible outcomes.

Options to Address Problem	***Potential Positive Outcomes if This Option Is Implemented***	***Potential Undesirable Outcomes if This Option Is Implemented***	***Is This Option a Good Choice?***
1. Tell your supervisor you are not competent to perform this task			
2. Ask your supervisor where you can get more information on this topic			
3. Ask your classmates or friends for help			
4. Try to remain calm and just "wing it" the day of the group			
5. Search for information resources			
Other options:			

What Relevant Resources Will You Use? (e.g., specific people to contact, book titles, websites, particular articles)	***Action Plan for Each Resource (e.g., specific library databases, Internet URLs, process for obtaining written materials/ videos, contact phone numbers)***
1.	
2.	
3.	
4.	
5.	

Learning Activity 3-7: Administering a Standardized Test

Imagine you are completing your Level II fieldwork and are expected to administer a particular standardized test to meet objectives for fieldwork. You have not learned about this assessment in school and have not yet seen it used on fieldwork. You would like to implement the standardized test properly so that you will pass fieldwork. Consider how you might approach this dilemma. For this exercise, choose a standardized assessment with which you are not familiar. You might ask one of your academic instructors or your fieldwork educator for access to a standardized test such as one that assesses particular development in children, visual motor skills, or coordination. Consider the following:

Name of Assessment: ______________________________

1. What steps can you take to become more knowledgeable about this test?
   1.
   2.
   3.
   4.
   5.
2. What kinds of information does this test provide? ______________________________
   ____
3. Indicate three possible conditions that this test might be used for:
   1.
   2.
   3.
4. Indicate the age range appropriate for use with this test: ______________________________
5. Is this test valid and reliable? ______Yes ______ No
6. Indicate the type of setting where this test may be administered (e.g., quiet room with privacy, rehab gym, playground, classroom): ______________________________
   ____
7. Indicate the general format for the assessment (e.g., interview, gross or fine motor activities, ADLs, visual, constructional, written responses): ______________________________
   ____
   ____
8. How much time is needed to administer this test? ______________________________

Learning Activity 3-7: Administering a Standardized Test (continued)

9. What is the format for providing instructions to the client?
____ Written instructions ____ Word-for-word verbal instructions ____ Paraphrase verbal instructions
____ Other

10. Indicate all the equipment or supplies you will need to gather to administer this test (e.g., table, paper, pencil, timer, blocks, leather-lacing project, occlusion board, etc.)
____
____

11. What possible factors may interfere with test administration?
____
____

12. Find three evidence-based articles that support or discourage the use of this assessment and cite them below:
1. ____
____
2. ____
____
3. ____
____

13. Indicate how the results of this assessment may relate to a client's occupational performance:
____
____

14. List three alternate standardized assessments that an OT can use to measure similar performance skills, client factors, or occupations as the assessment you chose for this exercise.
1. ____
____
2. ____
____
3. ____
____

Worksheet 3-7

Advocacy

Indicate if the following statements are true (T) or false (F).

1. T ___ F ___ It is redundant to join a state occupational therapy association if you are already a member of the American Occupational Therapy Association (AOTA).

2. T ___ F ___ Occupational therapy practitioners should advocate to help occupational therapy consumers receive the services they need.

3. T ___ F ___ An OT or occupational therapy student should join the AOTA primarily to receive the journals.

4. T ___ F ___ An OT cannot really do anything about changing a law that has an impact on occupational therapy.

5. T ___ F ___ Occupational therapy students are not able to meet with legislative staff regarding health care reform because students are not yet licensed professionals.

6. T ___ F ___ An OT can demonstrate advocacy by joining the AOTA.

7. T ___ F ___ Although advocacy is important to change laws, it does not affect reimbursement of occupational therapy.

8. T ___ F ___ Social media is not an effective method for advocacy because it is not a professional format.

9. T ___ F ___ Donating money is the most effective way to advocate.

10. T ___ F ___ One method to advocate for occupational therapy is by signing a petition.

11. T ___ F ___ It is difficult for an OT or occupational therapy student to know what to write in a letter to legislators regarding current issues affecting occupational therapy.

12. T ___ F ___ Advocacy only affects federal issues.

13. T ___ F ___ The AOTA can contribute directly to political candidates.

14. T ___ F ___ Advocacy cannot affect state regulatory issues, such as occupational therapy scope of practice and continuing competency requirements, because state legislators create the laws.

15. T ___ F ___ An issue requiring occupational therapy advocacy is fair and equal access to health care.

Worksheet 3-8

Teamwork

1. Which of the following jobs is most important in a hospital?
   A. Nurse
   B. Housekeeper/janitor
   C. Occupational therapy practitioner
   D. Health information system manager

2. The desired goal of conflict resolution is primarily which of the following?
   A. Getting a raise
   B. Meeting goals in a client's intervention plan
   C. Meeting yearly personal goals
   D. A mutually beneficial situation for parties involved

3. The three rehabilitation department heads (physical, occupational, and speech therapy) are meeting to create a new mission statement for the rehabilitation department. On an average day, the physical therapy department provides 100 client sessions, the occupational therapy department provides 50, and the speech department provides 20. Which of the department heads should have the most say in what the mission statement should include?
   A. Physical therapy
   B. Occupational therapy
   C. Physical therapy and occupational therapy
   D. Physical therapy, occupational therapy, and speech therapy

4. An OT and PT are treating different clients at the same time in the rehabilitation gym. No other staff is present in the room. The OT observes a client giving the other therapist a hard time. The client is calling the PT names and is complaining loudly about the care received. As the OT is finishing up with her own client, what primary course of action should she take?
   A. Ask the PT if there is anything the OT can do to help
   B. Get the rehabilitation director
   C. Do not interfere with the PT and client interaction
   D. Tell the PT's client that the negative behavior is not appropriate

5. During their daily supervision meeting, an OTA and OT collaborated about a particular client and determined the client needs supervision for safe functional ambulation at home. The therapist asked the OTA to represent occupational therapy at a rehabilitation team meeting later that day with that client's PT, nurse, and social worker to discuss the client's discharge plan. During the meeting, the PT disagreed with the OTA that the client is unsafe. What should the OTA do first?
   A. Tell the team that the PT is wrong
   B. Provide examples of the client's unsafe behavior
   C. Defer to the PT because the PT has more expertise regarding ambulation training
   D. Go get the OT

Learning Activity 3-8: Interprofessional Collaboration

Considering various practice settings, list several ways in which each of the following professional disciplines or support staff may have a direct impact on an occupational therapy practitioner's role, function, or efficiency for safe and effective client care.

1. Social worker
   Example: Orders the durable medical equipment that the OT or OTA recommends for client's home
2. Dietary staff
   Example: Provides food for occupational therapy meal preparation training
3. Biomedical equipment technologist
4. Health records personnel
5. Physical therapist
6. Speech and language pathologist
7. Nursing staff
8. Housekeeper/janitor
9. Direct care worker
10. Teacher
11. Other:
12. Other:

Reprinted with permission from Morreale, M. J. (2015). *Developing clinical competence: A workbook for the OTA*. Thorofare, NJ: SLACK Incorporated.

Worksheet 3-9

Team Members

For each of the practice settings indicated in the following chart, list additional health team members who might collaborate to provide direct care/specialized services to clients or family/caregivers.

Early Intervention/School	***Behavioral Health Setting***
1. *OT/OTA*	1. *OT/OTA*
2.	2.
3.	3.
4.	4.
5.	5.
6.	6.
7.	7.
8.	8.
9.	9.
10.	10.
Home care	***Rehabilitation Hospital***
1. *OT/OTA*	1. *OT/OTA*
2.	2.
3.	3.
4.	4.
5.	5.
6.	6.
7.	7.
8.	8.
9.	9.
10.	10.

Reprinted with permission from Morreale, M. J. (2015). *Developing clinical competence: A workbook for the OTA*. Thorofare, NJ: SLACK Incorporated.

Learning Activity 3-9: Emerging Practice Areas

Use the AOTA website (www.aota.org) to search for emerging niches in the six primary areas of occupational therapy practice (AOTA, 2013d). When you have completed the following chart, indicate which of the niches you might consider working in as an area of practice and explain why you chose it.

Practice Area	*Choose Two Emerging Niches*	*Indicate Age Range Served*	*Type of Setting (e.g., school, client's home)*	*Kinds of Interventions (e.g., groups, environmental modifications, consultation)*
Children and youth	1. 2.			
Health and wellness	1. 2.			
Mental health	1. 2.			
Productive aging	1. 2.			
Rehabilitation and dis-ability	1. 2.			
Work and industry	1. 2.			

Adapted from Morreale, M. J. (2015). *Developing clinical competence: A workbook for the OTA*. Thorofare, NJ: SLACK Incorporated.

Worksheet 3-10

Emerging Methods and Settings of Service Delivery

With changes in technological options and the United States health care system in general, many opportunities exist for occupational therapy practitioners to provide services to those who are underserved or can benefit from the holistic approach to health and well-being that is espoused by the profession.

This worksheet challenges your knowledge of new methods of service delivery and new practice arenas for occupational therapy practitioners.

1. Benefits of telehealth are numerous and include which one of the following according to the AOTA position paper "Telehealth" (AOTA, 2013f)?
   A. Save the expense of travel for clients living far from health care facilities
   B. Increase caseload of therapist through enhanced efficiency of service delivery
   C. Provide more expedient access to care for those in rural areas
   D. Enhance opportunities for therapists who are unable to drive or who prefer to work from home

2. As a model of health care delivery, telehealth includes all but one of the following types of service.
   A. Health care
   B. Health information
   C. Health education
   D. Health literacy

3. Telehealth is considered to be which one of the following types of service delivery?
   A. Direct service
   B. Indirect service
   C. Consultation
   D. Hands free

4. Telehealth services can be provided in a synchronous or asynchronous manner. Examples of synchronous technology include all but which of the following?
   A. Telephone
   B. Video recordings
   C. Voice over Internet
   D. Video teleconferencing

5. Primary care settings are described as those that:
   A. Are the first medical facilities visited by newborns
   B. Are identical to family medicine practices
   C. Are practices that focus on prevention and disease management
   D. Are located in hospital emergency departments

Worksheet 3-10 (continued)

Emerging Methods and Settings of Service Delivery

6. An occupational therapist working in a primary care setting would likely:
   A. Work with clients post-cerebrovascular accident (CVA) to assist them with regaining ADL independence
   B. Provide school-based services to children after primary care physician referral
   C. Discuss home safety with a client who reports a recent fall in her home to the primary care physician
   D. Set up transportation services for elderly clients to enable independent trips to the pharmacy to pick up needed medications

7. The Affordable Care Act supports primary care models of health care as part of the Triple Aim, which is interested in:
   A. Improving the care experience for individuals, improving populations' health, and lessening per capita care costs
   B. Improving the individual experience of care and that of the health care provider to ensure a cost-efficient delivery of service
   C. Improving health of populations with a focus on preventing disease in those who are invested in taking personal responsibility for their quality of life and well-being
   D. Reducing per capita cost of care, improving the experience of care, and ensuring the ethical and moral practice of medicine

Indicate whether the following statements are true (T) or false (F):

8. Primary care is the provision of integrated, accessible health care that addresses clients' personal health care needs, includes the establishment of sustained partnerships with clients, and provides clinical practice within the context of family and community. ________

9. When employed in a primary care setting, occupational therapy services will greatly resemble those provided in an outpatient rehabilitation setting. ______

10. Assisting clients to establish healthful habits and routines will be a responsibility of the OT in a primary care setting of the future. _____

11. The administration of occupational therapy through telehealth technology is not covered by all third-party payers. ________

12. Occupational therapists can evaluate and treat clients remotely through telehealth technology. This includes hands-on interventions completed by an individual who is physically with the client as instructed by the therapist remotely. _______

Answers to Chapter 3 Worksheets

Worksheet 3-1: Roles and Responsibilities

An OTA performs occupational therapy services under the supervision of an OT (AOTA, 2010b, 2014a). The OTA collaborates with the OT to perform delegated responsibilities and aspects of client care for which the OTA has service competency, are within the scope of ethical occupational therapy practice, and adhere to federal, state, and facility guidelines (AOTA, 2010b, 2014a, 2014d, 2015). Most answers that follow are based on *Guidelines for Supervision, Roles, and Responsibilities During the Delivery of Occupational Therapy Services* (AOTA, 2014a), *Scope of Practice* (AOTA, 2014d), and *Standards of Practice for Occupational Therapy* (AOTA, 2010b). Additional pertinent references are noted in the chart as appropriate.

	Task	OT	OTA
1.	Instruct client in a home exercise program	*	*
2.	Develop the occupational therapy intervention plan	*	
3.	Determine whether a client performs a cooking task safely	*	*
4.	Gait Training *This is typically the role of physical therapy, although occupational therapy can support function* (AOTA, 2013e)		
5.	Teach positioning techniques to a parent of a child with cerebral palsy	*	*
6.	Upgrade an exercise program	*	*
7.	Determine discharge from occupational therapy	*	
8.	Respond to a referral to occupational therapy	*	
9.	Implement occupational therapy interventions	*	*
10.	Teach one-handed shoe-tying	*	*
11.	Complete the occupational therapy initial evaluation report independently	*	
12.	Administer a standardized assessment	*	*
13.	Interpret initial evaluation results	*	
14.	Fabricate an orthotic device	*	*
15.	Customize a resident's wheelchair with specialized inserts	*	*
16.	Administer superficial thermal modalities as the sole client intervention during a session *A physical agent modality is not considered occupational therapy unless it is followed up by additional therapeutic intervention to improve function* (AOTA, 2012b)		
17.	Document occupational therapy intervention	*	*
18.	Provide intervention to a home care client	*	*
19.	Instruct client in workplace ergonomics	*	*
20.	Provide specialized instruction in self-care	*	*
21.	Help a student put on boots for recess *Anyone can help a child don boots. However, if the occupational therapy practitioner is implementing an occupational therapy intervention plan, such as teaching self-care skills or working on client factors such as bilateral integration or balance, then that would be considered skilled occupational therapy* (Morreale & Borcherding, 2013)		
22.	Develop goals for an Individualized Education Program (IEP)	*	
23.	Assess transfer skills	*	*
24.	Provide occupational therapy in a neonatal intensive care unit (AOTA, 2006)	*	
25.	Attain certification in hand therapy (Hand Therapy Certification Commission [HTCC], 2013)	*	
26.	Attain AOTA board certification in pediatrics (AOTA, 2013a)	*	

	Task	OT	OTA
27.	Attain AOTA specialty certification in low vision (AOTA, 2013a)	*	*
28.	Make recommendations to a teacher regarding compensatory techniques for a student receiving occupational therapy services	*	*
29.	Delegate aspects of an occupational therapy initial evaluation	*	
30.	Write short-term goals in a treatment note as a substep toward implementing an established intervention plan	*	*
31.	Update a client's intervention plan	*	
32.	Write a discharge report independently	*	
33.	Adapt an ADL device to improve a client's self-care performance	*	*
34.	Assess range of motion using a goniometer	*	*
35.	Teach nursing staff how to apply a client's orthotic device	*	*
36.	Provide a handout on cardiac precautions *Anyone can give a client a brochure or handout. This is not considered skilled occupational therapy unless followed up by skilled instruction or practice* (Morreale & Borcherding, 2013).		
37.	Supervise a rehabilitation aide	*	*
38.	Supervise a volunteer in the occupational therapy department	*	*
39.	Supervise a Level I OTA student (ACOTE, 2012; AOTA, 2007)	*	*
40.	Supervise a Level II OTA student (ACOTE, 2012; AOTA, 2012a)	*	*
41.	Supervise a Level I OT student (ACOTE, 2012; AOTA, 2007)	*	*
42.	Supervise a Level II OT student (ACOTE, 2012; AOTA, 2012a)	*	
43.	Lead an occupational therapy group in a behavioral health setting	*	*
44.	Observe a child color a picture *Simply watching someone do an activity is not skilled occupational therapy. However, if the occupational therapy practitioner was assessing the child's performance skills, such as balance, coordination, or safety, then that could be considered a skilled service* (Morreale & Borcherding, 2013).		
45.	Recommend durable medical equipment upon client's discharge home	*	*
46.	Assess a client's orientation to person, place, and time	*	*
47.	Inform nursing staff about a client's report of pain	*	*
48.	Provide an in-service to the rehabilitation staff about an evidence-based practice article	*	*
49.	Assess vital signs	*	*
50.	Attend a team meeting to discuss a client's care and progress	*	*

Worksheet 3-2: Supervision

1. C. Steve has mutual responsibility to ensure that he receives appropriate supervision levels (AOTA, 2014a). He should go through the proper chain of command and discuss his concerns with his supervising OT first. The therapist may not be aware that Steve has those concerns. If Steve and his occupational therapy supervisor are not able to come to a satisfactory arrangement, he might then seek help from the rehabilitation director. Although Steve could ask his colleagues about their level of supervision, their needs may not be relevant to Steve's, and it could also be perceived negatively as complaining or gossiping. Thus, it is best to speak to the therapist directly.
2. A. It is not ethical for Leila to perform those assessments because they clearly require supervision based on Leila's student status, lack of knowledge, and inexperience (AOTA, 2014a, 2015). Because Leila has already discussed her concerns with the fieldwork educator without a satisfactory resolution, the next step is to ask her academic

fieldwork coordinator to intervene. As a student, it would not be appropriate in this instance to go over her supervisor's head and speak to the rehabilitation director before contacting the academic fieldwork coordinator.

3. D. If the OTA is merely expressing legitimate concerns, firing the OTA would not be an appropriate response. An OT should not "force" an OTA to perform a delegated task that the OTA believes will cause harm to the client (AOTA, 2014a, 2015). However, the therapist should have an honest and open discussion with the OTA to explain why this intervention is appropriate and provide evidence-based resources to alleviate the OTA's concerns. They might also establish a professional development plan for the OTA to obtain further information as needed for this diagnosis or intervention.
4. C. It is not ethical for the OT to delegate a skilled occupational therapy task to an aide. However, an aide can ask a client to fill out a form that the OT will review with the client later. All the other answers require professional judgment and knowledge and are not appropriate for the aide to perform (AOTA, 2014a; Morreale & Borcherding, 2013).
5. A. It is not appropriate for a volunteer to review client charts because this would violate confidentiality. Teaching a client how to use adaptive equipment is skilled intervention that is not appropriate to delegate to a volunteer or aide (AOTA, 2014a). It is appropriate for a volunteer to assist with preparing equipment—in this case, cutting out pieces of hook and loop fastener that the occupational therapy practitioners can apply to orthotic devices.

Worksheet 3-3: Student Supervision

Suggestions to improve this interaction:

1. The OT should use people-first language (e.g., "client who had a stroke" or "client with a diagnosis of CVA," rather than saying "stroke patient" or "CVA patient").
2. The client is not an assist level. The OT should indicate that the client requires moderate assistance rather than he is an assist level (Morreale & Borcherding, 2013).
3. The OT is not adhering to appropriate guidelines for supervision, which is unethical (AOTA, 2014a, 2015).
4. Clearly, the OT should be providing direct supervision for a task that may be a safety concern and for which the student has not demonstrated competency.
5. If the OT cannot provide the appropriate supervision for this task, the OT could suggest another intervention the student can implement with this client that is not a safety concern for Mr. Betta (e.g., grooming while sitting up in bed).
6. The OT could offer reasonable alternatives for the transfer, such as having another staff member either demonstrate the client transfer or assist the student with the transfer.
7. The occupational therapy student should demonstrate clinical reasoning and try to determine the adaptive equipment needed for a client with a stroke rather than just asking her supervisor to provide the information.
8. The OT does not effectively acknowledge the student's concerns.

Worksheet 3-4: Cultural Competence

1. D. As a health professional, an OT should respect the sociocultural background of the client and not discriminate based on Carl's sexual orientation (AOTA, 2010b, 2014b, 2014c, 2015; Robins, 2006). An OT is also expected to educate family and significant others as needed to facilitate the discharge process (AOTA, 2010b). The therapist can have personal religious values or beliefs but must demonstrate cultural sensitivity, set aside personal judgment or bias, and treat the client with dignity and respect. It would be disrespectful, uncomfortable, and embarrassing for the client and his partner to discuss the therapist's personal beliefs or to offer to pray for their redemption. The therapist should also discuss ethical conflicts or concerns with the occupational therapy supervisor to become more culturally competent.
2. B. It is important to respect the client's cultural and religious beliefs and not insist that the client perform tasks that violate his morals (AOTA, 2010b, 2014b, 2014c, 2015; Royeen & Crabtree, 2006). If there is no male occupational therapy practitioner on staff who could work on bathing with this client, the OT should instead work on the relevant skills needed for bathing, such as ROM, activity tolerance, or balance. Although it is not appropriate to ask another discipline to provide skilled occupational therapy, collaboration with other team

members is helpful. However, the therapist might first determine whether training the client's wife for this task or simply having the client's wife present in the room would make a difference in allowing the therapist to work on bathing with this client.

3. D. When implementing meal preparation interventions, it is helpful for an OT to discuss food choices with the client ahead of time because the client may have allergies, dislikes, or cultural considerations. Observant followers of the Orthodox sect of Judaism normally follow kosher guidelines, which prohibit pork products and the consumption of meat and dairy products together at meals (Goldsmith, 2006). Also, realize that special plates, utensils, and food preparation methods may be needed, such as certified kosher foods for consumption and utensils wrapped in plastic. Further information regarding kosher guidelines can be found at http://www.jewfaq.org/kashrut.htm.
4. C. It is important to respect Parita's deep-rooted cultural beliefs and consider the traditional clothing that she will wear upon discharge from the facility (AOTA, 2010b, 2014c, 2015). However, it is still important to note the safety hazard and document any client education provided along with the need for supervision or assistance. Perhaps the client will allow the garment to be pinned or modified to minimize the hazard effectively, and attempts at this should also be documented. The OT should also discuss the concern with the PT, who has the expertise to assess what other mobility devices might be appropriate and safer for Parita to use at this time.
5. B. In this case, the OT should first recommend that the client discuss the medical necessity of the exercises with his religious leader as there may be special dispensation for activities needed to improve an individual's health. However, it is important to respect the client's cultural and religious beliefs and not insist that the client perform tasks that violate his faith (AOTA, 2010b, 2014c, 2015; Royeen & Crabtree, 2006).
6. C. Rosary beads are prayer beads associated with Catholicism, not Judaism. A, B, and D are incorporated into Jewish rituals for males along with other special items, such as wearing thread fringes and a yarmulke head covering (Goldsmith, 2006).
7. A. A vegan does not eat or use animal products, so plant-based craft materials are the most appropriate (Merriam-Webster, 2013). B, C, and D would not be good choices for this client because they consist of animal-based products (wool, eggs, and leather). String or cord used for a dream-catcher or lacing project is also a safety concern for this patient.
8. A. A primary goal for clients with severe pain is to decrease pain for improved quality of life and occupational performance. In this case, the client's perception is that she now has markedly decreased pain, which is the desired outcome. The OT should respect the client's cultural belief regarding a healing service or other cultural remedies (Royeen & Crabtree, 2006). It would not be useful to disagree or argue with this client. Education or appropriate intervention would be needed for any cultural practices that are truly harmful.
9. B. For Catholics, Good Friday is a holy day requiring abstinence from meat and fasting for adults (of certain ages); limited food is allowed and exceptions may be made for a person's health (Richert, 2013).
10. B. Because this client's communication style may be cultural, an OT must be careful not to jump to other conclusions (Asher, 2006). The therapist's observations should be discussed with the other team members. Perhaps alternate communication methods, such as a journal entry or art project, may be more appropriate for this client to express his emotions more easily.

Worksheet 3-5: Cultural Competence—More Practice

1. D. The OT needs to establish rapport. Using a strong term such as *obese* could make the client defensive, insecure, or untrusting. The therapist should avoid value judgments and not insinuate that the client cannot be a good mother because of her size. Answer B is incorrect because the children have not yet exceeded normal weight ranges. In this case, it is best to gently, and in a nonjudgmental manner, discuss possible services the client can benefit from.
2. C. Answers A and B may embarrass the client. Answer D is not the most tactful and may make the client uncomfortable. Answer C is a positive response that respects the client's cultural tenets.
3. C. It is important to respect the client's cultural beliefs, such as gender roles (AOTA, 2014c; Royeen & Crabtree, 2006). Of course, any practices that are truly harmful would need to be addressed. Calling the father sexist is judgmental and inappropriate. However, the OT might discuss the extra stress that a child's disability can create and that his wife may need extra help.

4. A. Clearly, the family does not want to place their loved elder in a nursing home because this would go against their cultural beliefs. The therapist could encourage the family members to discuss concerns they may have regarding their ability to care for Huan, so that strategies can potentially be recommended. The team should provide the appropriate support and resources to enable the client to remain safely at home for as long as medically possible. Because of the client's severe medical problems, it is not feasible for him to ambulate or attend an adult day care program outside of the home.
5. D. Physical contact such as hugs, social touching, or shaking hands with an unrelated member of the opposite sex would likely violate this client's religious boundaries.

Worksheet 3-6: Attaining Service Competency

1. B. For a client who requires maximum assistance for transfers, a facility might have policies in place requiring that a second person assist or a mechanical lift be used to avoid injury. The OT should ensure safety for herself and her client and always follow the facility's policy and procedures. Although the OT could perform a different intervention or ask other disciplines to perform the transfer, competence in transfers is an essential function of this therapist's job. The OT needs to learn how to perform transfers safely and should discuss a plan with the OT's supervisor. Although resources such as books and the Internet are useful, formal instruction and supervised hands-on-practice would be the most beneficial.
2. C. The entry-level OT should be able to perform the intervention without the supervisor directly present because there are no surgical precautions, the interventions are basic and very clear, and the client outcome appears stable. The entry-level OT should review the client's health documentation in the chart and use resources to obtain information about the diagnosis. However, the therapist should contact the occupational therapy supervisor if he has further significant concerns or questions rather than proceeding with treatment.
3. D. Because of the student's inexperience and the length of time that has passed since her skills class, the primary course of action should be for the student to practice making an orthosis with an occupational therapy practitioner at that site before attempting to fabricate an orthosis on a client (under the direct supervision of the fieldwork educator and, if allowed by that state and other regulatory agencies). Of course, the student may also review a textbook and use Internet resources.
4. D. Using a variety of resources will be the most useful for learning.
5. B. Health care, including occupational therapy, is always evolving as new evidence emerges, society changes, and new laws are passed. An occupational therapy practitioner has a responsibility for ongoing professional development while practicing occupational therapy (AOTA, 2010a).
6. A. NBCOT provides an extensive listing of activities that may be used to meet professional development requirements for recertification (NBCOT, 2011). Answer A is not one of the approved activities (at time of publication of this book).

Worksheet 3-7: Advocacy

The AOTA website (www.aota.org) contains an Advocacy & Policy section that explains the role and functions of the American Occupational Therapy Association Political Action Committee (AOTPAC) and delineates current state and federal issues and proposed legislation affecting occupational therapy. The AOTA Legislative Action Center (part of the Advocacy and Policy section) describes AOTA's advocacy efforts and suggests ways that individuals can get involved (AOTA, 2013b).

1. T ___ F _*_ It is redundant to join a state occupational therapy association if you are already a member of American Occupational Therapy Association (AOTA).

   State associations collaborate with AOTA to address that area's state and local issues affecting occupational therapy. Both have unique member benefits, resources, and networking opportunities (AOTA, 2013c).
2. T _*_ F ___ Occupational therapy practitioners should advocate to help occupational therapy consumers receive the services they need.

   The principle of justice is addressed in the Code of Ethics (AOTA, 2015).

3. T ___ F _*_ An OT or occupational therapy student should join the AOTA primarily to receive the journals.

   Although the journals are a useful benefit, membership includes other important benefits, such as advocacy, professional and career resources, the website, and discounts, to name a few (AOTA, 2013c).

4. T ___ F _*_ An OT cannot really do anything about changing a law that has an impact on occupational therapy.

   The AOTA website lists a variety of ways that occupational therapy practitioners can help influence public policy (AOTA, 2013b).

5. T ___ F _*_ Occupational therapy students are not able to meet with legislative staff regarding health care reform because students are not yet licensed professionals.

   Students can participate in AOTA's Capitol Hill Day or, as constituents, can contact their elected representatives (AOTA, 2013b).

6. T _*_ F ___ An OT can demonstrate advocacy by joining the AOTA.

   Membership dollars help support advocacy efforts (AOTA, 2013c).

7. T ___ F _*_ Although advocacy is important to change laws, it does not affect reimbursement of occupational therapy.

   Legislation, such as the Individuals With Disabilities Education Act (IDEA), Medicaid and Medicare regulations (e.g., Prospective Payment System, Medicare B therapy cap), directly affect health care access and/or reimbursement of occupational therapy services. Advocacy can influence public policy and how individual lawmakers vote (AOTA, 2013b).

8. T ___ F _*_ Social media is not an effective method for advocacy because it is not a professional format.

   Social media can spread the word regarding issues. Also, online petitions can be useful.

9. T ___ F _*_ Donating money is the most effective way to advocate.

   Monetary donations certainly help support advocacy activities. However, other ways to help include volunteering, writing letters, calling elected representatives, meeting with legislative staff, and networking with other professionals and organizations. The AOTA Legislative Action Center, in the Advocacy and Policy section of the AOTA website, delineates current issues and ways that individuals and groups can advocate (AOTA, 2013b).

10. T _*_ F ___ One method to advocate for occupational therapy is by signing a petition.

    Petitions let elected officials know what issues are important to constituents.

11. T ___ F _*_ It is difficult for an OT or occupational therapy student to know what to write in a letter to legislators regarding current issues affecting occupational therapy.

    The AOTA Legislative Action Center has sample letters that occupational therapy practitioners may copy and send to legislators regarding specific current issues affecting occupational therapy (AOTA, 2013b).

12. T ___ F _*_ Advocacy only affects federal issues.

    Advocacy can also influence local and state policy issues. State occupational therapy associations collaborate with the AOTA to advocate for issues such as state occupational therapy licensure laws, access to health care, rights of people with disabilities, and reimbursement for covered health services in that state (e.g., Medicaid, Workers' Compensation, Early Intervention).

13. T ___ F _*_ AOTA can contribute directly to political candidates.
Funds must be contributed through a political action committee (AOTPAC, 2008).

14. T ___ F _*_ Advocacy cannot affect state regulatory issues, such as occupational therapy scope of practice and continuing competency requirements, because state legislators create the laws.
Advocacy can influence state policy issues and how individual lawmakers vote. State occupational therapy associations collaborate with AOTA to advocate for issues such as a state's OT licensure regulations, access to health care, and rights of people with disabilities (AOTA, 2013b).

15. T _*_ F ___ An issue requiring occupational therapy advocacy is fair and equal access to health care.
The principle of justice is addressed in the Code of Ethics (AOTA, 2015).

Worksheet 3-8: Teamwork

1. This is really a trick question as *every* job is extremely important in health care. Besides direct client services that health professionals provide, other employees, such as support staff, cleaning staff, food service workers, health information technology personnel, and other disciplines, are essential to keeping clients safe, equipment working properly, and the facility running smoothly. Think about what would happen if bathrooms, medical devices, and operating rooms were not cleaned, the electronic documentation system was not working, food was not prepared, or the facility could not send bills to insurance companies for care implemented.
2. D. When several parties do not agree initially on an issue, the best result is a mutually beneficial situation in which the parties have negotiated and each party feels satisfied with the final outcome or compromise. OTs often encounter workplace situations that require peaceful, practical solutions. Some issues that may cause conflict include compensation and benefits, productivity levels, frequency and amount of supervision, a client's care plan, personality conflicts with colleagues or clients, vacation schedules, and office space.
3. D. If the mission statement represents the entire rehabilitation department, the three department heads should have equal input.
4. A. The best course of action is to first ask the PT if he needs any help with anything. The PT can then decide if the OT can intervene in some way or the situation warrants contacting the rehabilitation director. The client may have cognitive problems or a history of violence that the PT knows about, but the OT does not. Of course if the OT feels that the therapist or anyone else is in imminent danger, then the OT should take action according to the facility's policies and procedures for emergencies or security issues.
5. B. It is not productive to criticize or embarrass the team member. The OTA should first tactfully provide specific examples of the client's unsafe behavior so that the team can understand the client's need for supervision. It is important to do what is in a client's best interest. In this case, if the OTA knows the client is truly unsafe, the OTA has an obligation to speak up. If concerns or lack of consensus remain, the OTA can ask the OT to intervene if necessary. Realize that, in some settings, to meet requirements for particular third-party payers such as Medicare, the OTA can attend, but cannot take the place of an OT being present at designated meetings with the physician and rehabilitation team.

Worksheet 3-9: Team Members

The team members listed in the following table may not be present in every setting or you might find that other disciplines are also necessary for client care.

Early Intervention/School	***Behavioral Health Setting***
1. OT/OTA 2. PT/PTA 3. Speech therapist 4. Child development specialist 5. School nurse 6. Teacher/special educator 7. Teacher's aide 8. Psychologist 9. Blind mobility specialist 10. Social worker/guidance counselor 11. Adaptive physical education teacher 12. Vocational rehabilitation counselor	1. OT/OTA 2. Psychiatrist 3. Nurse 4. Social worker 5. Recreation therapist 6. Dance therapist 7. Music therapist 8. Art therapist 9. Direct care worker 10. Dietician 11. Pharmacist 12. Rehabilitation counselor
Home care	***Rehabilitation Hospital***
1. OT/OTA 2. PT/PTA 3. Speech therapist 4. Physician/physician's assistant 5. Nurse 6. Home health aide 7. Social worker 8. Dietician 9. Clergy 10. Respiratory therapist 11. Pharmacist	1. OT/OTA 2. PT/PTA 3. Speech therapist 4. Audiologist 5. Nurse 6. Physician/physician's assistant 7. Certified nursing assistant 8. Social worker 9. Rehabilitation counselor 10. Orthotist/prosthetist 11. Respiratory therapist 12. Recreation therapist 13. Assistive technology specialist 14. Exercise physiologist 15. Dietician 16. Pharmacist 17. Clergy

Worksheet 3-10: Emerging Methods and Settings of Service Delivery

References: AOTA, 2013f, 2014e.

1. C. *AOTA's Position Paper "Telehealth" (AOTA, 2013f) focuses on the benefit of providing more expedient access to care for those in rural areas, although other benefits may also be realized.*
2. D
3. A. *Telehealth is considered a direct service delivery model. The use of telehealth technology can include teleconsultation* (AOTA, 2013f).
4. B. *Synchronous telehealth services are delivered in real-time through interactive technology* (AOTA, 2013f).
5. C
6. C
7. A. AOTA, 2014e.

True or False:

8. Primary care is the provision of integrated, accessible health care that addresses clients' personal health care needs, includes the establishment of sustained partnerships with clients, and provides clinical practice within the context of family and community. T (AOTA, 2013f)
9. When employed in a primary care setting, occupational therapy services will greatly resemble those provided in an outpatient rehabilitation setting. F
10. Assisting clients to establish healthful habits and routines will be a responsibility of the OT in a primary care setting of the future. T
11. The administration of occupational therapy through telehealth technology is not covered by all third-party payers. T
12. Occupational therapists can evaluate and treat clients remotely through telehealth technology. This includes hands-on interventions completed by an individual who is physically with the client as instructed by the therapist remotely. T

Chapter 3 References

Accreditation Council for Occupational Therapy Education. (2012). 2011 Accreditation Council for Occupational Therapy Education (ACOTE) Standards. *American Journal of Occupational Therapy, 66*(Suppl. 6), S6–S74.

American Occupational Therapy Association. (2006). Specialized knowledge and skills for occupational therapy practice in the neonatal intensive care unit. *American Journal of Occupational Therapy, 60,* 659–668.

American Occupational Therapy Association. (2007) COE Guidelines for an occupational therapy fieldwork experience—Level I. Retrieved from http://aota.org/Educate/EdRes/Fieldwork/LevelI/38248.aspx?css=print

American Occupational Therapy Association. (2010a). Standards for continuing competence. *American Journal of Occupational Therapy, 64* (Suppl. 6), S103–S105.

American Occupational Therapy Association. (2010b). Standards of practice for occupational therapy. *American Journal of Occupational Therapy, 64*(Suppl. 6), S106–S111.

American Occupational Therapy Association. (2012a) Fieldwork level II and occupational therapy students: A position paper. *American Journal of Occupational Therapy, 66*(Suppl. 6), S75–S77.

American Occupational Therapy Association. (2012b). Physical agent modalities. *American Journal of Occupational Therapy, 66*(Suppl. 6), S78–S80.

American Occupational Therapy Association. (2013a). AOTA certification: Board and specialty certification. Retrieved from http://www.aota.org/Practitioners/ProfDev/Certification.aspx?css

American Occupational Therapy Association. (2013b). Legislative Action Center. Retrieved from http://capwiz.com/aota/home

American Occupational Therapy Association. (2013c). Member benefits overview. Retrieved from http://www.aota.org/AboutAOTA/Membership/Overview.aspx

American Occupational Therapy Association. (2013d). Practice. Retrieved from http://www.aota.org/Practice.aspx

American Occupational Therapy Association. (2013e). Q & A: Gait assessment for falls risk. Retrieved from http://www.aota.org/Practitioners/Resources/Scope-of-Practice-QA/Gait-Assessment.aspx

American Occupational Therapy Association. (2013f). Telehealth. *American Journal of Occupational Therapy, 67*(Suppl. 6), S69–S90.

American Occupational Therapy Association. (2014a). Guidelines for supervision, roles, and responsibilities during the delivery of occupational therapy services. *American Journal of Occupational Therapy, 68*(Suppl. 3), S16–S22.

American Occupational Therapy Association. (2014b). Occupational therapy's commitment to nondiscrimination and inclusion. *American Journal of Occupational Therapy, 68*(Suppl. 3), S23–S24.

American Occupational Therapy Association. (2014c). Occupational therapy practice framework: Domain and process, 3rd edition. *American Journal of Occupational Therapy, 68*(Suppl. 1), S1–S48.

American Occupational Therapy Association. (2014d). Scope of practice. *American Journal of Occupational Therapy, 68*(Suppl. 3), S34–S40.

American Occupational Therapy Association. (2014e). The role of occupational therapy in primary care. *American Journal of Occupational Therapy, 68*(Suppl. 3), S25–S33.

American Occupational Therapy Association. (2015). Occupational therapy code of ethics (2015). *American Journal of Occupational Therapy*, 69 (Suppl. 3), 6913410030. http://dx.doi.org/10.5014/ajot.2015.696S03

American Occupational Therapy Association Political Action Committee [AOTPAC]. 2008. AOTPAC fact sheet. Retrieved from http://www.aota.org/Practitioners/Advocacy/AOTPAC/About/36338.aspx?FT=.pdf

Asher, A. (2006). Asian Americans. In M. Royeen, & J. L. Crabtree (Eds.), *Culture in rehabilitation: From competency to proficiency* (pp. 151–180). Upper Saddle River, NJ: Pearson Education.

Goldsmith, M. C. (2006). Understanding Judaism and Jewish Americans. In M. Royeen & J. L. Crabtree (Eds.), *Culture in rehabilitation: From competency to proficiency* (pp. 203–217). Upper Saddle River, NJ: Pearson Education.

Hand Therapy Certification Commission. (2013). Eligibility requirements. Retrieved from http://htcc.org/certify/test-information/eligibility-requirements

Merriam-Webster. (2013). *Merriam-Webster dictionary.* Retrieved from http://www.merriam-webster.com/dictionary/vegan

Morreale, M. J. (2015). *Developing clinical competence: A workbook for the OTA.* Thorofare, NJ: SLACK Incorporated.

Morreale, M. J., & Borcherding, S. (2013). *The OTA's guide to documentation: Writing SOAP notes* (3rd ed.). Thorofare, NJ: SLACK Incorporated.

National Board for Certification in Occupational Therapy. (2011). NBCOT® professional development units (PDU) activities chart. Retrieved from http://www.nbcot.org/pdf/renewal/pdu_chart.pdf

Richert, S. P. (2013). About.com Catholicism guide: Can Catholics eat meat on Good Friday? Retrieved from http://catholicism.about.com/od/catholicliving/f/Meat_Good_Fri.htm

Robins, S. (2006). Understanding sexual minorities. In M. Royeen & J. L. Crabtree (Eds.), *Culture in rehabilitation: From competency to proficiency* (pp. 357–376). Upper Saddle River, NJ: Pearson Education.

Royeen, M., & Crabtree, J. L. (Eds.). (2006). *Culture in rehabilitation: From competency to proficiency.* Upper Saddle River, NJ: Pearson Education.

Chapter 4

Applying Fundamental Principles

The worksheets and learning activities presented in this chapter address fundamental language and principles for occupational therapy practice. These topics include an overview of the American Occupational Therapy Association (AOTA) official documents and multiple exercises to test your understanding of the *Occupational Therapy Practice Framework: Domain and Process* (2014b). Other topics presented in this chapter include activity/occupational analysis, grading and adapting, frames of reference, intervention planning, and the basics of evidence-based practice, such as research methodology and statistics. Answers to worksheet exercises are provided at the end of the chapter.

Contents

Morreale, M. J., & Amini, D.
The Occupational Therapist's Workbook for Ensuring Clinical Competence (pp. 121-163).

Learning Activity 4-1: Official Documents of the American Occupational Therapy Association

The AOTA creates official documents that are used to guide practice or to set forth the tenets of the association about specific topics. This activity reviews the locations of the various documents and assists in recall of the purposes of each.

Visit the practice section of the AOTA website (www.aota.org) and locate the categories of Official Documents (AOTA, 2014c).

Activity: List the documents that you find under the following categories:

Ethics

Guidelines

Position Papers

Standards

Statements

Worksheet 4-1

Using AOTA Official Documents

1. Which of the following is the World Health Organization document referenced in the *Occupational Therapy Practice Framework*?
   A. International Classification of Functioning, Disability and Health (ICF)
   B. International Classification of Diseases (ICD)
   C. Health Insurance Portability and Accountability Act (HIPAA)
   D. Current Procedural Terminology (CPT)

2. An occupational therapist (OT) re-entering practice after a long absence is unsure as to whether an occupational therapy assistant (OTA) can still be delegated aspects of an initial evaluation. The therapist plans to review relevant licensure laws and regulations and utilize AOTA resources. Of the following choices, which would be the most useful to provide an answer to the therapist's question?
   A. Occupational Therapy Code of Ethics
   B. Standards of Practice
   C. Occupational Therapy Practice Framework
   D. Guidelines for Documentation of Occupational Therapy

3. An OT is unsure as to whether she has an obligation to treat a client whose personal behaviors conflict with the OT's religious beliefs. Which of the following documents would be most useful to help with making this decision?
   A. Guidelines for Supervision Roles and Responsibilities During the Delivery of Occupational Therapy Services
   B. The Role of Occupational Therapy in Primary Care
   C. Scope of Practice
   D. Occupational Therapy Code of Ethics.

4. Which of the following AOTA Official Documents is not categorized by AOTA as a position paper?
   A. Scope of Practice
   B. Obesity and Occupational Therapy
   C. Occupational Therapy and the Promotion of Health and Well-Being
   D. Complementary and Alternative Medicine

5. In regard to Official Documents, which of the following areas of practice does the AOTA describe in a position paper?
   A. Wound management
   B. Scholarship in occupational therapy
   C. Disaster preparedness
   D. Cognitive rehabilitation

Worksheet 4-1 (continued)

Using AOTA Official Documents

6. Which of the following documents best describes the array of services that occupational therapy practitioners provide?
   A. Standards of Practice
   B. Guidelines for Supervision Roles and Responsibilities During the Delivery of Occupational Therapy Services
   C. Scope of Practice
   D. Occupational Therapy Code of Ethics.

7. An OTA would like to develop a professional development plan. Of the following choices, which would be the most useful resource?
   A. Standards of Practice
   B. Guidelines for Supervision Roles and Responsibilities During the Delivery of Occupational Therapy Services
   C. The Importance of Occupational Therapy Assistant Education to the Profession
   D. Standards for Continuing Competence

8. An OT is unsure as to whether an aide can be delegated a particular task. He plans to review relevant licensure laws and regulations and utilize AOTA resources. Of the following choices, which would be the most useful for making this decision?
   A. Guidelines for Supervision Roles and Responsibilities During the Delivery of Occupational Therapy Services
   B. Scope of Practice
   C. Standards for Continuing Competence
   D. Standards of Practice

9. An occupational therapy manager is developing a new occupational therapy evaluation form for clients admitted to a rehabilitation hospital. Which of the following documents is likely the least useful resource for creating this form?
   A. Occupational Therapy Practice framework
   B. Accreditation Council for Occupational Therapy Education (ACOTE) Standards and Interpretive Guide
   C. Guidelines for Documentation of Occupational Therapy
   D. Standards of Practice

10. An OT working in a step-down acute care unit is deciding whether to ask an OTA to assist with some of the evaluations. Which of the following documents would be most useful in helping the therapist to make this decision?
    A. Guidelines for Supervision Roles and Responsibilities During the Delivery of Occupational Therapy Services
    B. The Role of Occupational Therapy in Primary Care
    C. The Standards for Continuing Competence
    D. The Importance of Occupational Therapy Assistant Education to the Profession

Worksheet 4-2

Occupational Therapy Practice Framework—Domain and Process

Originally created in 2002 and most recently updated in 2014, the *Occupational Therapy Practice Framework: Domain and Process* (also referred to as the *Framework*; AOTA, 2014b) is the guiding practice document of the profession of occupational therapy in the United States. This worksheet will enhance your recall of several important concepts found within the *Framework*.

Members of the AOTA can download a copy of the Framework at the AOTA website (www.aota.org). The document can also found in the March/April 2014 issue of the *American Journal of Occupational Therapy* (AJOT) or for sale through the AOTA Press.

For each of the following statements, indicate whether they are true (T) or false (F).

1. ______ A definition of occupational therapy adopted from the Model Practice Act can be found in the Preface of the *Framework*.
2. ______ Several definitions for occupation can be found within the *Framework*.
3. ______ The *Framework* provides a unique definition of occupation.
4. ______ The *Framework* is divided into three distinct sections, the domain, the process, and the outcomes.
5. ______ The *Framework* supports a top-down approach to intervention.
6. ______ The concept of the therapeutic use of self is found in the domain of the *Framework*.
7. ______ The process of occupational therapy is described as having three parts: the occupational profile, the standards of service, and the analysis of occupation.
8. ______ Purposeful activities are described as one type of intervention within the *Framework*.
9. ______ The domain of occupational therapy includes performance patterns, occupations, performance skills client factors, and environment and context.
10. ______ The overarching statement of the *Framework* is "Supporting health and participation in life through engagement in occupation."

Worksheet 4-3

Occupational Therapy Practice Framework—Activities and Occupations

A person's daily occupations as described in the *Framework* comprise a variety of activities (AOTA, 2014b). However, some activities may not fit neatly into a single occupational category; identification of the occupation being described depends on the perspective of the individual or population's interests and needs (AOTA, 2014b). For example, baking bread may be classified as part of an instrumental activity of daily living (IADL; meal preparation), a leisure activity for someone whose hobby is baking, or it may be considered social participation or volunteer work if a group is making challah bread for a religious service or a fundraising event. Indicate which area(s) of occupation that each of the activities listed that follow belong to, according to your personal interests, values, and roles. Also, list additional 10 activities that you personally do in a typical day or week and categorize them.

Client Activity	***ADLs***	***IADLs***	***Play***	***Leisure***	***Work***	***Education***	***Rest and Sleep***	***Social Participation***
Baking bread								
Cleaning contact lenses								
Taking the train to get to a job								
Donning an orthosis								
Playing hopscotch with others								
Attending religious services								
Making a collage for an occupational therapy class assignment								
Watching TV to fall asleep								
Feeding the household cat or dog								
Listening to music								
Preparing a resume								
Walking to the dinner table								
Taking a nap								
Babysitting a younger sibling								
Organizing school papers into folders								
Volunteering at a hospital gift shop								
Attending a bridal shower or bachelor party								
Paying bills								
Getting to next class on time								
Knitting a sweater to wear								
Using contraception								
Setting an alarm clock								

Client Activity	*ADLs*	*IADLs*	*Play*	*Leisure*	*Work*	*Education*	*Rest and Sleep*	*Social Participation*
Reading e-mails								
Taking vitamins								
Sewing a button back on a shirt								
Planting flowers in the yard								
Writing a performance review for a staff member								
Navigating a wheelchair in the home								
Dressing a Barbie doll								
Exercising at the gym								
Calling 911 when smelling smoke								
Eating lunch with colleagues								

My Activities	*ADLs*	*IADLs*	*Play*	*Leisure*	*Work*	*Education*	*Rest and Sleep*	*Social Participation*

Worksheet 4-4

Differentiating Client Factors and Performance Skills

For each of the following sentences, indicate whether it represents a *client factor* (F) or *performance skill* (S) according to the *Occupational Therapy Practice Framework* (2014b). Remember that *conditions* arise from deficiencies in underlying structures and functions and may affect occupational performance.

1. ______ The client who had shoulder surgery achieved left arm abduction to 160°.
2. ______ The resident is able to manipulate knitting needles with both hands.
3. ______ The client has intact short-term memory.
4. ______ The client admitted to the acute psychiatric unit today has signs and symptoms consistent with severe depression.
5. ______ The client has a pain level of 7 today per the 10-point visual analog scale.
6. ______ The client demonstrates good dynamic standing balance when pulling up his pants.
7. ______ The student remained calm when another student bumped into him.
8. ______ The client sitting in the power wheelchair has poor lymphatic drainage, causing 1+ edema in his right leg.
9. ______ The client has a below-knee amputation.
10. ______ The child playing hopscotch is able to hop on one leg four times without falling.
11. ______ During a family intervention, the client stated agreement with need to attend sobriety meetings.
12. ______ The infant demonstrates a positive Babinski sign.
13. ______ The client at risk for thrombosis is using an intermittent compression pump on her legs when lying in her hospital bed.
14. ______ The client with autism is exhibiting tactile defensiveness during art class.
15. ______ The client achieved a right grip strength of 100 pounds when using a dynamometer.
16. ______ The child with asthma has difficulty using her inhaler properly.
17. ______ The client would benefit from paraffin to help loosen stiff finger joints.
18. ______ Because of increased tone in the client's fingers, the OT premolded the orthotic device on her own hand to prevent difficulty when making a resting pan orthosis.
19. ______ The resident can roll from side to side using bed rails.
20. ______ The client has the condition of Bell's palsy, which is creating difficulty with her ability to coordinate chewing.

Worksheet 4-5

Differentiating Client Factors and Performance Skills—More Practice

For each of the following sentences, indicate whether it represents a *client factor* (F) or a *performance skill* (S) according to the *Occupational Therapy Practice Framework* (2014b). Remember that *conditions* arise from deficiencies in underlying structures and functions and may affect occupational performance.

1. _______ The student uses a static tripod grasp when writing.
2. _______ The client needed to rest after standing to cook at the stove.
3. _______ The client with schizophrenia hears voices in his head.
4. _______ The client was able to tear open the package of potato chips.
5. _______ The client lying in bed has unilateral neglect.
6. _______ The client's resting blood pressure of 160/95 resulted in the OT contacting the client's physician.
7. _______ The client demonstrates an improvement in muscle strength from Fair to Good for left elbow flexion.
8. _______ The client is able to don and doff his protective fracture brace independently.
9. _______ The client is able to carry a 10-pound grocery bag from her car to the kitchen.
10. _______ The client is unable to cut her toenails because she has difficulty bending.
11. _______ The client's scaphoid fracture needed 6 months to heal completely.
12. _______ The client's gray hair and wrinkles make her appear older than she really is.
13. _______ The resident cannot push up with his arms to perform a sliding board transfer.
14. _______ The client is incontinent of urine secondary to a prolapsed bladder.
15. _______ The client with chemical dependency endures the side effects of withdrawal.
16. _______ The client's loss of protective sensation in his feet is a safety concern due to his diabetes.
17. _______ The child with dyspraxia did not fall today while running in gym class.
18. _______ The resident asked for a calendar to help her remember her therapy appointments.
19. _______ The client diagnosed with an anxiety disorder chooses not to attend occupational therapy group today.
20. _______ The client with a nut allergy cannot be exposed to peanut butter.

Worksheet 4-6

Habits, Rituals, Routines, and Roles

For each of the following activities, indicate whether it is a habit, ritual, routine, or role, according to the *Occupational Therapy Practice Framework* (AOTA, 2014b).

1. ____________________ Always decorating the tree on Christmas Eve.
2. ____________________ A family has a tradition of making s'mores over the fire whenever camping.
3. ____________________ Flossing every time after brushing teeth.
4. ____________________ Taking care of the family pet before leaving for work.
5. ____________________ Saying a prayer when lighting candles on the Sabbath.
6. ____________________ Reading a bedtime story after the child's nightly bath and tucking him into bed.
7. ____________________ A daughter who is caring for an elderly parent with dementia.
8. ____________________ Smoking a cigarette right after dinner.
9. ____________________ Buckling a seat belt before driving.
10. ____________________ Shaking hands when meeting someone new.
11. ____________________ The woman who enjoys gardening is known as having a "green thumb."
12. ____________________ Identifying as a Roman Catholic and joining the church choir.
13. ____________________ A young musician is proficient at playing a piano.
14. ____________________ Kissing your spouse when he or she comes home from work.
15. ____________________ An avid bingo player.
16. ____________________ Making breakfast and packing your child's lunch before driving him to school.
17. ____________________ Completing your shift as a volunteer firefighter.
18. ____________________ A mother helping the teacher by accompanying the child's class on a field trip.
19. ____________________ Saying prayers at the gravesite on the 1-year anniversary of the deceased's date of death.
20. ____________________ Hanging up your coat when you come home.

Learning Activity 4-2: Performance Patterns

This exercise is designed to help you identify performance patterns in your own life.

Habits: Complete the table that follows with a list of habits you have. Identify each of your habits as useful, dominating, or impoverished (Dunn, 2000) and the effect of your habits on occupational performance.

Habits	***Categorize Each Habit as Useful, Dominating, or Impoverished***	***Indicate Whether This Habit Supports or Hinders Occupations***	***Describe the Habit's Effect on Your Occupational Performance***
Example: Biting nails	*Dominating*	*Hinders*	*May affect ability to dress up and appear well groomed or feel confident with appearance. Can also impede ability to do activities requiring nails, such as peeling off a sticker, scratching an itch, or opening a bobby pin.*
1.			
2.			
3.			
4.			
5.			
6.			

Learning Activity 4-2: Performance Patterns (continued)

Rituals: Considering a holiday you celebrate or a religion that you identify with, list five associated rituals that you perform.

Rituals	*Holiday or Religion*
1.	
2.	
3.	
4.	
5.	

Routines: List five routines that you perform in a typical day or week and the associated occupations.

Routines	*Associated Occupation*
1.	
2.	
3.	
4.	
5.	

Roles: List five of your personal roles and identify the associated occupations.

Roles	*Associated Occupation*
1.	
2.	
3.	
4.	
5.	

Learning Activity 4-3: Activity/Occupational Analysis

To complete the activity in Figure 4-1, first create an image in your mind of an activity or occupation that you are doing now or have done in the past. As you analyze the activity, consider all of the following aspects as delineated in the *Occupational Therapy Practice Framework* (AOTA, 2014b). A useful resource for learning the activity analysis process is Thomas's (2012) book *Occupation-Based Activity Analysis*, which also contains various detailed forms.

Activity/Occupational Analysis

Activity or occupation:

Relevance and meaning to (you) the client:

Activity Demands:

- Objects used and their properties:

  Materials:

  Tools:

  Equipment:

- Space Demands:
- Social Demands:

Occupation

Link your activity to one or more of the following occupations and explain application.

ADL ______________________________

IADL______________________________

Education ______________________________

Work ______________________________

Play ______________________________

Leisure ______________________________

Social participation ______________________________

Rest and sleep ______________________________

Figure 4-1A. Activity/occupational analysis form (page 1).

Learning Activity 4-3: Activity/Occupational Analysis (continued)

Performance Skills

Indicate which of the following skill areas are required and how/why.

Skill Area	Is This Skill Area Used for This Activity?	Describe Skill Required
Motor		
Process		
Social Interaction		

Client Factors

Indicate which of the following factors are used when you complete the activity and if they are also required to do this activity.

- ***Values, beliefs, and spirituality***

  Values (principles, standards, qualities considered worthwhile or desirable by the client who holds them) __________ __________

  Used through this activity   Required to do this activity

  Beliefs (Cognitive content held as true) ______ ________

  Used   Required

  Spirituality ______ ________

  Used   Required

- ***Body Functions*** (mark if used in this activity and mark again if required by this activity. For example, the function of tasting may be used during a cooking activity, but may not be required to complete the activity)
  - o **Mental functions** (affective, cognitive, perceptual)

    Specific mental functions (used/required):

    High-level cognitive ________ ________

    Attention ________ ________

    Memory ________ ________

    Perception ________ ________

    Thought ________ ________

    Sequencing complex movement ________ ________

    Emotional ________ ________

    Experience of self and time ________ ________

    Global mental functions (used/required):

    Consciousness ________ ________

    Orientation ________ ________

    Temperament and personality ________ ________

    Energy and drive ________ ________

    Sleep (physiological process) ________ ________

Figure 4-1B. Activity/occupational analysis form (page 2).

- **Sensory functions and pain** (used/required):

  Seeing and related functions including acuity, stability and visual field functions ________ ________

  Hearing functions ________ ________

  Vestibular functions ________ ________

  Taste functions ________ ________

  Proprioceptive functions ________ ________

  Smell functions ________ ________

  Touch functions ________ ________

  Temperature and pressure ________ ________

  Sensations of pain ________ ________

- **Neuromusculoskeletal and movement related functions** (used/required):

  Functions of joint and bones

  Mobility of joints ________ ________

  Stability of joints ________ ________

  Muscle power ________ ________

  Muscle endurance ________ ________

  Muscle tone ________ ________

  Motor reflexes ________ ________

  Involuntary movement reactions ________ ________

  Control of voluntary movement ________ ________

  Gait pattern ________ ________

Describe how this activity may affect or be affected by mood, outlook, and self-efficacy or if this activity will affect those areas.

____

____

How does this activity relate to quality of life or have meaning to this client?

____

____

Contexts and environment

Identify as appropriate.

Context	**Supports Activity**	**Barrier to Activity**	**Neither (check)**
Physical			
Social			
Cultural			
Personal			
Temporal (time of day, year, season)			
Virtual			

Figure 4-1C. Activity/occupational analysis form (page 3).

Worksheet 4-7
Grading and Adapting

For each of the statements that follow, indicate whether the intervention is an example of grading (G) or adapting (A).

1. ______ To manage clothing without assistance during toileting, the OT suggested that the client use elastic waist pants rather than pants with fastenings.
2. ______ During yesterday's intervention session, the OT asked a client diagnosed with social anxiety to make a phone call to a pizzeria to ask the cost of a large pizza. Today, they went to the pizzeria together so that the client could place an order for two slices of pizza.
3. ______ The OT had the child use a button board with smaller buttons than previously to work on three-point pinch.
4. ______ The OT attached a brake extension to a wheelchair for the client with left hemiplegia.
5. ______ The OT asked a client diagnosed with traumatic brain injury to bake refrigerated dough cookies last week, then attempted to have her make cookies using a boxed mix today.
6. ______ The OT suggested that the child with hand weakness practice handwriting for 5 minutes daily this week and 10 minutes daily next week.
7. ______ The OT taught the client to use a calendar to remember appointments.
8. ______ To help improve decision-making skills, the OT gave the client diagnosed with depression a choice of only two craft projects yesterday and a choice of three projects today.
9. ______ The OT instructed the client with chronic obstructive pulmonary disease (COPD) to sit during ironing when she returns home.
10. ______ The OT had the client with bilateral integration problems roll out dough with a rolling pin during last week's session. Today the therapist had the client mix dough ingredients with her dominant hand while holding onto a bowl with the nondominant hand.
11. ______ The OT asked the OTA to attach a zipper pull to the student's backpack.
12. ______ The OT told the parents that the toddler could now eat semisoft foods in addition to pureed food.
13. ______ The OT discontinued the client's forearm-based thumb spica orthosis today and issued a hand-based thumb spica orthosis.
14. ______ The OT instructed the caregiver to purchase an electric kettle with an automatic shut off for the client with early-stage dementia.
15. ______ The OT instructed the client in use of a pill organizer to help her remember to take her medication.
16. ______ The OT determined that the client diagnosed with a Colles fracture could initiate light therapy putty exercises today.
17. ______ The OT worked on the client's wheelchair mobility by having him wheel his wheelchair outdoors today.
18. ______ The OT asked the teacher to allow the first-grader to eat raisins or granola at his desk to minimize fidgeting during class.
19. ______ The OT gave the client with schizophrenia a structured leisure worksheet because the client could not come up with three desired leisure tasks when initially asked.
20. ______ As the client with cancer was at risk for infection outdoors, the OT instructed the family to set up an indoor windowsill garden.

Learning Activity 4-4: Grading—Preparing Breakfast (Traumatic Brain Injury)

Your client is a 35-year-old female recovering from a traumatic brain injury. She has difficulty performing IADLs (e.g., meal preparation and laundry) due to deficits in organization, problem solving, and safety, but does not have any impairment in range of motion (ROM), strength, or endurance.

For the occupation of preparing breakfast, put the following food choices in order of preparation difficulty (easier to harder) for this client scenario. Indicate the activity demands that make each task easier or harder. Compare your answers for this exercise to your answers for Learning Activity 4-5. Is your order of difficulty the same or different?

A. Scrambled eggs and bacon
B. Frozen breakfast sandwich
C. Cereal and milk
D. Smoothie (made from scratch)
E. Hard-boiled eggs
F. Frozen waffles
G. Toast
H. Pancakes (using a mix)
I. Yogurt
J. Fresh fruit salad (apple, grapes, melon)

List Tasks in Order of Difficulty From Easier to Harder	*Activity Demands*
1.	
2.	
3.	
4.	
5.	
6.	
7.	
8.	
9.	
10.	

Learning Activity 4-5: Grading—Preparing Breakfast (Rheumatoid Arthritis)

Your client is a 65-year-old female with severe rheumatoid arthritis. She has difficulty managing clothing fastenings and performing home management tasks due to multiple joint contractures in both hands and inability to make a full fist or perform tip pinch.

For the occupation of preparing breakfast, put the following food choices in order of preparation difficulty (easier to harder) for this client scenario. Indicate the activity demands that make each task easier or harder. Compare your answers for this exercise to your answers for Learning Activity 4-4. Is your order of difficulty the same or different?

A. Scrambled eggs and bacon
B. Frozen breakfast sandwich
C. Cereal and milk
D. Smoothie (made from scratch)
E. Hard-boiled eggs
F. Frozen waffles
G. Toast
H. Pancakes (using a mix)
I. Yogurt
J. Fresh fruit salad (apple, grapes, melon)

List Tasks in Order of Difficulty From Easier to Harder	*Activity Demands*
1.	
2.	
3.	
4.	
5.	
6.	
7.	
8.	
9.	
10.	

Worksheet 4-8

Grading and Adapting—Making Coffee

List ways to grade and adapt the occupation of making coffee by indicating various modifications for the activity demands designated at the top of each column.

Activity Demand: Task Material—Coffee	***Activity Demand: Required Action of Opening Coffee Container***	***Activity Demand: Required Action of Measuring Coffee***	***Activity Demand: Required Action of Heating the Water/Brewing Coffee***
Example: *Instant coffee*	Example: *Can of coffee requiring use of a can opener*	Example: *Use a measuring spoon*	Example: *Boil water in tea kettle using stove*

Reprinted with permission from Morreale, M. J. (2015). *Developing clinical competence: A workbook for the OTA*. Thorofare, NJ: SLACK Incorporated.

Worksheet 4-9

Grading and Adapting—Laundry

List the sequence of steps to wash clothes and various ways to grade and adapt each step.

Sequence of Steps to Perform the Occupation of Laundry	**_Grade/Adapt Task Methods_**	**_Grade/Adapt Task Materials_**
Example: *Carry a laundry basket full of clothes to washer*	Example: *Place dirty clothes directly in machine when getting changed*	Example: *Use a rolling laundry cart; use a laundry bag*

Reprinted with permission from Morreale, M. J. (2015). *Developing clinical competence: A workbook for the OTA.* Thorofare, NJ: SLACK Incorporated.

Worksheet 4-10

Frames of Reference

Frames of reference (FOR) or practice models (the terms are often used interchangeably) are an important part of the clinical reasoning process. Understanding the underlying theory that supports a particular frame of reference and applying that frame appropriately based on the needs and interests of the client ensures an evidence-based approach to care. Read the activity scenarios that follow and determine which frame of reference best fits the theory underlying the activity selection. Additional exercises regarding frames of reference and practice models specific to mental health and pediatric practice areas can be found in Chapters 8 and 10.

Frames of reference

Biomechanical
Rehabilitation
Neurodevelopmental theory (NDT: adult or child)
Sensory integration
Cognitive behavioral
Psychodynamic
Behavioral
Occupational science/occupational performance/occupation based/Model of Human Occupation (MOHO)
Cognitive rehabilitation
Task-oriented approach

Activities

1. To get a person to take a shower, a reward of his liking is provided. Therapist works with client to ensure that he gathers necessary bath items and plans appropriately for after bath grooming and dressing. ____________
2. A client with limited elbow extension (straightening) is given a weaving activity to complete based on her request and interest in creating handmade placemats and wall hangings. Client is instructed to pull yarn to length that encourages both elbow extension and flexion during activity. Activity is to be completed for a minimum of 4 hours per day, spaced at appropriate intervals. ____________
3. Client with poor memory for phone numbers brings cell phone to clinic along with important phone numbers. Therapist and client work together to add phone numbers to speed dial on phone. Therapist and client then create a small "cheat sheet" with names and speed dial numbers that will be pasted to the back of the phone and made into wallet size card. ____________
4. A child who is unable to feed herself due to the effects of athetoid cerebral palsy is provided with a Winsford feeder. The therapist teaches the child and her mother how to use the device. Child is now able to complete feeding after setup. ____________
5. A child who had difficulty sitting straight in his chair and paying attention in class is provided with activities during therapy, such as bouncing on therapy ball, propelling self in scooter board along the floor, and catching bean bags in hands while swinging in a net swing. ____________
6. A woman is so fearful of getting into a car crash that she is unable to leave the house to go to work. The therapist presents her with credible statistics regarding the likelihood that she will be involved in a car accident. The therapist also works with client to determine alternate means of transportation and determine how these will be used for the client to get to work every day and on time. She will be supported by the companionship of an occupational therapist during first several days of using alternative transportation and eventually driving herself. ____________
7. Client is unable to participate in desired leisure activities because of fatigue associated with chemotherapy. The OT works with the client to determine which activities he would like to participate in and helps him to brainstorm on various ways to complete the activities in a way that the fatigue does not interfere. ____________

Worksheet 4-10 (continued)
Frames of Reference

8. Adult man with flaccid upper extremity from a stroke is placed in a "weight-bearing" position intended to normalize tone in extremity. In addition, he is given tactile cues that assist his body in knowing how to sit in a more symmetrical way when in his wheelchair. ________________
9. A 6-month-old child with cerebral palsy is placed in a developmental position known as "prone on elbows" to provide needed weight bearing into shoulder girdle. This technique is theorized to assist the brain with learning "normal movement patterns." ________________
10. A depressed individual is asked to draw a picture representing her feelings for the day. The picture is analyzed to determine her underlying feelings in an effort to help her to understand how her unconscious is dealing with various life challenges. Theory states that when she becomes aware of her underlying issues, she will be able to come to terms with her reactions and change her thinking to decrease the depressive symptoms. ________________
11. A child with poor handwriting is given fine motor coordination activities to work on in an attempt to enhance his motor control. The activities include clothespin pinching, putty squeezing, and marble picking up and harboring in hand. ________________
12. A client who sustained a stroke and who now has moderate weakness of her left upper extremity is given interesting tasks such as cleaning CD-ROMs that she must complete using both hands in a naturalistic manner. She is to clean 25 CDs to complete the task. ________________

Intervention Planning Tips

To help with decision making when choosing a model of practice or frame of reference (FOR), O'Brien (2014) suggests that the therapist reflect on the guiding questions outlined in Box 4-1.

Box 4-1.

Guiding Questions to Consider When Deciding on a Model of Practice or Frame of Reference

Setting	Does this model of practice or FOR fit within the setting?
Population	Does this model of practice or FOR address the needs of the population being treated?
Basic principles	What is the theory of this model of practice or FOR, and does it make sense for the population being treated? Is this model of practice or FOR congruent with occupational therapy practice? Is there adequate research to support the theory and principles?
Evidence	Has the research supported the use of this model of practice or FOR and, if so, with which population? Does this model of practice or FOR support cost-effective intervention? Are the assessment tools associated with this model of practice or FOR well designed and clinically relevant? Is there documentation that this model of practice or FOR can improve the occupations of clients? Is this model of practice or FOR congruent with occupational therapy core values and beliefs?
Assessment and evaluation	What assessments or tests are compatible with the model of practice or FOR? Are the assessments standardized, reliable, and valid? Does the model of practice or FOR provide reliable measures for assessment and evaluation?
Practical considerations	Does the clinic or site have the equipment necessary to competently use this model of practice or FOR?
Clinical expertise	Is the practitioner adequately trained to use the associated techniques or assessment tools? How much training is necessary?

Reprinted with permission from O'Brien, J. (2014). Intervention planning. In K. Jacobs, N. MacRae, & K. Sladyk (Eds.), *Occupational therapy essentials for clinical competence* (2nd ed., pp. 295–307). Thorofare, NJ: SLACK Incorporated.

Worksheet 4-11

When to Use Evidence-Based Practice

Practitioners should always ensure that their clinical decision making is based on the best available evidence, which includes results from critically analyzed research, their knowledge and expertise, and client preferences. This worksheet includes case situations that may or may not require the use of evidence-based practice (EBP) to undertake. Indicate whether each of the following instances will require the practitioner to consider best available evidence.

1. _______ Agreeing with the client's choice of outfit for the day
2. _______ Choosing to use or not use hip precautions with a frail client 8 weeks status post hip arthroplasty
3. _______ Agreeing to provide an adapted aid to allow the client with swallowing precautions to eat the outside of a chocolate-filled lollipop
4. _______ Starting a 6-week modified constraint-induced movement therapy (mCIMT) regimen with a client who has left upper extremity weakness status post cerebrovascular accident
5. _______ Per the physician's order, completing an ultrasound treatment on a client with significant sensory loss
6. _______ Using a standard vs a sports wheelchair to transport a 50-year-old male client to therapy when both are available in the rehabilitation hospital
7. _______ Scheduling clients for therapy sessions
8. _______ Using a neurodevelopmental treatment (NDT) approach with a 6-year-old child with right hemiplegia
9. _______ Suggesting that a teacher use an Apple iPad vs a Samsung tablet with a child diagnosed with autism spectrum disorder when both items are available in the classroom.
10. _______ Assessing a client using the nine-hole peg test to determine readiness to return to work.

Worksheet 4-12

Starting With Evidence

When investigating the best available evidence to support client interventions, it is important to distinguish among journal, trade journal, and magazine articles. Journal articles are typically referred to as *scholarly*, trade journals are written for professionals in a particular field, but are not research-related, and magazine articles are usually considered *popular* and do not rely on any type of peer review process. In the world of occupational therapy, there are a host of journals from which a practitioner may find strong evidence to support interventions. Some examples include the *American Journal of Occupational Therapy* (AJOT), the *Canadian Journal of Occupational Therapy* (CJOT), and *OTJR: Occupation, Participation and Health* (OTJR), as well as journals that are dedicated to specialty areas within occupational therapy and others that are not specific to the profession, but can certainly inform practice, such as the *Journal of the American Medical Association* (JAMA).

Complete the chart below to differentiate key features between these sources of information.

	Journal	Trade Journal	Magazine
Examples of publications	*AJOT, CJOT, OTJR, JAMA*	*ADVANCE for Occupational Therapy Practitioners, Today in OT*	
How publications are titled			Titles that focus on population for whom the publication is created
Appearance of publications in print		Printed version may be covered and contain pages printed on newsprint or standard paper. Cover often contains a picture that highlights contents. Listing of contents, trademark title and date of publication found. Advertisements and job ads found throughout that are focused on the targeted topic	
Appearance of publications online			Subscription may or may not be required based on nature of publication. Brightly illustrated with possible menu of contents. Articles are often hyperlinked and are accessed through hyperlinks from other sources.
Authors of contents	Researchers, scholars, those with advanced degrees and training within topic area		
Where to find online			Google name of magazine, name of professional interviewed, or name of topic
References cited			No citations typical
Language		Written for professionals in the United States; not typically translated	
Audience			Laypeople and professionals

Adapted from Colorado State University. (2013). *Popular Magazines vs. Trade Magazines vs. Scholarly Journals*. Retrieved from http://lib.colostate.edu/howto/poplr.html

Learning Activity 4-6: Levels of the Evidence

Evidence-based practice (EBP) requires the use of the best available evidence to support professional decision making with regard to assessments and interventions. Randomized controlled trials (RTCs) are considered the "gold standard" of research methodology. However, EBP does not always rely on RTCs; other types of evidence can also provide rationale when used with practitioner expertise and the desires of the client.

This learning activity asks you to define and differentiate between various levels of evidence and to provide examples of each. Use an Evidence Pyramid (State University of New York, 2014a) or other resource describing levels of evidence as a reference while completing this activity. Helpful resources for novice researchers can be found on websites of various university libraries, such as State University of New York Downstate Medical Center's Evidence Based Medicine Tutorial (State University of New York, 2014b). However, online access to a university's research databases and scholarly materials is typically only available to those affiliated with the particular institution.

Levels of Evidence From Highest to Lowest Quality	Define Level of Evidence	Examples of Where This Level of Evidence Is Found	Challenges Associated With Use of This Level of Evidence

Worksheet 4-13

Reading Primary Source Studies

Knowing when to seek evidence and being able to identify reputable sources of evidence are just the beginning of applying the evidence to practice. Appraisal of the findings of a study are paramount to knowing whether the evidence is worthwhile and indicated for your client. A practitioner can seek primary source studies or those that have been appraised by others (secondary source studies). Secondary source studies can be found under headings such as systematic reviews, meta-analyses, critically appraised papers (CAPs), and critically appraised topics (CATs). The Cochrane Collaboration (www.cochrane.org) is a well-known group that appraises medical research to assist with understanding the validity of a body of work. This worksheet challenges your knowledge of key points that a practitioner should be aware of when reviewing primary source studies.

1. Which of the following best describes the term *primary source*?
   A. The author that created the original work
   B. A published research paper that is not being read as part of a critical appraisal
   C. A research paper that was not published
   D. The first month that a paper is printed in a journal

2. When determining whether a study was completed according to the gold standard of evidence, you would expect it to be based on which type of design?
   A. Case study
   B. Single subject design
   C. Survey research
   D. Randomized control trial

3. Which of the following terms is used to indicate that the number of participants involved in a study was large enough to ensure clinical significance?
   A. Subjects
   B. Power
   C. Weakness
   D. *N*

4. Before choosing a research paper (primary or secondary) to inform a clinical decision, what should a practitioner have?
   A. A medical library or electronic database to ensure access to the paper
   B. A patient who has the disorder described in the paper
   C. A research question that matches the topic of the paper
   D. A list of at least 50 search terms

5. Which of the following statements indicates that a paper is not a quantitative study?
   A. Practice beliefs and choices of novice OTs
   B. Outcomes of mCIMT, a systematic review
   C. Functional outcomes using NDT, a RCT
   D. A survey of functional performance after OT intervention

Worksheet 4-14

Statistical Tests

Most occupational therapy practitioners are not statisticians, nor should they need be. However, when looking for quality primary evidence to support a clinical decision, the OT should be able to determine whether study results are based on meaningful statistical analysis. Figure 4-2 delineates the steps in quantitative and qualitative research. The following worksheet will review some of the basic statistical tests and terms used in medical research.

Matching: Match the parametric (based on normal distribution) statistical test with the description that best matches.

1. Two-sample (unpaired) t-test ________
2. One-sample (paired) t-test ________
3. One-way analysis of variance using total sum of squares (F test) ________
4. Two-way analysis of variance ________
5. Product-moment correlation coefficient (Pearson's r) ________

a. Three or more sets of observations are made on a single sample
b. Compares two independent samples drawn from the same population
c. Tests the influence and interaction of two difference covariates when three or more sets of observations are made on a single sample
d. Compares two sets of observations on a single sample
e. Assesses the strength of the straight-line association between two continuous variables

Matching: Match the nonparametric version of the parametric tests with the example that best describes its application.

1. Mann-Whitney U test ________
2. Wilcoxon matched pairs test ________
3. Analysis of variance by ranks (Kruskall-Wallis test) ________
4. Two-way analysis of variance by ranks ________
5. Spearman's rank correlation coefficient ________

a. To assess and to determine the extent of functional limitations related to severity of cerebrovascular accident (CVA) in a client with a stroke
b. To determine whether dressing abilities improve in a client with a stroke after one, two, or three sessions of occupational therapy
c. To determine whether handwriting abilities improve in a child with hemiplegia after one, two, or three sessions of occupational therapy and also determine whether there is a difference between males and females
d. To compare ROM of wrist extension before and after a school-based craft activity
e. To compare range of motion measurements of clients after completion of a cooking task and those completing a dressing task

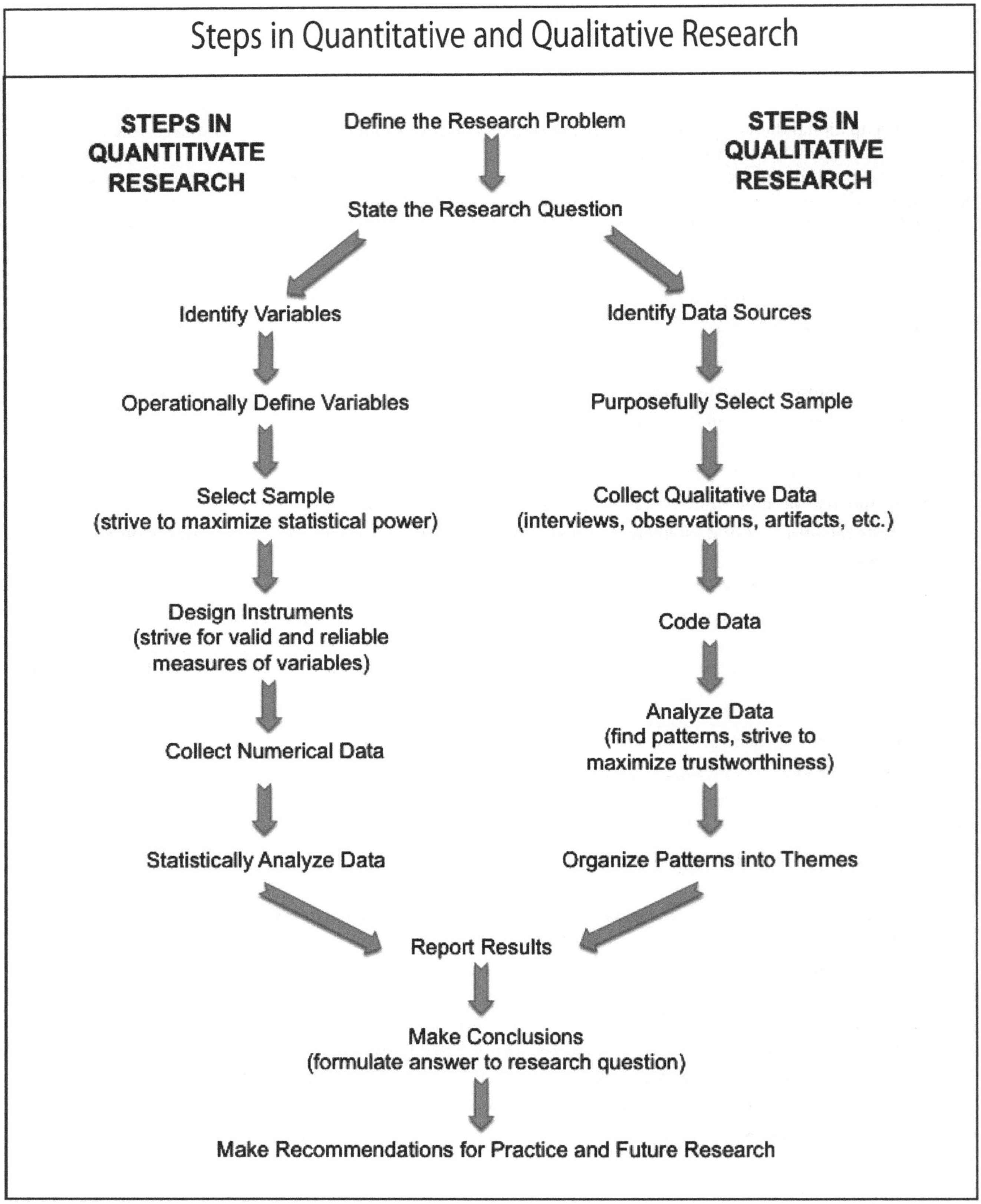

Figure 4-2. Steps in quantitative and qualitative research. (Reprinted with permission from Bell, S. [2015]. Understanding research. In K. Sladyk & R. Ryan [Eds.], *Ryan's occupational therapy assistant: Principles, practice issues, and techniques* [5th ed., pp. 556–570]. Thorofare, NJ: SLACK Incorporated.)

Learning Activity 4-7: Case Study—Evidence-Based Practice

Earl Elderlee, a 75-year-old retired carpenter, sustained a right CVA 6 days ago. He was recently admitted to an inpatient rehabilitation center with the goal of returning home. He is widowed and currently lives in a first-floor garden apartment. His only child, a son aged 50, lives 3,000 miles away. Before his illness, Mr. Elderlee was independent in driving. He also enjoyed walking his dog, attending Major League baseball games, occasionally going to a local casino, and fixing things for his friends. Mr. Elderlee now has left facial droop, slurred speech, and dysphagia requiring a pureed diet and liquids with a nectar consistency. He exhibits impulsivity since his stroke and has moderate left neglect and poor spatial relations. Passive ROM (PROM) of the nondominant left upper extremity is within normal limits, but subluxation is present at the glenohumeral joint. The left upper extremity is starting to develop some voluntary motion, but Mr. Elderlee can only actively lift his arm half way. He is just starting to develop a gross grasp but cannot fully maintain grasp on objects or manipulate them. He has absent protective sensation in the left hand, functional strength in his left lower extremity, and good dynamic balance. However, Mr. Elderlee requires minimal assistance to transfer and ambulate using a hemi-walker due to his decreased safety awareness. He also requires moderate assistance for self-care ADLs.

To assist you in developing an appropriate intervention plan based on the evidence, choose one of the following categories, and complete the questions that follow.

Constraint-induced movement therapy
Mirror therapy
Upper extremity orthotic intervention
Task-oriented approach
Neurodevelopmental treatment (e.g., Bobath, Brunnstrom, proprioceptive neuromuscular facilitation [PNF])
ADL retraining
Functional mobility training
IADL retraining
Driver rehabilitation
Facilitating leisure participation
Approaches to minimize unilateral neglect
Electrical stimulation
Sensory retraining
Cognitive/perceptual retraining
Therapeutic use of computer or video games/Wii

Category chosen: ____

Brief definition of category:

How does your topic relate to this client's occupational performance?

Search the professional literature for research related to your topic and this client. Locate and include the citations for the following:

A case report: ____________________

Five peer-reviewed research study articles (primary source) published within the past 5 years:

1. ____________________

2. ____________________

3. ____________________

4. ____________________

5. ____________________

Meta-analysis or systemic review published within the past 5 years ____________________

What does your previous clinical experience (what you were taught in school or observed in Level I or Level II fieldwork) tell you about the choice you made?

____

What are the client's thoughts regarding the technique that you have chosen? Does this technique fit well with his lifestyle? Does it support your client's goals?

____

On the basis of the evidence you located, what methods for your assigned category would you use or not use for this client?

____

Answers to Chapter 4 Worksheets

Worksheet 4-1: Using AOTA Official Documents

Reference: AOTA (2014c).

1. A. The *Occupational Therapy Practice Framework* was written in part to be consistent with terminology used by the World Health Organization's *International Classification of Functioning, Disability and Health* (AOTA, 2014b).
2. B. This document delineates specific clinical practice requirements for OTs and OTAs for evaluation, intervention, and outcomes (AOTA, 2010b).
3. D. This document delineates core concepts such as altruism, equality, and client dignity and guiding principles such as beneficence and justice (AOTA, 2015).

4. C
5. A
6. C. This document describes the general kinds of services occupational therapy practitioners provide. Answers A, B, and D address other aspects of practice (AOTA, 2014d).
7. D. (AOTA, 2010a.)
8. A. This document provides specific guidelines for the kinds of tasks that may or may not be delegated to an aide (AOTA, 2014a).
9. B. The ACOTE Standards are criteria used for OT and OTA academic programs (AOTA, 2012).
10. A

Worksheet 4-2: Occupational Therapy Practice Framework—Domain and Process

Reference: AOTA, 2014b.

1. ___T___ A definition of occupational therapy adopted from the Model Practice Act is found in the Preface of the *Framework*.
2. ___T___ Several definitions for occupation can be found within the *Framework*.
3. ___T___ The *Framework* provides a unique definition of occupation.
4. ___F___ The *Framework* is divided into three distinct sections, the domain, the process, and the outcomes.

   The Framework comprises two distinct sections: the domain and the process:
5. ___T___ The *Framework* supports a top-down approach to intervention
6. ___F___ The concept of the therapeutic use of self is found in the domain of the *Framework*.

   In a change from previous versions, the third edition of the Framework *classifies "The Therapeutic Use of Self" as part of the Process.*
7. ___F___ The Process of OT is described as having three parts: the occupational profile, the standards of service, and the analysis of occupation.

   The process of OT has three parts: evaluation, intervention, and targeting of outcomes.
8. ___F___ Purposeful activities are described as one type of intervention within the *Framework*.

   The Framework *does not refer to activities as being* purposeful. *Interventions of this type are referred to as* occupations *or* activities.
9. ___T___ The domain of OT includes performance patterns, occupations, performance skills, client factors, and environment and context.
10. ___F___ The overarching statement of the *Framework* is "Supporting health and participation in life through engagement in occupation."

    The overarching statement is: "Achieving, health, well-being and participation in life through engagement in occupation."

Worksheet 4-3: Occupational Therapy Practice Framework—Activities and Occupations

Some items fit neatly into one category, whereas other activities may be placed into several categories depending on the particular context and one's personal values, interests, or roles (AOTA, 2014b). For example, reading e-mail can be a work-related task, a leisurely way to pass time, or considered a means of social communication. Thus, your classifications may be slightly different from the ones indicated on the next page.

Client Activity	***ADLs***	***IADLs***	***Play***	***Leisure***	***Work***	***Education***	***Rest and Sleep***	***Social Participation***
Baking bread		*		*				
Cleaning contact lenses	*							
Taking the train to get to a job		*						
Donning an orthosis	*							
Playing hopscotch with others			*					*
Attending religious services								*
Making a collage for an occupational therapy class assignment						*		
Watching TV to fall asleep				*			*	
Feeding the household cat or dog		*						
Listening to music				*				
Preparing a resume					*			
Walking to the dinner table	*							
Taking a nap							*	
Babysitting a younger sibling		*			*			*
Organizing school papers into folders						*		
Volunteering at a hospital gift shop					*			*
Attending a bridal shower or bachelor party								*
Paying bills		*						
Getting to next class on time						*		
Knitting a sweater to wear				*				
Using contraception	*							*
Setting an alarm clock							*	
Reading e-mails				*	*			*
Taking vitamins		*						
Sewing a button back on a shirt		*						
Planting flowers in the yard		*						
Writing a performance review for a staff member					*			
Navigating a wheelchair in the home	*							
Dressing a Barbie doll			*					
Exercising at the gym		*		*				
Calling 911 when smelling smoke		*						
Eating lunch with colleagues				*	*			*

Worksheet 4-4: Differentiating Client Factors and Performance Skills

According to the *Occupational Therapy Practice Framework* (2014b), client factors are what the client *has* (e.g., anatomical and physiological structures and functions), whereas performance skills (motor, social interaction, and process skills) are what the client *does* (e.g., observable actions). For example, ROM and strength are client factors that affect motor performance skills, such as reaching to put cans in a cabinet or bending to tie shoes. As another example, having vocal nodules or brain lesions may affect communication skills, such as the ability to modulate voice, talk on the telephone, or say a prayer. Realize that some things that are observable such as Bell's palsy or edema may be considered *conditions*, not client factors. Conditions typically arise from deficiencies in underlying structures and functions such as impaired facial nerves, brain lesions, impaired sensory processing, or poor lymphatic drainage and can affect occupational performance.

1. __F__ The client who had shoulder surgery achieved left arm abduction to 160°.
2. __S__ The resident is able to manipulate knitting needles with both hands.
3. __F__ The client has intact short-term memory.
4. __F__ The client admitted to the acute psychiatric unit today has signs and symptoms consistent with severe depression.
5. __F__ The client has a pain level of 7 today per the 10-point visual analog scale.
6. __S__ The client demonstrates good dynamic standing balance when pulling up his pants.
7. __S__ The student remained calm when another student bumped into him.
8. __F__ The client sitting in the power wheelchair has poor lymphatic drainage causing 1+ edema in his right leg.
9. __F__ The client has a below-knee amputation.
10. __S__ The child playing hopscotch is able to hop on one leg four times without falling.
11. __S__ During a family intervention, the client stated agreement with need to attend sobriety meetings.
12. __F__ The infant demonstrates a positive Babinski sign.
13. __F__ The client at risk for thrombosis is using an intermittent compression pump on her legs when lying in her hospital bed.
14. __F__The client with autism is exhibiting tactile defensiveness during art class.
15. __F__ The client achieved a right grip strength of 100 pounds when using a dynamometer.
16. __S__ The child with asthma has difficulty using her inhaler properly.
17. __F__ The client would benefit from paraffin to help loosen stiff finger joints.
18. __F__ Due to increased tone in the client's fingers, the OT premolded the orthotic device on her own hand to prevent difficulty when making a resting pan orthosis.
19. __S__ The resident can roll from side to side using bed rails.
20. __S__ The client has the condition of Bell's palsy, which is creating difficulty with her ability to coordinate chewing.

Worksheet 4-5: Differentiating Client Factors and Performance Skills—More Practice

According to the *Occupational Therapy Practice Framework* (2014b), client factors are what the client *has* (e.g., anatomical and physiological structures and functions) whereas performance skills (motor, social interaction, and process skills) are what the client *does* (e.g., observable actions). For example, the client factors of sensation and vision affect motor skills such as putting a key in a lock or cutting vegetables safely. As another example, the client factors of self-concept and emotional regulation affect process skills such as desire to live and waiting one's turn patiently. Realize that some things that are observable or measurable such as pain or edema may be considered *conditions*, not client factors. Conditions such as depression, hypertension, allergies, frequent colds, or fracture nonunion may arise due to deficiencies in underlying structures or functions such as chemical imbalance, impaired cardiac function, blocked vessels, or a poor immune system and may affect occupational performance.

1. __S__ The student uses a static tripod grasp when writing.
2. __S__ The client needed to rest after standing to cook at the stove.
3. __F__ The client with schizophrenia hears voices in his head.
4. __S__ The client was able to tear open the package of potato chips.
5. __F__ The client lying in bed has unilateral neglect.
6. __F__ The client's resting blood pressure of 160/95 resulted in the OT contacting the client's physician.
7. __F__ The client demonstrates an improvement in muscle strength from Fair to Good for left elbow flexion.
8. __S__ The client is able to don and doff his protective fracture brace independently.
9. __S__ The client is able to carry a 10-pound grocery bag from her car to the kitchen.
10. __S__ The client is unable to cut her toenails because she has difficulty bending.
11. __F__ The client's scaphoid fracture needed 6 months to heal completely.
12. __F__ The client's gray hair and wrinkles make her appear older than she really is.
13. __S__ The resident cannot push up with his arms to perform a sliding board transfer.
14. __F__ The client is incontinent of urine secondary to a prolapsed bladder
15. __S__ The client with chemical dependency endures the side effects of withdrawal.
16. __F__ The client's loss of protective sensation in his feet is a safety concern due to his diabetes.
17. __S__ The child with dyspraxia did not fall today while running in gym class.
18. __S__ The resident asked for a calendar to help her remember her therapy appointments.
19. __S__ The client diagnosed with an anxiety disorder chooses not to attend occupational therapy group today.
20. __F__ The client with a nut allergy cannot be exposed to peanut butter.

Worksheet 4-6: Habits, Rituals, Routines, and Roles

For each of the following activities, indicate whether it is a habit, ritual, routine or role. (AOTA, 2014b)

1. *Ritual.* Always decorating the tree on Christmas Eve.
2. *Ritual.* A family has the tradition of making s'mores over the fire whenever camping.
3. *Habit.* Flossing every time after brushing teeth.
4. *Routine.* Taking care of the family pet before leaving for work.
5. *Ritual.* Saying a prayer when lighting candles on the Sabbath.
6. *Routine.* Reading a bedtime story after the child's nightly bath and tucking him into bed.
7. *Role.* A daughter who is caring for an elderly parent with dementia.
8. *Habit.* Smoking a cigarette right after dinner.
9. *Habit.* Buckling a seat belt before driving.
10. *Ritual.* Shaking hands when meeting someone new.
11. *Role.* A woman who enjoys gardening is known as having a "green thumb."
12. *Role.* Identifying as a Roman Catholic and joining the church choir.
13. *Role.* A young musician is proficient at playing a piano.
14. *Habit.* Kissing your spouse when he or she comes home from work.
15. *Role.* An avid bingo player.

16. *Routine.* Making breakfast and packing your child's lunch before driving him to school.
17. *Role.* Completing your shift as a volunteer firefighter.
18. *Role.* A mother helping the teacher by accompanying the child's class on a field trip.
19. *Ritual.* Saying prayers at the gravesite on the 1-year anniversary of the deceased's date of death.
20. *Habit.* Hanging up your coat when you come home.

Worksheet 4-7: Grading and Adapting

For each of the statements that follow, indicate whether the intervention is an example of grading (G) or adapting (A).

1. __A__ To manage clothing without assistance during toileting, the OT suggested that the client use elastic waist pants rather than pants with fastenings.
2. __G__ During yesterday's intervention session, the OT asked a client diagnosed with social anxiety to make a phone call to a pizzeria to ask the cost of a large pizza. Today they went to the pizzeria together so that the client could place an order for two slices of pizza.
3. __G__ The OT had the child use a button board with smaller buttons than previously to work on three-point pinch.
4. __A__ The OT attached a brake extension to a wheelchair for the client with left hemiplegia.
5. __G__ The OT asked a client diagnosed with traumatic brain injury to bake refrigerated dough cookies last week then attempted to have her make cookies using a boxed mix today.
6. __G__ The OT suggested that the child with hand weakness practice handwriting for 5 minutes daily this week and 10 minutes daily next week.
7. __A__ The OT taught the client to use a calendar to remember appointments.
8. __G__ To help improve decision-making skills, the OT gave the client diagnosed with depression a choice of only two craft projects yesterday and a choice of three projects today.
9. __A__ The OT instructed the client with chronic obstructive pulmonary disease to sit during ironing when she returns home.
10. __G__ The OT had the client with bilateral integration problems roll out dough with a rolling pin during last week's session. Today the OT had the client mix dough ingredients with her dominant hand while holding onto a bowl with the nondominant hand.
11. __A__ The OT asked the OTA to attach a zipper pull to the student's backpack.
12. __G__ The OT told the parents that the toddler could now eat semisoft foods in addition to pureed food.
13. __G__ The OT discontinued the client's forearm-based thumb spica orthosis today and issued a hand-based thumb spica orthosis.
14. __A__ The OT instructed the caregiver to purchase an electric kettle with an automatic shut off for the client with early-stage dementia.
15. __A__ The OT instructed the client in use of a pill organizer to help her remember to take her medication.
16. __G__ The OT determined that the client diagnosed with a Colles fracture could initiate light therapy putty exercises today.
17. __G__ The OT worked on the client's wheelchair mobility by having him wheel his wheelchair outdoors today.
18. __A__ The OT asked the teacher to allow the first-grader to eat raisins or granola at his desk to minimize fidgeting during class.
19. __A__ The OT gave the client with schizophrenia a structured leisure worksheet because the client could not come up with three desired leisure tasks when initially asked.
20. __A__ As the client with cancer was at risk for infection outdoors, the OT instructed the family to set up an indoor windowsill garden.

Worksheet 4-8: Grading and Adapting (Making Coffee)

Here are some suggestions, although you may come up with other ideas. Consider which modifications are needed for motor difficulties vs cognitive impairment.

Activity Demand: Task Materials (Coffee)	***Activity Demand: Required Action of Opening Coffee Container***	***Activity Demand: Required Action of Measuring Coffee***	***Activity Demand: Required Action of Heating the Water/Brewing Coffee***
Example: *Instant coffee*	Example: *Can of coffee requiring use of a can opener*	Example: *Use a measuring spoon*	Example: *Boil water in teakettle using stove*
• Whole coffee beans • Coffee "tea-bags" • Specific type of coffee (decaffeinated vs regular, espresso-type coffee, flavored) • Bottle of liquid iced coffee • Ground coffee	• Jar with lid • Tear off pouch • Cut pouch with scissors • Paper wrapper • Box/carton (pods) • Screw cap/bottle top • Can of coffee with a metal/foil pull-off lid • Can of coffee with a plastic lid • Place coffee in another container or bag • Carafe/thermos (containing hot coffee)	• Single-serve instant coffee packet • Pods/K-cups (Keurig) • Premeasured drip coffee package • Have family member premeasure and place in plastic bags or containers	• Microwave water • Electric kettle/hot pot with/without automatic shutoff • Automatic drip coffee maker with/without automatic shutoff • Programmable machine family member can preset • Espresso/cappuccino machine • K-Cup machine (Keurig) • Electric percolator • Stovetop glass percolator • Stovetop metal percolator (espresso) • French press

Worksheet 4-9: Grading and Adapting—Laundry

List the sequence of steps to wash clothes and ways to grade and adapt each step. You may come up with other suggestions.

Sequence of Steps	***Grade/Adapt Task Methods***	***Grade/Adapt Task Materials***
Example: *Carry a laundry basket full of clothes*	Example: *Place dirty clothes directly in machine when getting changed*	Example: *Use a rolling laundry cart* *Use a laundry bag*
• Check pockets before putting clothes in laundry basket	• Post visual reminders	• Wear clothing without pockets
• Sort items (by color, materials, delicate, hand wash)	• Post list of instructions • Sit instead of stand	• Use a divided laundry cart
• Open machine lid/door and put appropriate amount of items in machine	• Take clothes to dry cleaner • Use a laundry service • Use a hamper or basket to determine correct amount of laundry to put in machine • Sit instead of stand	• Use a reacher • Use a front-loading vs a top-loading machine • Use a coin-operated machine

Sequence of Steps	Grade/Adapt Task Methods	Grade/Adapt Task Materials
• Open detergent containers and measure detergent, fabric softener, bleach (pour into cap, use scoop measure)	• Use premeasured detergent or pods • Use markings on caps	• Premeasured detergent/pods • Use dispenser-type bottle • Laundry detergent sheets • Powder versus liquid • Dryer sheets • Use a different measuring device • Purchase items from Laundromat vending machine • Use small-sized containers
• Put detergent, bleach, softener in proper machine dispensers and close lid	• Label dispensers clearly	• Pod or detergent sheet vs liquid or powder • Use an "all-in-one" product • Use small-sized containers
• Set proper cycles temp, delicate/heavy-duty, fabric softener, extra rinse, and turn machine on	• Post list of instructions • Label cycles clearly	• Use machine with more or less buttons or cycles • Push buttons, digital panel, or a dial
• Remember to take clothes out of washer	• Designate a consistent day and time to do laundry • Stay by machine to perform other tasks	• Machine with an audible signal • Use a timer
• Put clothes in dryer and set time/setting on dryer	• Sit instead of stand • Hang up clothes instead • Post list of instructions	• Clothesline • Drying rack • Use a reacher • Use a machine with fewer buttons or cycles
• Remember to take clothes out of dryer and put away	• Store clothing close to washer and dryer	• Machine with an audible signal • Use a timer • Use a reacher

Worksheet 4-10: Frames of Reference

Suggested resource: Schell, Gillen, Scaffa, & Cohn, 2014.

1. To get a person to take a shower, a reward of his liking is provided. Therapist works with client to ensure that he gathers necessary bath items and plans appropriately for after-bath grooming and dressing. Behavioral
2. A client with limited elbow extension (straightening) is given a weaving activity to complete based on her request and interest in creating handmade placemats and wall hangings. Client is instructed to pull yarn to a length that encourages both elbow extension and flexion during activity. Activity is to be completed for a minimum of 4 hours per day, spaced at appropriate intervals. Occupational science/occupational performance/occupation-based/MOHO
3. Client with poor memory for phone numbers brings cell phone to clinic along with important phone numbers. Therapist and client work together to add phone numbers to speed dial on phone. Therapist and client then create a small "cheat sheet" with names and speed dial numbers that will be pasted to the back of the phone and made into a wallet-size card. Cognitive rehabilitation

4. A child who is unable to feed herself due to the effects of athetoid cerebral palsy is provided with a Winsford feeder (Northcoast Medical Inc.) The therapist teaches the child and her mother how to use the device. The child is now able to complete feeding after setup. *Rehabilitation*
5. A child who had difficulty sitting straight in his chair and paying attention in class is provided with activities during therapy such as bouncing on therapy ball, propelling self in scooter board along the floor, and catching bean bags in hands while swinging in a net swing. *Sensory integration*
6. A woman is so fearful of getting into a car crash that she is unable to leave the house to go to work. The therapist presents her with credible statistics regarding the likelihood that she will be involved in a car accident. The therapist also works with client to determine alternate means of transportation and determine how these will be used for the client to get to work every day and on time. She will be supported by the companionship of an occupational therapist during first several days of using alternative transportation and eventually driving herself. *Cognitive behavioral*
7. Client is unable to participate in desired leisure activities because of fatigue associated with chemotherapy. The OT works with the client to determine which activities he would like to participate in and helps him to brainstorm on various ways to complete the activities in a way that the fatigue does not interfere. *Occupational science/occupational performance/occupation-based/MOHO*
8. Adult man with flaccid upper extremity from a stroke is placed in a "weight-bearing" position intended to normalize tone in extremity. In addition, he is given tactile cues that assist his body in knowing how to sit in a more symmetrical way when in his wheelchair. *NDT, Bobath*
9. A 6-month-old child with cerebral palsy is placed in a developmental position known as "prone on elbows" to provide needed weight bearing into shoulder girdle. This technique is theorized to assist the brain with learning "normal movement patterns." *NDT, Bobath*
10. A depressed individual is asked to draw a picture representing her feelings for the day. The picture is analyzed to determine her underlying feelings in an effort to help her to understand how her unconscious is dealing with various life challenges. Theory states that when she becomes aware of her underlying issues, she will be able to come to terms with her reactions and change her thinking to decrease the depressive symptoms. *Psychodynamic*
11. A child with poor handwriting is given fine motor coordination activities to work on in an attempt to enhance his motor control. The activities include clothespin pinching, putty squeezing, and marble picking up and harboring in hand. *Biomechanical*
12. A client who sustained a stroke and now has moderate weakness of her left upper extremity is given interesting tasks, such as cleaning CD-ROMs, that she must complete using both hands in a naturalistic manner. She is to clean 25 CDs to complete the task. *Task-oriented approach*

Worksheet 4-11: When to Use Evidence-Based Practice

1. _____ Agreeing with the clients' choice of outfit for the day. *(This decision does not require supportive evidence if the outfit will not impair the ability of the client to participate in treatment.)*
2. __X__ Choosing to use or not use hip precautions with a frail client 8 weeks status post hip arthroplasty.
3. __X__ Agreeing to provide an adapted aid to allow the client with swallowing precautions to eat the outside of a chocolate-filled lollipop.
4. __X__ Starting a 6-week-long modified constraint-induced therapy (mCIMT) regimen with a client who has left upper extremity weakness status post cerebrovascular accident.
5. __X__ Per the physician's order, completing an ultrasound treatment on a client with significant sensory loss.
6. _____ Using a standard vs a sports wheelchair to transport a 50-year-old male client to therapy when both are available in the rehabilitation hospital. *(Because both are simply used as a means to transport the client to a therapy session, it will not affect efficiency or efficacy of therapy itself.)*
7. _____ Scheduling clients for therapy sessions. *(Although an important concept, this is not a situation in which supportive evidence is required; it is typically a decision made with consideration of multiple and changeable variables.)*
8. __X__ Using an NDT approach with a 6-year-old child with right hemiplegia.

9. _____ Suggesting that a teacher use an Apple iPad versus a Samsung tablet with a child diagnosed with autism spectrum disorder when both items are available in the classroom. *(Because both devices are available and are equivalent technology, the decision to use one over the other can be made based on therapist preference alone.)*

10. __X__ Assessing a client using the nine-hole peg test to determine readiness to return to work.

Worksheet 4-12: Starting With Evidence

	Journal	*Trade Journal*	*Magazine*
Examples of publications	*AJOT, CJOT, OTJR, JAMA*	*ADVANCE for Occupational Therapy Practitioners, Today in OT*	*Women's Health, Men's Health, Healthcare News*
How publications are titled	Most often has the word "journal" in the title	May refer to a specific profession or diagnostic category	Titles that focus on population for whom the publication is created
Appearance of publications in print	Printed cover and pages are typically made with shiny paper, pictures not typically present, graphics include trademarked title, date, and volume of issue and summary list of contents. Very few, if any, advertisements or job ads. If found, they are subtle or located in the back of the journal.	Printed version may be covered and contain pages printed on newsprint or standard paper. Cover often contains a picture that highlights contents. Listing of contents, trademark title, and date of publication found. Advertisements and job ads found throughout that are focused on the targeted topic	Printed cover created to market to the target population. Pictures on cover are standard as are eye-catching listing of contents. Paper can vary; many various advertisements found throughout. Job ads not found.
Appearance of publications online	May require subscription, username, and password	Found at a specific URL. Typically no cost but may require creation of an account. Brightly colored, multiple illustrations, links to various sections and resources.	Subscription may or may not be required based on nature of publication. Brightly illustrated; possible menu of contents. Articles are often hyperlinked and may be accessed through hyperlinks from other sources.
Authors of contents	Researchers, scholars, those with advanced degrees and training within topic area	Professionals within the target group or other similar groups	Freelance writers or writers working for magazine. Professionals are interviewed and quoted but not typically authors.
Where to find online	May be accessed through professional databases (PubMed, Google Scholar, CINAHL, EBSCO) or university libraries	Google, Google Scholar, Google name of trade journal/organization	Google name of magazine, name of professional interviewed, or name of topic.
References cited	Scholarly journal articles, textbooks, government or organizational papers	May not include citations. May include those found in journals, but this is not typical.	Typically there are no citations.

Language	Written for advanced readers. May be translated.	Written for professionals in the United States; not typically translated	Written for laypeople, not translated if accessed within United States
Audience	Researchers, scholars, professionals	Professionals	Laypeople and professionals

Adapted from Colorado State University (2013). *Popular Magazines vs. Trade Magazines vs. Scholarly Journals.* Retrieved from http://lib.colostate.edu/howto/poplr.html

Worksheet 4-13: Reading Primary Source Studies

Suggested resource: Greenhalgh, 2010.

1. B
2. D
3. B
4. C
5. A

Worksheet 4-14: Statistical Tests

Suggested resource: Greenhalgh, 2010.
Match the parametric (based on normal distribution) statistical test with the description that best matches.

1. Two-sample (unpaired) t-test __b__
2. One-sample (paired) t-test __d__
3. One-way analysis of variance using total sum of squares (F test) __a__
4. Two-way analysis of variance __c__
5. Product-moment correlation coefficient (Pearson's r) __e__
   a. Three or more sets of observations are made on a single sample
   b. Compares two independent samples drawn from the same population
   c. Tests the influence and interaction of two difference covariates when three or more sets of observations are made on a single sample
   d. Compares two sets of observations on a single sample
   e. Assesses the strength of the straight-line association between two continuous variables.

Match the nonparametric version of the parametric tests with the example that best describes its application.

1. Mann-Whitney U test __e__
2. Wilcoxon matched pairs test __d__
3. Analysis of variance by ranks (Kruskall-Wallis test) __b__
4. Two-way analysis of variance by ranks __c__
5. Spearman's rank correlation coefficient __a__
   a. To assess and to determine the extent of functional limitations related to severity of cerebrovascular accident (CVA) in a client with a stroke
   b. To determine whether dressing abilities improve in a client with a stroke after one, two, or three sessions of occupational therapy
   c. To determine whether handwriting abilities improve in a child with hemiplegia after one, two, or three sessions of occupational therapy and also determine whether there is a difference between males and females
   d. To compare range of motion of wrist extension before and after a school-based craft activity
   e. To compare range of motion measurements of clients following completion of a cooking task and those completing a dressing task.

Chapter 4 References

Accreditation Council for Occupational Therapy Education. (2012). 2011 Accreditation Council for Occupational Therapy Education (ACOTE®) Standards. *American Journal of Occupational Therapy, 66*(Suppl. 6), S6–S74.

American Occupational Therapy Association. (2010a). Standards for continuing competence. *American Journal of Occupational Therapy, 64*(Suppl. 6), S103–S105.

American Occupational Therapy Association. (2010b). Standards of practice for occupational therapy. *American Journal of Occupational Therapy, 64*(Suppl. 6), S106–S111.

American Occupational Therapy Association. (2014a). Guidelines for supervision, roles, and responsibilities during the delivery of occupational therapy services. *American Journal of Occupational Therapy, 68*(Suppl. 3), S16–S22.

American Occupational Therapy Association. (2014b). Occupational therapy practice framework: Domain and process (3rd ed.). *American Journal of Occupational Therapy, 68*(Suppl. 1), S1–S48.

American Occupational Therapy Association. (2014c). Official Documents. Retrieved from http://www.aota.org/Practice/Manage/Official.aspx

American Occupational Therapy Association. (2014d). Scope of practice. *American Journal of Occupational Therapy, 68*(Suppl. 3), S34–S40.

American Occupational Therapy Association. (2015). Occupational therapy code of ethics (2015). *American Journal of Occupational Therapy,* 69 (Suppl. 3), 6913410030. http://dx.doi.org/10.5014/ajot.2015.696S03.

Bell, S. (2015). Understanding research. In K. Sladyk & R. Ryan (Eds.), *Ryan's occupational therapy assistant: Principles, practice issues, and techniques* (5th ed., pp. 556–570). Thorofare, NJ: SLACK Incorporated.

Colorado State University. (2013). *Popular Magazines vs. Trade Magazines vs. Scholarly Journals.* Retrieved from http://lib.colostate.edu/howto/poplr.html

Dunn, W. (2000). Habit: What's the brain got to do with it? *OTJR: Occupation, Participation and Health, 20*(Suppl. 1), S6–S20.

Greenhalgh, T. (2010). *How to read a paper: The basics of evidence based medicine* (4th ed.). Hoboken, NJ: Wiley-Blackwell.

Morreale, M. J. (2015). *Developing clinical competence: A workbook for the OTA.* Thorofare, NJ: SLACK Incorporated.

Morreale, M. J., & Borcherding, S. (2013). *The OTA's guide to documentation: Writing SOAP notes* (3rd ed.). Thorofare, NJ: SLACK Incorporated.

O'Brien, J. (2014). Intervention planning. In K. Jacobs, N. MacRae, & K. Sladyk (Eds.), *Occupational therapy essentials for clinical competence* (2nd ed., pp. 295–307). Thorofare, NJ: SLACK Incorporated.

Schell, B. A. B., Gillen, G., Scaffa, M. E., & Cohn, E. (Eds.). (2014). *Willard and Spackman's occupational therapy* (12th ed.). Philadelphia: Lippincott, Williams & Wilkins.

State University New York Downstate Medical Center. (2014a). Guide to research methods: The Evidence Pyramid. Retrieved from http://library.downstate.edu/EBM2/2100.htm

State University New York Downstate Medical Center. (2014b). Downstate Medical Center's Evidence Based Medicine Tutorial. Brooklyn, NY. Retrieved from http://library.downstate.edu/EBM2/contents.htm

Thomas, H. (2012). *Occupation-based activity analysis.* Thorofare, NJ: SLACK Incorporated.

Chapter 5

Incorporating Activities and Occupations

Occupational therapy practitioners use a variety of methods and interventions to facilitate occupational performance and role competence, maintain health and wellness, and improve quality of life (American Occupational Therapy Association [AOTA], 2014). Depending on the client's unique circumstances, the intervention plan may include approaches such as developing or remediating specific client factors and performance skills; modifying the task, environment, or performance patterns; or compensating for lost function (AOTA, 2014). Although preparatory interventions can also be an important part of a client's intervention plan, these methods and tasks should supplement, but never replace, activities and occupations (AOTA, 2014). Occupational therapy practitioners must use a holistic approach that incorporates meaningful "real-life" interventions that address or support the client's therapeutic goals for occupational engagement (AOTA, 2014). Activities and occupations are emphasized in this chapter, along with select preparatory methods and tasks that also contribute to occupational performance (e.g., client/family education and training; provision of adaptive equipment, durable medical equipment (DME), assistive technology; therapeutic exercises). Note that space limitations allow for only select initial evaluation data to be presented here. A "real" evaluation would include more complete information, such as the specific aspects of occupations needing assistance and the various factors, contexts, or performance skills hindering or supporting occupational performance. Answers to worksheet exercises are provided at the end of the chapter.

Contents

Morreale, M. J., & Amini, D.
The Occupational Therapist's Workbook for Ensuring Clinical Competence (pp. 165-204).

Worksheet 5-1

Teaching-Learning Process (Total Hip Replacement)

Elaine, a client in acute care, is a 65-year-old female who underwent left total hip replacement (THR) surgery (posterolateral approach) 2 days ago. She currently has non-weight-bearing status for her affected leg and her secondary diagnoses include hypertension (HTN) and hyperlipidemia. Elaine was evaluated by an occupational therapist (OT) yesterday and received preliminary instruction in total hip precautions. The therapist noted that, although the client's upper extremity function and cognition are intact, the client requires moderate assistance to transfer using a rolling walker. The expected discharge plan is for Elaine to go to a short-term rehabilitation facility 3 days from now then eventually return home. The therapist is planning to teach the client lower body dressing techniques today. Consider the process for implementing this intervention session, such as equipment/supplies needed, methods of instruction, and sequence of steps that the therapist should use for the occupation of dressing.

1. Where will the session take place? ____________________
2. What is the anticipated length of session? ____________________
3. What equipment/supplies will the OT need to bring to the session? ____________________
____
____

   Besides gathering equipment and supplies, what are several things the OT should do before entering the client's room? ____________________
____
____

4. List the general steps of how the session should be implemented:
   1. *Perform hand hygiene and use* ____________________ *as indicated*
   2. *Greet client and explain* ____________________
   3.
   4.
   5.
   6.
   7.
   8.
   9.
   10.
   11.
   12.
   13.
   14.
   15.

In what ways, if any, might the OT implement the intervention session differently if the client was 90 years old and diagnosed with early-stage Alzheimer's disease?

Learning Activity 5-1: Teaching-Learning Process (Carpal Tunnel Syndrome)

Ben is a 35-year-old computer programmer diagnosed with carpal tunnel syndrome (CTS) in his dominant right hand. He is otherwise in good health. Ben was evaluated by an OT at an outpatient clinic 3 days ago. The following is some information taken from the initial evaluation report:

Chief complaint: Ben reports he has been experiencing decreased hand strength and increased pain, numbness, and tingling in his right thumb, index, and long fingers for the past 4 months.

Activities of daily living (ADLs)/instrumental ADLs (IADLs): Ben's symptoms are creating difficulty with sleeping, job performance, his daily exercise routine at the gym, and yard maintenance.

Pain: Right hand reported as 7/10

Sensation: Right hand:

2-point discrimination: 8 mm index and long fingers, 5 mm ring and small fingers

Phalen's test: Positive, eliciting numbness/tingling at 15 seconds.

Semmes-Weinstein monofilament test: 4.31 volar thumb, index, and long fingers, 3.61 radial aspect of palm and dorsal tips of index and ring fingers. 2.83 remainder of hand

Active range of motion (AROM): BUE WNL

Strength	***Right Hand***	***Left Hand***
Grip	78 lb	98 lb
3-point pinch	20 lb	28 lb
Lateral pinch	28 lb	30 lb
Tip pinch	17 lb	22 lb

After completing Ben's evaluation, the OT fabricated and issued a volar wrist immobilization orthosis for Ben to wear at work, nighttime, and during heavy tasks. Today Ben has his first follow-up appointment, and the therapist will be working with Ben to start teaching him median nerve gliding exercises, tendon gliding exercises, and ergonomics for work. Consider the process for implementing these interventions such as equipment/supplies needed, specific methods of instruction, and sequence of steps that the OT should follow. Incorporate several activities needed for Ben's desired level of job performance.

1. Where will the session take place? ______________________________
2. What is the anticipated length of session? ______________________________
3. What equipment/supplies will the OT need to gather for the therapy session? ______________________________

   ____

   ____

4. Use resources to locate specific instructions/pictures for the nerve and tendon gliding exercises and ergonomic recommendations for which Ben will need instruction.

5. List the general sequence of how the OT should implement all of Ben's interventions for today, including several activities needed for his job:
   1. *Perform hand hygiene*
   2. *Greet Ben and explain* ______________________________

Learning Activity 5-1: Teaching-Learning Process (Carpal Tunnel Syndrome) (continued)

3.

4.

5.

6.

7.

8.

9.

10.

11.

12.

13.

14.

15.

How do the tendon and nerve gliding exercises relate to Ben's occupational performance?

Worksheet 5-2

Intervention Categories

Indicate if each of the following is a true (T) or false (F) statement regarding the categorization of interventions used in occupational therapy.

1. ________ Creating a wrist immobilization orthosis for a client 6 weeks post wrist fracture is a preparatory task.
2. ________ The application of therapeutic ultrasound is considered an activity.
3. ________ Completing upper extremity weight bearing by having the client lean on a table within the therapy gym where other clients and practitioners are working is a group intervention.
4. ________ Picking up beanbags with a reacher and placing them into a bucket is a preparatory task.
5. ________ Making dinner after a trip to the grocery store to purchase ingredients is an activity.
6. ________ Brushing teeth in the middle of the afternoon is an activity.
7. ________ Getting up in the morning and going to work is an occupation.
8. ________ Completing a wheelchair fitting with a client is a preparatory method.
9. ________ Running a lunch-hour eating activity with three clients is a group intervention.
10. ________ Instructing a client in how to button with a button hook is considered training.

For those interventions that were answered *false*, indicate the category of intervention that would make the statement *true*.

Statement number	Correct category of intervention
________________	______________________________
________________	______________________________
________________	______________________________
________________	______________________________
________________	______________________________

Worksheet 5-3

Cerebrovascular Accident Interventions

Marvin, a 62-year-old male diagnosed with left cerebrovascular accident (CVA), was just admitted to a subacute rehabilitation facility. Marvin retired from his postal worker job 2 years ago, got divorced last year, and lived alone independently before his stroke. Here is some information taken from Marvin's occupational therapy evaluation report:

ADL: Requires moderate assistance for self-care and transfers

Upper Extremity (UE) Status:

Hand dominance: Right

ROM: PROM WNL BUE

Strength: RUE flaccid, LUE WFL

Sensation: Intact protective sensation RUE

Communication: Demonstrates dysarthria, but understands and follows three-step verbal commands

Balance and mobility: Weakness noted in trunk and right lower extremity. Dynamic sitting and standing balance are fair. While seated in wheelchair, client tends to lean to the right and slide forward with a posterior pelvic tilt. He requires moderate assistance to ambulate using mobility device.

Which of the following equipment, adaptive devices, or modalities are likely appropriate for an occupational therapy practitioner to use with Marvin at this time to address his primary deficits? Assume that interventions would include, not only the provision of a particular piece of equipment or DME, but actual instruction and practice in its use.

1. ______ Rocker knife
2. ______ Nonslip matting
3. ______ Built-up utensils
4. ______ Plate guard
5. ______ Walker
6. ______ Power wheelchair
7. ______ Electric razor
8. ______ Sock aid
9. ______ Therapy putty
10. ______ Exercise bands
11. ______ Pulleys
12. ______ Vest restraint
13. ______ Wheelchair arm support
14. ______ Soap-on-a-rope
15. ______ Wash mitt
16. ______ Soap/shampoo dispenser
17. ______ Long-handle sponge
18. ______ Tub seat/bench
19. ______ Hot pack to right shoulder
20. ______ Paraffin to right hand
21. ______ Constraint-induced movement therapy (CIMT)
22. ______ Teach self-range of movement (ROM)
23. ______ Lapboard
24. ______ Large pegboard
25. ______ Nine-hole peg test

Worksheet 5-4

Total Hip Replacement Interventions

Anna is a 74-year-old female who underwent left hip replacement surgery (posterolateral approach) 5 days ago for degenerative joint disease (DJD) that was causing severe left hip pain. She was admitted to a skilled nursing facility yesterday for short-term rehabilitation, with an expected discharge plan to return home in several weeks. Anna's medical history includes HTN, type 2 diabetes, and vitamin B_{12} deficiency. She never married, retired from her teaching job at age 62, and has lived alone independently in senior housing for the past 9 years. Doctor's orders state that Anna is not yet allowed to bear any weight on her left lower extremity. At present, Anna requires minimal assistance to transfer and ambulate short distances and is unable to perform lower body dressing and bathing because of her total hip precautions. Both upper extremities exhibit good range of motion and muscle strength of fair plus. The intervention plan for Anna includes goals for modified independence in lower body bathing, dressing, and transfers; and also to increase upper extremity muscle strength by half a muscle grade to support ADL independence.

Which of the following equipment, adaptive devices, or techniques are likely appropriate for an occupational therapy practitioner to use with Anna at this time to address her primary deficits? Assume that interventions would include not only the provision of a particular piece of equipment or DME, but actual instruction and practice in its use.

1. ________ Raised toilet seat
2. ________ Adduction cushion
3. ________ Built-up utensils
4. ________ Commode
5. ________ Crossing legs to tie shoes
6. ________ Walker
7. ________ Power wheelchair
8. ________ Long-handle shoehorn
9. ________ Sock aid
10. ________ Hot pack to left hip
11. ________ Paraffin to left hand
12. ________ Teach stair climbing with crutches
13. ________ Wheelchair arm support
14. ________ Exercise bands
15. ________ Quad cane
16. ________ Elastic shoelaces
17. ________ Wedge cushion for wheelchair
18. ________ Reacher
19. ________ Long-handle sponge
20. ________ Tub seat/bench
21. ________ Leg lifter
22. ________ CIMT
23. ________ Sliding board
24. ________ Buttonhook
25. ________ Hospital bed for home

Worksheet 5-5

Improving Basic and Instrumental Activities of Daily Living Occupations

1. An OT is working with a client on functional ambulation in the kitchen so that the client can prepare meals safely. The client uses a walker because of a left femur fracture and partial weight-bearing status. Which of the following is the correct sequence for using the walker:
   A. Advance walker, then weak leg, then strong leg
   B. Advance weak leg, then walker, then strong leg
   C. Advance walker, then strong leg, then weak leg
   D. Advance strong leg, then weak leg, then walker

2. A client admitted to an inpatient rehabilitation hospital has a diagnosis of bilateral below-knee amputations and is not a candidate for prostheses. He is independent in sliding board transfers, but his wheelchair will not be able to fit through his bathroom doorway at his small, ranch-style home. The OT should instruct the client in use of which of the following to enable him to perform toileting independently at home?
   A. Raised toilet seat and grab bar
   B. Commode
   C. Power mobility scooter
   D. Platform walker

3. An OT is working on transfer training with a client who uses a walker and is diagnosed with Parkinson's disease. When having the client transfer from a chair to a standing position, the OT should instruct the client to do which of the following?
   A. Keep client's knees close together
   B. Hold onto a transfer belt around OT's waist
   C. Lean forward over client's center of gravity
   D. Have client use his arms to push up from walker

4. A client in acute care is diagnosed with a right CVA. His left upper extremity is flaccid, and he exhibits fair dynamic standing balance, left neglect, and impulsivity. One of the client's goals is to achieve independence in shaving. Which of the following would best facilitate the client's shaving performance?
   A. Sitting on edge of bed using a bedside table (with mirror) and a safety razor
   B. Standing at sink using electric razor
   C. Sitting in a chair at the sink using electric razor
   D. Sitting in a chair at the sink using a safety razor

5. A client diagnosed with amyotrophic lateral sclerosis (ALS) is working with an OT to improve self-feeding skills. The client has good trunk control, but exhibits weakness of the intrinsic hand muscles and oral musculature. To best facilitate feeding skills, the OT should place the client in which of the following positions?
   A. Sitting in a chair and using an electronic feeding device
   B. Sitting in a chair with chin slightly tucked
   C. Sitting in a chair with neck hyperextended
   D. Sitting in a chair with client's pelvis in a posterior tilt

Worksheet 5-5 (continued)

Improving Basic and Instrumental Activities of Daily Living Occupations

6. A 5-year-old child with a developmental delay is having difficulty donning a coat due to motor planning difficulties with bringing the coat around her back. Which primary method would best help the child become independent in donning her coat?
   A. Use an over-the-head method to don coat
   B. Use mirroring technique
   C. Write down step-by-step instructions
   D. Use a larger size coat

7. An OT is teaching energy conservation techniques to a female client who has a diagnosis of chronic obstructive pulmonary disease (COPD), uses portable oxygen, and fatigues easily. The client is able to ambulate short distances using a rolling walker. Which of the following instructions would be most useful for homemaking?
   A. Use a barbeque grill instead of having to bend when using the oven broiler
   B. Use a tub seat when bathing
   C. Exhale before picking up a laundry basket, then inhale while placing it on top of dryer
   D. Use a flat sheet rather than a fitted sheet

8. An OT is working with a client who is diagnosed with a complete C-4 spinal cord injury. Assuming the therapist is competent in all the following tasks, which would be the least appropriate intervention for this client?
   A. Instruct client in use of a mouth stick to operate computer keyboard
   B. Instruct client in functional mobility using a sip-and-puff wheelchair
   C. Instruct client in use of environmental controls to operate TV
   D. Instruct client in use of hand controls for driving

9. An OT is working with a male client who is diagnosed with a complete C-6 spinal cord injury. Which of the following would be the least appropriate intervention for this client?
   A. Instruct client in use of a button hook
   B. Instruct client in adaptive shaving techniques
   C. Instruct client in use of a wrist-driven hinge orthosis for feeding
   D. Instruct client in wheelchair pushups to relieve pressure while sitting

10. An OT is working with a client who is diagnosed with a complete C-7-8 spinal cord injury. Which of the following would be the least appropriate intervention for this client?
   A. Instruct client in light meal preparation
   B. Instruct client in functional mobility using a power wheelchair
   C. Instruct client in wheelchair push-ups to relieve pressure while sitting
   D. Instruct client in use of a padded bench/chair for bathing

Worksheet 5-6

Total Knee Replacement Interventions

Harvey is a 70-year-old male who underwent right total knee replacement (TKR) surgery 3 days ago and was subsequently admitted to a subacute rehabilitation facility yesterday. Harvey lives with his wife in a fourth-floor apartment, with elevator access, in a naturally occurring retirement community. Before admission, he worked part-time as a sales clerk in a home improvement store and was independent in all ADLs, including driving. Expected discharge to home is in 1 week. Here is some information taken from Harvey's occupational therapy evaluation report:

Weightbearing Status: PWB right lower extremity

ROM: BUE WFL, right knee extension lacks 10 degrees and flexion is limited to 75 degrees.

Strength: BUE WFL

Pain: Right knee pain reported as 4/10 at rest and 7/10 when standing

Functional mobility and transfers: Client needs minimal assistance sit ←→ stand and contact guard assistance to ambulate using a walker.

Activity Tolerance: Activity tolerance for standing is limited to approximately 5 minutes due to post-surgical knee pain and stiffness

ADL: Requires minimal assistance for lower-body bathing and moderate assistance to place underwear and pants over right foot and to don right sock and shoe.

Which of the following equipment, adaptive devices, or interventions are likely appropriate for an occupational therapy practitioner to use with Harvey at this time to address his deficits? Assume that interventions would include not only the provision of a particular piece of equipment or DME but actual instruction and practice in its use.

1. ___ Raised toilet seat
2. ___ Tub seat/bench
3. ___ Pillow under right knee when lying in bed
4. ___ Buttonhook
5. ___ Long handle shoehorn
6. ___ Commode
7. ___ Hot pack to right knee
8. ___ Elastic shoelaces
9. ___ Sock aid
10. ___ Reacher
11. ___ Beanbag toss activity while seated on mat
12. ___ Ambulation using parallel bars
13. ___ Squatting exercises to increase knee ROM
14. ___ Using ambulation device while obtaining items from refrigerator
15. ___ Standing to make a sandwich
16. ___ Power wheelchair mobility training
17. ___ Pegboard activity
18. ___ Cone stacking activity with wrist weights
19. ___ Standing at bathroom sink to shave with electric razor
20. ___ Ambulating up and down the hallway

Worksheet 5-7

Activities as Interventions—Using a Menu

Occupational therapy practitioners work with clients who have brain injuries, intellectual disabilities, mental health conditions, or problems with social interaction. It is beneficial to incorporate activities and occupations during therapy sessions as an effective means to increase the client's occupational performance. For this exercise, determine 10 ways in which a menu can be used in occupational therapy to improve specific mental functions, process skills, or social interaction skills needed for various occupations by role-playing (using a take-out menu or the menu on a restaurant website), going to the on-site cafeteria, or visiting another eating establishment in the community. List the occupation category, client factor/performance skill being addressed, along with the specific intervention task and methods of implementation. Two examples are provided.

Occupation	***Client Factor/Performance Skill to Be Addressed***	***Specific Intervention Activity***	***Method (e.g., role-play, menu choices, educate client)***
IADL—financial management	*Improve calculation skills*	*Select an appetizer, entrée, and dessert, which total less than $20 before tax and tip*	*Choose items from menu* *Teach math skills*
IADL—health management	*Demonstrate healthy food choices* *Improve problem solving*	*Choose an entrée and side dish that are not deep-fried*	*Choose items from menu* *Educate client regarding healthy versus unhealthy foods and emotional eating (e.g., comfort foods)*

Reprinted with permission from Morreale, M. J. (2015). *Developing clinical competence: A workbook for the OTA*. Thorofare, NJ: SLACK Incorporated.

Learning Activity 5-2: Activities as Interventions—Using a Newspaper

Occupational therapy practitioners work with clients who have brain injuries, intellectual disabilities, mental health conditions, or problems with social interaction. It is beneficial to incorporate activities and occupations during therapy sessions as an effective means to increase the client's occupational performance. For this exercise, determine 10 ways in which a newspaper can be used in occupational therapy to improve specific mental functions or process skills needed for various occupations. For each of your tasks, determine how it might change the task demands if you were to use a "real" newspaper vs a web-based newspaper. List the occupation category, client factor/performance skill being addressed, along with the specific intervention activity. Two examples are provided.

Occupation	***Client Factor/Performance Skill to Be Addressed***	***Specific Intervention Activity***	***A "Real" Newspaper vs a Web-Based Newspaper***
Leisure participation	*Improve scanning/visual field awareness*	*Scan page to find TV schedule for a specific time of day*	*A "real" newspaper opened up provides a much larger area for scanning*
IADL—community mobility	*Improve problem solving and topographical orientation*	*Read a restaurant review and then figure out directions to get there*	*A web-based newspaper may have a link for directions to the restaurant*

Reprinted with permission from Morreale, M. J. (2015). *Developing clinical competence: A workbook for the OTA*. Thorofare, NJ: SLACK Incorporated.

Learning Activity 5-3: Activities as Interventions—Using a Food Circular

Occupational therapy practitioners work with clients who have brain injuries, intellectual disabilities, mental health conditions, or problems with social interaction. It is beneficial to incorporate activities and occupations during therapy sessions as an effective means to increase the client's occupational performance. For this exercise, determine 10 ways in which a food sale circular can be used in occupational therapy to improve specific mental functions, process skills, or social interaction skills needed for occupational performance. List the occupation category, client factor/performance skill being addressed, along with the specific intervention activity. Two examples are provided.

Occupation	***Client Factor/Performance Skill to Be Addressed***	***Specific Intervention Activity***
IADL—shopping and financial management	*Improve categorization skills*	*Match a stack of coupons to items that are listed in the food circular*
IADL—shopping *Social participation*	*Improve assertiveness skills*	*Request a rain check for an advertised sale item that is not in stock*

Reprinted with permission from Morreale, M. J. (2015). *Developing clinical competence: A workbook for the OTA*. Thorofare, NJ: SLACK Incorporated.

Worksheet 5-8

Improving Basic and Instrumental Activities of Daily Living Occupations—More Practice

1. A client diagnosed with dysphagia has dietary restrictions that allow only pureed foods and liquids with a nectar consistency. The client also exhibits fair upper extremity muscle strength. Which of the following primary methods is appropriate for the OT to implement when teaching this client feeding skills?
   A. Position client sitting in a chair and provide a straw to sip plain apple juice
   B. Position client sitting in a chair and provide a large-handled spoon to eat cream of tomato soup
   C. Position client sitting in a chair and provide a built-up spoon to eat scrambled eggs
   D. Position client in a chair, instruct in chin tuck and provide a two-handled cup to drink plain milk

2. An OT is working in a rehabilitation hospital with a 72-year-old client who sustained a right CVA 2 weeks ago. The client is beginning to demonstrate some limited motor return for left scapula and glenohumeral motions, but exhibits subluxation at the glenohumeral joint. The client also requires moderate assistance to transfer to the bed, wheelchair, and toilet. Which of the following devices is most appropriate for the therapist to use at this time to address the client's upper extremity deficits?
   A. Airplane orthosis
   B. Arm trough
   C. Pulleys
   D. Therapy putty

3. An OT is working with a 52-year-old client who exhibits left upper and lower extremity hemiplegia. The client requires assistance for self-care tasks and is presently unable to perform functional ambulation independently. Which of the following devices is probably the least useful for the therapist to recommend at this time?
   A. Plate guard
   B. Handheld shower head
   C. Rolling walker
   D. Buttonhook

4. An OT is working with a client who has a diagnosis of right macular degeneration. To help compensate for deficits associated with this condition, the therapist should recommend which of the following devices?
   A. Hearing aid
   B. Magnifying glass
   C. Sock assist
   D. Forearm-based thumb spica orthosis

5. An OT is working with an older adult who lives alone. The client is diagnosed with a vestibular problem that is creating safety concerns. To help compensate for deficits associated with this condition, which of the following devices is most useful for the therapist to recommend?
   A. Use a tub seat when bathing
   B. Install a fire alarm that uses strobe lights
   C. Use rubber-soled backless slippers when performing functional ambulation at home
   D. Pull up from walker when transferring sit to stand

Worksheet 5-8 (continued)

Improving ADL and IADL Occupations—More Practice

6. An OT is working with an older adult who lives alone and is diagnosed with bilateral presbycusis. To help compensate for deficits associated with this condition, which of the following devices is most useful for the therapist to recommend?
   A. Reacher
   B. Elevated toilet seat
   C. Sock assist
   D. Telephone amplifier

7. An OT is working with a male client who has severe COPD and sustained a Colles fracture of his dominant right arm. The client's cast was removed last week, and he has difficulty grasping and manipulating objects. Which of the following interventions is most appropriate for the therapist to implement at this time to improve the client's hand function?
   A. Exercising with pulleys
   B. Fluidotherapy
   C. Buttoning a shirt
   D. Sanding and staining a wood birdhouse

8. An OT's primary role in hospice care is which of the following?
   A. Teach bed mobility and transfers
   B. Fabricate orthotic devices and teach proper positioning
   C. Design interventions to support occupational engagement
   D. Improve upper body strength

9. A 32-year-old client with a hand amputation has an upper limb prosthesis classified as a passive terminal device. During prosthetic training, which of the following is most appropriate for an OT to have the client do with the prosthetic hand?
   A. Perform sensory activities to help distinguish hot and cold water
   B. Perform sensory activities to help distinguish sharp from dull objects
   C. Attempt to use it as a gross assist
   D. Test the battery before attempting a functional task

10. A 45-year-old client with an upper extremity amputation is learning how to use his myoelectric prosthesis. During prosthetic training, which of the following is most appropriate for an OT to have the client do with the prosthetic hand?
   A. Attempt to pick up a foam cup
   B. Perform sensory activities to help distinguish hot and cold
   C. Practice isolated finger motion for buttoning a shirt
   D. Perform finger to palm translation using coins

Worksheet 5-9
Fracture Interventions

Abe, a 64-year-old male sustained a scaphoid fracture in his dominant right upper extremity secondary to a motor vehicle accident as a passenger. The cast was removed 2 days ago, and Abe was referred to outpatient occupational therapy. The prescription states: "OT for RUE P/AROM, PAMs PRN, and ADL/IADL retraining; 3 times weekly for 4 weeks." Here is some information taken from Abe's occupational therapy evaluation report:

Medical History: Parkinson's disease, DJD left hip, and history of kidney stones.

Prior level of function: Lives with wife in a garden apartment. Retired 4 years ago from his job teaching high school science. Client was independent in ADLs and IADLs except for driving, which he stopped 1 year ago due to Parkinson's effects.

Edema: None noted in RUE

Pain: Right wrist reported as 6/10

Sensation: Intact

UE ROM:

Bilateral resting tremors noted.

LUE: WNL.

RUE: Shoulder and elbow WNL

Forearm pronation 0/76, supination 0/54

Wrist flexion 0/42, extension 0/32, ulnar deviation 0/14, radial deviation 0/8

Client presents with moderate stiffness in right hand, inability to flex fingers to touch palm, opposition only to index finger.

Functional mobility and transfers: Client able to perform functional ambulation and transfers independently with slightly increased time. Reports pain in left hip when standing (5/10).

ADL/IADL: Since his injury, client reports difficulty performing activities requiring grip or fine motor skills, such as managing clothing fastenings, shaving, brushing teeth, eating, writing, performing home maintenance.

The intervention plan for Abe includes goals to increase right wrist and hand ROM/strength to enable modified independence in self-care ADLs. Which of the following equipment, adaptive devices, or adapted techniques may be appropriate for an occupational therapy practitioner to use with Abe during therapy during the first 2 weeks to address his primary deficits? Assume that interventions would include not only the provision of a particular piece of equipment or DME, but actual instruction and practice in its use.

1. ___ Built-up pen
2. ___ Pegboard
3. ___ Built-up utensils
4. ___ Arm pushups while sitting on mat
5. ___ Universal cuff
6. ___ Paraffin to right hand
7. ___ Sock aid
8. ___ Retrograde massage
9. ___ Vigorous stretching to wrist
10. ___ Elastic shoelaces
11. ___ MP extension resting hand orthosis
12. ___ Wash mitt
13. ___ Practice transfers using a raised toilet seat
14. ___ Sensory retraining
15. ___ Towel scrunching with fingers
16. ___ Shoes with Velcro closures
17. ___ Hot pack to wrist
18. ___ Hot pack to left hip
19. ___ Pulleys
20. ___ Walker

Worksheet 5-10

Chronic Obstructive Pulmonary Disease Interventions

Frank is a 72-year-old male residing with his wife, who has dementia, in an assisted living facility. He recently experienced an exacerbation of chronic obstructive pulmonary disease (COPD), was subsequently admitted to an acute care hospital for 3 days, and then was transferred to a rehabilitation hospital where he is currently. Frank worked as a painter, but had to retire at age 58 due to respiratory ailments. In addition to the medications needed to address his respiratory problems, Frank has been taking Coumadin (warfarin) since being diagnosed with atrial fibrillation 2 years ago. Before this recent hospitalization, Frank continued to drive a car, could manage self-care ADLs with increased time, and used a rollator walker when not in his room. At present, Frank is on portable oxygen. He needs minimal assistance to perform transfers, moderate assistance to complete lower body bathing and dressing, and cannot stand for more than 2 minutes without shortness of breath. Upper extremity ROM is within normal limits (WNL).

Which of the following equipment, adaptive devices, or interventions are likely appropriate for an occupational therapy practitioner to use with Frank at this time to improve performance skills and client factors needed to enable return to his residence? Assume that interventions would include not only the provision of a particular piece of equipment or DME, but actual instruction and practice in its use.

1. ___ Raised toilet seat
2. ___ One-arm drive wheelchair
3. ___ Instruction in joint protection
4. ___ Buttonhook
5. ___ Sanding and painting wood
6. ___ Commode
7. ___ Hot pack to shoulders
8. ___ Safety razor
9. ___ Exercise bands
10. ___ Reacher
11. ___ Ergonomics for yard work
12. ___ Standing while playing a game
13. ___ Energy conservation for doing laundry
14. ___ Using ambulation device while getting clothes from dresser
15. ___ Standing to cook at stove
16. ___ Pursed-lip breathing
17. ___ Long-handle shoehorn
18. ___ Sawing and staining wood to make a picture frame
19. ___ Teaching stair climbing
20. ___ Shampoo and soap dispenser in shower

Worksheet 5-11

Meal Preparation Adaptations

Carmen is a 65-year-old homemaker who sustained a left CVA 2 weeks ago. She lives with her husband in a private home and was fully independent in all ADLs before this illness. At present, Carmen's cognition appears to be intact, but she exhibits Broca aphasia and right hemiparesis. Her dominant right upper extremity is beginning to exhibit minimal motor return but is essentially nonfunctional except for some gross stabilization of objects. The client also demonstrates modified independence for functional ambulation using a hemi-walker. However, Carmen is unsafe when bending to reach for objects in lower kitchen cabinets. Her activity tolerance for standing is approximately 4 minutes. In each of the boxes in the following chart, list several suggestions indicating how the cooking tasks could be adapted to help enable safe and independent performance.

Adaptive Equipment and Compensatory Methods	***Scrambled Eggs***	***Bacon***	***Fresh Fruit Salad (apple, grapes, pear, strawberries)***	***Pancakes***
Required tools/equipment (list adaptive equipment or compensatory methods)	Example: *Use a nonstick pan for easier cleanup*			
Required supplies (food items)	Example: *Use a cooking spray to grease pan*			
Required actions and timing	Example: *Sit, rather than stand, at stove*			

Reprinted with permission from Morreale, M. J. (2015). *Developing clinical competence: A workbook for the OTA*. Thorofare, NJ: SLACK Incorporated.

Learning Activity 5-4: Prehension Patterns

Fill in the following table below with functional activities completed by both adults and children that involve use of the listed prehension patterns and are associated with the occupations delineated in the *Occupational Therapy Practice Framework* (AOTA, 2014).

	ADL	IADL	Work	Play	Leisure	Rest and Sleep	Education	Social Participation
Cylindrical Grasp: **(Adult)**	*Example: Holding onto a grab bar during a toilet transfer*	*Example: Opening the microwave door in order to heat a frozen dinner*	*Example: A carpenter using a hammer*	———	*Example: Shaking maracas to music*	*Example: Pulling on a pull cord to turn on the bedroom ceiling fan*	*Example: Holding a ruler*	*Example: Holding a racquet to play tennis with a partner*
Cylindrical Grasp **(Child)**	*Example: Holding a bottle to drink*	*Example: Mixing cookie batter with a wooden spoon*	———	*Example: Using a jump rope*	———	*Example: Grasping the arm of a stuffed animal*	*Example: Pulling on a rope to hoist the flag for the Pledge of Allegiance*	*Example: Playing tug of war*
Cylindrical Grasp **(Adult)**								
Cylindrical Grasp **(Child)**								
Spherical Grasp **(Adult)**								
Spherical Grasp **(Child)**								
Hook Grasp **(Adult)**								
Hook Grasp **(Child)**								

Learning Activity 5-4: Prehension Patterns (continued)

	ADL	IADL	Work	Play	Leisure	Rest and Sleep	Education	Social Participation
Disk Grasp (Adult)								
Disk Grasp (Child)								
3-Point Pinch (Adult)								
3-Point Pinch (Child)								
Lateral Pinch (Adult)								
Lateral Pinch (Child)								
Tip Pinch (Adult)								
Tip Pinch (Child)								

Learning Activity 5-5: Assistive Technology

Assistive technology encompasses a wide range of adaptations and modifications made to the environment that assist an individual in participating in desired activities and occupations. Assistive technology can be of a "no-tech" or "low-tech" nature, for which ordinary or simple, low-cost solutions are adequate; "moderate tech," for which inexpensive technological solutions are required; or "high tech," in which more expensive and sophisticated solutions are required to enable participation (Case-Smith & O'Brien, 2010; Schoonover, Levan, & Argabrite Grove, 2006).

The exercises that follow provide a simple case that highlights the need for an environmental adaptation for a client. Consider the use of a low-tech or no-tech, moderate-tech, and high-tech solution for the client described.

Example:

Gina is not able to turn on the lights in her home due to C6 quadriparesis.

A low-tech solution would be: *Replace standard light switches with decorator toggle plate switches.*

A moderate-tech solution would be: *Replace light switches with motion sensitive wall switches.*

A high-tech solution would be: *Obtain an environmental control unit to be accessed with Gina's wheelchair joystick control.*

1. Ralph has difficulty seeing the screen on his computer due to severe cataracts.
   - Low-tech or no-tech solution:
   - Moderate-tech solution:
   - High-tech solution:

2. Gerald is unable to drive due to right hemiparesis.
   - Low-tech or no-tech solution:
   - Moderate-tech solution:
   - High-tech solution:

3. Julia is not able to communicate with other children at school due to dysarthria resulting from athetoid cerebral palsy.
   - Low-tech or no-tech solution:
   - Moderate-tech solution:
   - High-tech solution:

4. Jamie is falling behind in class because he has difficulty keeping up with written class assignments due to proximal weakness.
   - Low-tech or no-tech solution:
   - Moderate-tech solution:
   - High-tech solution:

5. Felicia has bilateral below-knee amputations and needs a method of transferring from her wheelchair to her bathtub.
   - Low-tech or no-tech solution:
   - Moderate-tech solution:
   - High-tech solution:

Worksheet 5-12

Supported Employment

Joe is a 20-year-old man with Down syndrome. He attends a supported employment program with the goal for him to work in a grocery store packing groceries. Joe does not have any physical limitations that would hinder his job performance. However, he does exhibit difficulty with time management and transitioning between activities. Joe needs to learn how to perform his job functions correctly, including interacting appropriately with customers. Consider the activity demands for a grocery packing job. Use a professional format to list six goals for Joe that relate to his employment and encompass the following categories.

Example: Joe will be able to complete grocery packing for three customers without asking when he can take a break, within 2 months.

1. Time management

2. Activity transition

3. Social interaction

4. Packing groceries (specific aspect)

5. Packing groceries (specific aspect)

6. Packing groceries (specific aspect)

Reprinted with permission from Morreale, M. J. (2014). *Developing clinical competence: A workbook for the OTA*. Thorofare, NJ: SLACK Incorporated.

Worksheet 5-13

Additional Interventions: Advocacy, Self-Advocacy, Education, and Training

Indicate whether each of the following sentences highlights an example of advocacy, self-advocacy, education, or training.

A. Advocacy
B. Self-Advocacy
C. Education
D. Training

1. The practitioner contacts the insurance company to provide rationale for the purchase of a power wheelchair for her client. ____________________
2. The practitioner provides the client's family with information regarding why a power wheelchair is the best choice for him considering the progressive nature of his diagnosis. ____________________
3. The client requests contact information about the National Institute of Mental Health to learn about the programs it provides. ____________________
4. The practitioner sets up a wheelchair obstacle course for the client and works with him until he is able to maneuver safely and independently with a sip-and-puff switch. ____________________
5. The practitioner provides an in-service to the staff of the skilled nursing facility demonstrating the correct way to place a resting pan orthosis on the hand of a client with a flaccid hand. ______________________________
6. The practitioner presents a preconference institute at the annual AOTA conference covering the topic of electrical modality application. ____________________
7. The practitioner attends a "Take Back the Night" fundraising event with her client who is the victim of domestic violence. ____________________
8. As part of an intervention session, the practitioner assists the client with an Internet search of organizations that provide services for individuals who have sustained brain injury. ____________________
9. The rural-based practitioner votes for a congressional representative who supports telehealth initiatives. ____________________
10. The practitioner reviews the tools and techniques required to don socks using hip precautions. ____________________

Learning Activity 5-6: Community Mobility and Driving Rehabilitation

The freedom to move about within the community plays a significant role in our clients' abilities to participate in occupations of their choosing. When unable to freely and easily visit friends and relatives, go shopping, attend religious or cultural events, or simply have a change in scenery, one's independence and satisfaction with life can become significantly compromised. Driving and community mobility are listed as a component of the occupation of instrumental activities of daily living within the *Framework* (AOTA, 2014) and should be assessed and addressed as part of any occupational therapy evaluation. Both generalist and specialist practitioners have both an ethical and a professional obligation either to address deficits in community mobility (which may or may not include driving) or to refer to a practitioner who can (McGuire & Schold-Davis, 2012).

For each of the following areas of concern, consider the members of the population that comprise it and their needs. Identify one or more potential areas of concern and one or more occupational therapy strategies to address the concern(s).

Area of Concern	***Potential Concern***	***Occupational Therapy Strategy***
Teen driving	*Texting while driving without recognition of dangers posed*	*School-based group program geared to teens to address problem-solving skills, choice making, and identification of alternatives*
Developmental disabilities		
Early intervention (caregiver of a very young child)		
School system		
Sensory integration (individuals with sensory processing concerns)		
Physical disabilities		
Acute and subacute care		
Rehabilitation center and skilled nursing facilities		
Outpatient clinics		
Home- and community-based setting		

Learning Activity 5-6: Community Mobility and Driving Rehabilitation (continued)

Area of Concern	*Potential Concern*	*Occupational Therapy Strategy*
Low-vision population		
Mental health		
Older adults		
Cognitive decline		

Worksheet 5-14

Driving and Community Mobility

Indicate whether the following statements are true (T) or false (F).

1. ______ An occupational therapist can assist an older adult in making the decision to stop driving by conducting cognitive assessments to check attention, concentration, cognitive flexibility, and problem-solving skills.
2. ______ To address driving or other types of community mobility, an OT must be specialty certified.
3. ______ The Occupational Therapy Driver Off-Road Assessment is a battery of assessments that pinpoint areas to be addressed that relate to driving without going on the road.
4. ______ Your client reports that he has been driving since returning home after sustaining a CVA 4 weeks ago despite having no conversations with a health care provider about whether this is appropriate. As his occupational therapist, you should conduct a visual screening to determine whether he has sustained any loss of functional vision.
5. ______ An OT should tell hand therapy clients that they are not to drive under any circumstances unless they have a direct conversation with their physician.
6. ______ For many people, driving equates to being an independent adult. Having their license taken away can be devastating.
7. ______ When a family and physician believe that an older adult no longer has the cognitive status for safe driving, they must have the individual undergo a full driving evaluation to feel confident with their decision.
8. ______ Organizations such as the American Automobile Association (AAA), American Association of Retired Persons (AARP), the National Highway Traffic Safety Administration (NHTSA), and others have information and programs to assist older drivers.
9. ______ When an older adult has a driving license revoked, an OT should recommend that the individual take a cab to complete grocery shopping.
10. ______ OTs should be most concerned with the driving and community mobility status of adults and older adults because children have their parents to rely on.

Answers to Chapter 5 Worksheets

The worksheets in this chapter delineate only select interventions, which may not be appropriate for all clients with that condition. A client situation may also warrant other types of interventions or devices that are not included here.

Worksheet 5-1: Teaching-Learning Process (Total Hip Replacement)

Each intervention session will vary in terms of specific tasks performed and the order implemented depending on the client's medical status, level of function, doctor's orders, time frames, and client tolerance, among other factors, but here are some suggestions:

1. Where will the session take place? *Client's hospital room*
2. What is the anticipated length of session? *15 to 45 minutes as per client's tolerance*
3. What equipment/supplies will the OT need to bring to the session?
   - *Documentation materials (e.g., laptop/handheld device, paper, pen, documentation forms)*
   - *Adaptive equipment: sock aid, reacher, dressing stick, long shoehorn, elastic laces*
   - *Gloves/personal protective equipment for potential contact with blood or body fluids*
   - *Written client education materials*
   - *Ensure rolling walker is in room*
   - *Hospital scrubs for dressing practice if client does not have street clothes in room*
   - *As needed, stethoscope or other equipment to assess vital signs*
4. Besides gathering equipment and supplies, what are several things the OT should do before entering the client's room?
   1. *Review the occupational therapy evaluation report and intervention plan.*
   2. *Establish the therapist's schedule and coordinate time frames with the physical therapist (PT)/other disciplines as needed.*
   3. *Check client's chart for changes in medical status or new orders; review nursing and PT documentation and other sections as indicated.*
   4. *Obtain any further knowledge needed regarding this diagnosis or client's condition.*
   5. *Carefully consider any precautions/contraindications and safety concerns for this client and pertinent infection control issues.*
   5. *Double-check that this is the correct room and correct patient (e.g., check wrist band, verbally ask client).*
5. List the general steps of how the session should be implemented.
   1. *Perform hand hygiene and use personal protective equipment as indicated.*
   2. *Greet client and explain purpose of session (refer back to Chapter 1).*
   3. *Note any devices hooked up to client requiring caution during treatment, such as a catheter, monitor, or intravenous line.*
   4. *Take vital signs if part of protocol or as indicated during session.*
   5. *Review general total hip precautions and determine client understanding and carryover.*
   6. *Ensure bed brakes are locked and adjust bed rail as needed. Explain transfer procedure, then transfer client safely to a sitting position (edge of bed or into a chair depending on client's status and intervention plan) adhering to total hip precautions and using walker and safe client footwear if performing stand-pivot transfer.*
   7. *Explain/demonstrate use of adaptive devices for lower body dressing, one at a time.*
   8. *Following each explanation/demonstration, have client practice use of adaptive equipment to don lower body clothing/scrubs while adhering to precautions and providing assistance as needed. Incorporate use of walker and provide contact guard/physical assist when client stands to pull up clothing.*
   9. *Provide opportunities for problem solving and client feedback.*

10. *Determine whether client needs to practice using any of the devices a second time this session (or future sessions) or whether clothing needs to removed and hospital gown put back on.*
11. *Client may also don upper body clothing if indicated.*
12. *Transfer client back to bed or determine whether client should remain sitting in chair.*
13. *Make sure equipment is properly placed and client is comfortable, safe, and can reach call button.*
14. *Dispose of any personal protective equipment or used linens properly.*
15. *Wash hands.*
16. *Document according to facility time frame.*

Changes in the teaching-learning process for a 90-year-old client with early stage Alzheimer disease would depend on various factors, such as the client's prior level of function. Depending on the expected discharge plan, lower body dressing may or may not be a priority for this client (e.g., lived alone independently vs resided in a nursing home). If the client has age-related hearing loss or visual impairment, you might have to ensure that hearing aids are in place or large print educational materials are used. Processing may be slower, so the client may need greater task breakdown, additional opportunities to practice new skills, and memory aids. In addition, the client may require more rest breaks.

Worksheet 5-2: Intervention Categories

Suggested resource: AOTA, 2014.

1. __F__ Creating a wrist immobilization orthosis for a client 6 weeks post wrist fracture is a preparatory task. *Orthotic fabrication is a preparatory method.*
2. __F__ The application of therapeutic ultrasound is considered an activity. *(Ultrasound is a physical agent modality and is an intervention done "to" a client vs an activity completed "by" the client. Therefore, it is a preparatory method.)*
3. __F__ Completing upper extremity weight bearing by having the client lean on a table within the therapy gym where other clients and practitioners are working is a group intervention. *(A group intervention involves the practitioner working directly with two or more clients at the same time and completing the same activity.)*
4. __T__ Picking up beanbags with a reacher and placing them into a bucket is a preparatory task.
5. __F__ Making dinner after a trip to the grocery store to purchase ingredients is an activity. *(This is an example of the IADL of meal preparation, which is an occupation.)*
6. __T__ Brushing teeth in the middle of the afternoon is an activity.
7. __T__ Getting up in the morning and going to work is an occupation.
8. __T__ Completing a wheelchair fitting with a client is a preparatory method.
9. __T__ Running a lunch-hour eating activity with three clients is a group intervention.
10. __T__ Instructing a client in how to button with a buttonhook is considered training.

For those interventions that were answered *false*, indicate the category of intervention that would make the statement *true*.

Statement number	Correct category of intervention
1	Preparatory method
2	Preparatory method
3	One-on-one preparatory method intervention
5	Occupation

Worksheet 5-3: Cerebrovascular Accident Interventions

Suggested resources: Gillen, 2011; Logigian, 2015; Morawski & Padilla, 2012.

1. _*_ Rocker knife
2. _*_ Nonslip matting
3. ___ Built-up utensils *(Client is unable to use flaccid right hand and should not need built up utensils for his unaffected left hand.)*
4. _*_ Plate guard
5. ___ Walker *(This requires two hands, and client cannot grip walker with a flaccid hand. PT to determine when a hemi-walker is appropriate for client to use.)*
6. ___ Power wheelchair (*Client should be able to operate a manual wheelchair using his left arm and leg or a one-arm drive wheelchair.)*
7. _*_Electric razor
8. ___ Sock aid (*Client cannot use right hand, so it would be difficult to use this device one-handedly. It would probably be better to teach one-handed compensatory techniques.)*
9. ___ Therapy putty (*Cannot use with flaccid right hand.)*
10. ___ Exercise bands (*Cannot use with flaccid right upper extremity.)*
11. ___ Pulleys (*Using pulleys for passive ROM [PROM] to a flaccid upper extremity may overstretch joints/cause harm to the shoulder.)*
12. ___ Vest restraint (*A vest restraint is not appropriate. If Marvin is demonstrating poor posture in chair, then other, less restrictive alternatives should be tried, such as client education, verbal reminders, lateral cushions/supports, or a seatbelt that client can manage.)*
13. _*_ Wheelchair arm support
14. _*_ Soap-on-a-rope
15. _*_Wash mitt
16. _*_ Soap/shampoo dispenser
17. _*_ Long-handle sponge
18. _*_ Tub seat/bench
19. ___ Hot pack to right shoulder *(Not indicated for a flaccid extremity with no pain or PROM deficits. Also, cardiovascular status may not be stable.)*
20. ___ Paraffin to right hand *(Not indicated for a flaccid extremity with no pain or PROM deficits. Also, cardiovascular status may not be stable.)*
21. ___ CIMT (*Client does not have the requisite motor skills in his involved arm for this intervention as the arm is flaccid. Constraining the strong arm would not allow the client to perform any functional tasks at this time.)*
22. _*_ Teach self-ROM
23. ___ Lapboard *(This could be considered a restraint if the client is not able to remove it himself. Other alternatives should be tried first, such as a side arm support.)*
24. ___ Large pegboard *(Client's involved arm is flaccid, and this task would not be useful for the uninvolved arm. If the client had perceptual deficits, it could be used with the unaffected arm to work on specific perceptual skills, although a functional task would be more appropriate.)*
25. ___ Nine-hole peg test *(Client does not have any motor function in his involved dominant right upper extremity, so this test would not be a useful measure at this time.)*

Worksheet 5-4: Total Hip Replacement Interventions

Suggested resources: Coppard, Higgins, Harvey, & Padilla, 2012; Maher & Bear-Lehman, 2008; Gower & Bowker, 2015.

1. __*__ Raised toilet seat
2. ____ Adduction cushion *(Client needs an abduction cushion.)*
3. ____ Built-up utensils
4. __*__ Commode
5. ____ Crossing legs to tie shoes *(Unable to adduct hip due to surgical precautions.)*
6. __*__ Walker (*Generally the PT would determine whether this device is appropriate for gait training at this time. However, occupational therapy can support functional mobility and safety for occupational performance.*)
7. ____ Power wheelchair (*A manual wheelchair is typically more appropriate after hip replacement surgery.*)
8. __*__ Long-handle shoehorn
9. __*__ Sock aid
10. ____ Hot pack to left hip *(A hot pack is not indicated for acute postsurgical conditions, but a cold pack might be appropriate for pain and swelling. State regulation and facility policy delineate which disciplines may apply particular physical agents.)*
11. ____ Paraffin to left hand (*Not indicated for client's condition because no ROM deficits are noted.*)
12. ____ Teach stair climbing with crutches (*Teaching stair climbing is typically the role of the PT, although occupational therapy can support function. Crutches are not an appropriate mobility device for this client because of her age and functional level.*)
13. ____ Wheelchair arm support *(Client does not have unilateral neglect or ROM deficits.)*
14. __*__ Exercise bands *(Increasing upper body strength may be beneficial for walker use.)*
15. ____ Quad cane (*Cannot use with non-weight-bearing status.*)
16. __*__ Elastic shoelaces
17. ____ Wedge cushion for wheelchair (*This would provide excessive hip flexion. However, an elevated seat cushion would be appropriate.*)
18. __*__ Reacher
19. __*__ Long-handle sponge
20. __*__ Tub seat/bench
21. __*__ Leg lifter *(Useful to help lift involved lower limb when transferring to a tub bench or bed.)*
22. ____ CIMT *(This technique is useful for clients with neurological conditions [e.g., stroke] to improve upper limb function [Gillen, 2011]. Client does not have neurological impairment and has good voluntary motion in both upper extremities.)*
23. ____ Sliding board *(Instruction in stand-pivot transfers is a more appropriate method for this client and condition.)*
24. ____ Buttonhook *(Client has full AROM in both upper extremities and no coordination deficits are noted.)*
25. ____ Hospital bed for home *(Client has potential for good bed mobility and does not have another condition that would warrant use of a hospital bed, such as respiratory problems.)*

Worksheet 5-5: Improving Basic and Instrumental Activities of Daily Living Occupations

1. A. Minor & Minor (2010)
2. B. The client should be able to transfer independently onto the commode using a sliding board. A raised toilet seat is not useful because the client cannot enter the bathroom. Using a platform walker is not feasible. A power mobility scooter may not fit through the door or most likely will not be able to get close enough to the toilet for a sliding board transfer.
3. C. The client's knees should be apart to provide a wider base of support. A transfer belt could be placed around the client's waist, but not the therapist's. A walker is unstable as a device from which to push up, so this would be unsafe. The client needs to lean forward ("nose over toes") to facilitate rising from chair.
4. C. An electric razor is safer than a safety razor, which has sharp blades. Because the client has unilateral neglect and impulsivity, he needs to focus all his attention on the task at hand to best perform shaving. Standing would be more distracting in this case because the client would have to work to maintain his balance. However, realize there are instances when an occupational therapy practitioner would work on balance (or other client factors) and ADL performance simultaneously depending on the desired outcome for that session.
5. B. Clients should be as upright as possible when feeding. Neck hyperextension would hinder swallowing and could be unsafe (Winston & Loukas, 2014). Specialized swallowing techniques or alternate neck positions may be needed for some clients. If weakness is only evident in the hand intrinsic muscles, the client should be able to manage self-feeding with a universal cuff or adapted utensils.
6. A. The best strategy would be to teach an easier method, which, in this case, is over-the-head. While demonstration and written instructions could help, they are not the best option. A larger coat would still require the same sequence of motor planning.
7. D. Using a flat sheet as a bottom sheet entails less effort than using a fitted sheet. Although a tub seat is useful, it is not related to homemaking. It is contraindicated to use open flames (barbeque grill) around oxygen. The client should inhale before exertion and exhale during the exertion.
8. D. Driving is not feasible at this level, whereas the other interventions are appropriate (Fike, Pendleton, & Hewitt, 2015; Spinal Cord Injury Information Pages, 2013).
9. D. The triceps are not innervated at this level, but the client may be able to shift sideways to relieve pressure. Using a buttonhook and razor are feasible, but may require setup and use of a holder or a tenodesis grasp wrist-driven hinge orthosis (Fike et al., 2015; Spinal Cord Injury Information Pages, 2013).
10. B. The client is able to use a manual wheelchair at this level. The client should be able to perform many functional tasks, such as light meal preparation and bathing. Because the triceps are innervated at this level, the client should be instructed in wheelchair pushups to help relieve pressure while sitting (Fike et al., 2015; Spinal Cord Injury Information Pages, 2013).

Worksheet 5-6: Total Knee Replacement Interventions

Suggested resources: Coppard et al., 2012.

1. _*_ Raised toilet seat *(Could be useful.)*
2. _*_ Tub seat/bench
3. ___ Pillow under right knee when lying in bed *(A pillow under affected knee can contribute to a knee flexion contracture, which is undesirable.)*
4. ___ Buttonhook *(There are no upper extremity deficits noted.)*
5. _*_ Long-handle shoehorn
6. _*_ Commode
7. ___ Hot pack to right knee *(A hot pack is not indicated for acute postsurgical conditions but a cold pack might be appropriate for pain and swelling. State regulation and facility policy delineate which disciplines may apply particular physical agents.)*

8. _*_ Elastic shoelaces
9. _*_ Sock aid (*May not need, however.*)
10. _*_ Reacher
11. ___ Beanbag toss activity while seated on mat (*Sitting balance is not a problem.*)
12. ___ Ambulation using parallel bars (*This is typically a physical therapy intervention.*)
13. ___ Squatting exercises to increase knee ROM (*This is typically a physical therapy intervention, and knee may be unstable postoperatively.*)
14. _*_Using ambulation device while obtaining items from refrigerator (*Realize that, although activity tolerance for standing is an important goal for this client and condition, this activity may increase pain. The occupational therapy practitioner must decide whether the client would benefit more from a compensatory method, such as using a wheelchair or whether the client needs to work through the pain, depending on physician orders and the client's particular situation.*)
15. _*_ Standing to make a sandwich (*Realize that, although activity tolerance for standing is an important goal for this client and condition, this activity may increase pain. The occupational therapy practitioner must decide whether the client would benefit more from a compensatory method such as sitting on a chair at the kitchen counter or whether the client needs to work through the pain, depending on physician orders and the client's particular situation.*)
16. ___ Power wheelchair mobility training (*Power wheelchair is not needed.*)
17. ___ Pegboard activity (*No fine motor deficits indicated.*)
18. ___ Cone stacking activity with wrist weights (*Could possibly be used to increase endurance, but strength is already within functional limits, and client has other ADL priorities. Can use while standing to work on improving standing tolerance.*)
19. _*_ Standing at bathroom sink to shave with electric razor (*Realize that, although activity tolerance for standing is an important goal for this client and condition, this activity may increase pain. The occupational therapy practitioner must decide whether the client would benefit more from a compensatory method, such as sitting in a chair at the sink, or whether client needs to work through the pain, depending on physician orders and the client's particular situation.*)
20. ___ Ambulating up and down the hallway (*Ambulation training is typically a physical therapy intervention, although occupational therapy can support functional mobility for such occupations as safe navigation in the kitchen during meal preparation tasks.*)

Worksheet 5-7: Activities as Interventions—Using a Menu

Here are some suggestions, although you may come up with others. The methods listed here include the activity of role playing, but an occupational therapy practitioner should create opportunities to have clients perform real occupations, such as actually going to a restaurant.

Occupation	*Client Factor/Performance Skill to Be Addressed*	*Specific Intervention Activity*	*Method (e.g., role-play, menu choices, educate client)*
IADL—financial management	Improve calculation skills	Select an appetizer, entrée, and dessert, which total less than $20 before tax and tip	Choose items from menu Teach math skills
IADL—health management	Demonstrate healthy food choices Improve problem solving Improve coping skills	Choose an entrée and side dish that are not deep-fried	Choose items from menu Educate client regarding healthy vs unhealthy foods and emotional eating (e.g., comfort foods)
IADL—health management	Demonstrate healthy drinking choices Improve coping skills	Choose a beverage that does not contain alcohol or choose a beverage that will or will not add calories, depending on the client's dietary needs	Choose items from menu Educate client regarding healthy vs unhealthy beverage choices and emotional eating Role-play and suggest coping strategies
IADL—health management	Improve problem solving Improve safety awareness	Determine which items may contain allergens, such as nuts, dairy products, or gluten	Choose items from menu Educate client regarding hidden ingredients
Leisure participation Social participation	Improve decision-making skills	Within a 5-minute period, choose a beverage, entrée, and dessert without changing mind or choose a restaurant for the group to go to	Role-play and provide feedback
Leisure participation Social participation	Improve assertiveness skills	Ask the server for something not already on the table, such as a glass of water, extra napkins, or a condiment	Role-play and provide feedback
IADL—health management	Demonstrate healthy eating habits Improve assertiveness skills	Ask server how an item is prepared or ask for item to be specially prepared without butter, salt, or other ingredient	Role-play and provide feedback
ADL—feeding Social participation	Improve problem solving	Choose items that one can manage to eat without need for help or setup	Choose items from menu (e.g., finger foods or fish fillet that does not need to be cut) Educate regarding compensatory strategies
IADL—health management	Demonstrate healthy eating habits	Choose an appetizer, entrée, and beverage that total less or more than a specified amount of calories or sodium	Choose items from menu Educate client regarding healthy versus unhealthy foods and emotional response to food

Occupation	Client Factor/Performance Skill to Be Addressed	Specific Intervention Activity	Method (e.g., role-play, menu choices, educate client)
IADL—financial management	Improve calculation skills	Calculate tax and tip on specified items	Choose items from menu Teach math skills
IADL—financial management	Improve calculation skills	Determine change back from a $50 bill after selecting several items	Choose items from menu Teach math skills
IADL—financial management	Improve money management	Pay using exact change or perform credit card transaction properly	Role-play
Social participation	Improve interpersonal skills	Choose an appetizer or dessert that can be shared with the group	Choose items from menu Role-play and provide feedback

Worksheet 5-8: Improving Basic and Instrumental Activities of Daily Living Occupations—More Practice

1. B. Plain apple juice and milk are thin liquids that the client is not allowed to have. If thickeners were added to create a nectar consistency, they might be acceptable. Scrambled eggs are soft, but semisolid, and not considered to be pureed. It is essential to know what is acceptable or not acceptable for each client to eat. Clients may have dairy restrictions, food allergies, cultural considerations, or require special diets due to other medical concerns (e.g., a low-sodium or low-sugar diet).
2. B. Because the client must use a wheelchair, an arm trough may be helpful to support and protect the involved arm. An airplane orthosis is a shoulder immobilization orthotic device, which is not indicated for this condition. Pulleys may cause further damage to the shoulder if the arm is overstretched and the client also does not have the requisite grasp to manage this device or to use therapy putty with the left hand.
3. C. The client does not have the requisite function of the involved arm to hold onto a rolling walker. The other devices may be used to teach the client compensatory techniques for ADLs.
4. B. Macular degeneration is an eye disease. Only one of the choices relates to vision.
5. A. Vestibular problems may create vertigo or problems with balance. It is probably best that the client be seated while bathing. When going from sit to stand, the client should push up from the seated surface rather than pull up from a walker, which would be unsafe. Slippers without a back do not provide proper stability and may cause the foot to slide, possibly contributing to a fall. Although the client should have a fire alarm in the home, strobe lights are not needed.
6. D. Presbycusis is an age-related hearing loss. The only choice that relates to hearing is a telephone amplifier.
7. C. Due to the client's diagnosis of COPD, the OT should avoid activities that may create dust (such as Fluidotherapy and sanding) or fumes (staining wood). Although the use of pulleys may involve grasp, this device is not the best choice to facilitate hand function. A functional fine motor task, such as buttoning a shirt, is a better choice.
8. C. Although A, B, and D are possible interventions that an occupational therapy practitioner might provide to clients receiving hospice care, these interventions are not needed for every client. An occupational therapy practitioner considers each client individually to determine appropriate interventions to help support the client's desired or needed occupational roles and quality of life (AOTA, 2011).
9. C. An upper limb prosthesis classified as a passive terminal device does not have a battery. It is primarily used for cosmesis, but can possibly be used as a gross assist (Papdapoulos & Deverix, 2013; Vacek, 2015).
10. A. A myoelectric prosthesis can perform grasp, but does not have sensory function, isolated motion of digits, or the ability to perform in-hand manipulation. Training includes working on the ability to pick up various kinds of objects without damaging the objects (Papdapoulos & Deverix, 2013; Vacek, 2015).

Worksheet 5-9: Fracture Interventions

Suggested resources: Coppard et al., 2012; Skirven, Osterman, Fedorczyk, & Amadio, 2011.

1. _*_ Built-up pen
2. _*_ Pegboard *(However, it is better to perform functional activities, such as buttoning a shirt.)*
3. _*_ Built-up utensils
4. ___ Arm pushups while sitting on mat *(Contraindicated at this time. May cause excessive pressure on healing fracture.)*
5. _*_ Universal cuff
6. ___ Paraffin to right hand *(Tremors would create a safety concern for splashing paraffin or touching sides of unit.)*
7. ___ Sock aid *(Client does not have the necessary motor function in hand, and tremors also create more difficulty.)*
8. ___ Retrograde massage *(No edema present.)*
9. ___ Vigorous stretching to wrist *(Fracture may not yet be stable enough for vigorous stretching.)*
10. _*_ Elastic shoelaces
11. ___ MP extension resting hand orthosis *(Except for certain protocols [e.g., extensor tendon repair, MP joint replacement surgery], the hand generally should not be immobilized in MP extension because this is not a functional position.)*
12. _*_ Wash mitt
13. ___ Practice transfers using a raised toilet seat *(Client is already independent in transfers, although the OT may recommend this for the future.)*
14. ___ Sensory retraining *(Sensation is intact.)*
15. _*_ Towel scrunching with fingers
16. _*_ Shoes with Velcro closures
17. _*_ Hot pack to wrist
18. ___ Hot pack to left hip *(Client was referred for an upper extremity diagnosis. A referral to physical therapy may be warranted to address the client's hip pain.)*
19. ___ Pulleys *(Client's limited grip creates difficulty for holding the handle. Also, pulleys do not really address client's ROM deficits in hand and wrist.)*
20. ___ Walker *(Client is independent in ambulation. However, a referral to physical therapy may be warranted to determine whether an ambulation device is appropriate for this client to minimize hip pain.)*

Worksheet 5-10: Chronic Obstructive Pulmonary Disease Interventions

Resources: Peralta, Powell, & Plutschack, 2012.

1. _*_ Raised toilet seat
2. ___ One-arm drive wheelchair *(Client has use of both arms and legs and does not require use of this particular type of wheelchair.)*
3. ___ Instruction in joint protection *(Client does not have joint problems. Instruction on energy conservation would be more useful.)*
4. ___ Buttonhook *(No fine motor deficits noted.)*
5. ___ Sanding and painting wood *(Creates dust and fumes.)*
6. _*_ Commode
7. ___ Hot pack to shoulders *(No shoulder problems are noted, and heat is contraindicated for severe cardiopulmonary conditions.)*
8. ___ Safety razor *(Client is on blood thinners and should use an electric razor.)*
9. _*_ Exercise bands *(May be useful to increase strength and endurance.)*

10. _*_ Reacher
11. ___ Ergonomics for yard work *(Resides in assisted living facility.)*
12. _*_ Standing while playing a game *(Depending on the client's particular medical status and intervention plan, graded standing tasks may be useful to increase endurance.)*
13. ___ Energy conservation for doing laundry *(Resides in assisted living facility, so staff may do laundry.)*
14. _*_ Using ambulation device while getting clothes from dresser *(Graded functional mobility tasks may be useful to increase endurance. However, a compensatory method, such as performing task while seated in wheelchair, may be needed to enable independent performance of this occupation.)*
15. ___ Standing to cook at stove *(To increase endurance, this could be used as a purposeful activity, but meals are typically provided at an assisted living facility. Depending on the facility, client may be allowed to use a microwave or coffeemaker. However, a compensatory method, such as performing task while seated in wheelchair, may be needed to enable independent performance of this occupation.)*
16. _*_ Pursed-lip breathing
17. _*_ Long-handle shoehorn
18. ___ Sawing and staining wood to make a picture frame (*Creates dust and fumes, and client is also on blood thinners, making the saw unsafe.)*
19. ___ Teaching stair climbing *(This is typically the role of physical therapy.)*
20. _*_ Shampoo and soap dispenser in shower *(Eliminates reaching for bottles or lifting them.)*

Worksheet 5-11: Meal Preparation Adaptations

Here are some suggestions for adaptive equipment and compensatory techniques for this client, although you may come up with others. Realize that the dominant hand is unable to perform grasp. Built-up handled objects would not be needed for the nondominant hand.

Adaptive Equipment and Compensatory Methods	*Scrambled Eggs*	*Bacon*	*Fresh Fruit Salad (apple, grapes, pear, strawberries)*	*Pancakes*
Required tools/ equipment (list adaptive equipment or compensatory methods)	• Nonstick pan for easier cleanup • Can use a microwave instead of stove • Nonslip matting to secure bowl • Use a bowl with a handle to pour	• Can use a microwave instead of stove • Nonstick pan for easier clean up	• Adapted cutting board with nails • Nonslip matting • Apple-peeling device • Can use an egg slicer to slice berries	• Depending on method (e.g., frozen pancakes or using a mix) can use a toaster, toaster oven, microwave, electric griddle, or top of stove • If making batter, use nonslip matting to secure bowl • If making batter, use a bowl with a handle to pour or use a batter dispenser • Nonstick pan for easier cleanup

Adaptive Equipment and Compensatory Methods	***Scrambled Eggs***	***Bacon***	***Fresh Fruit Salad (apple, grapes, pear, strawberries)***	***Pancakes***
Required supplies (food items)	• Cooking spray to grease pan • Liquid eggs in a carton • Frozen prepared eggs	• Precooked store-bought bacon in dairy section • Store-bought bacon bits	• Precut bags of fruit in frozen food or refrigerated section of supermarket • Canned fruit • Precut fresh fruit from a grocery store/salad bar	• Pancakes from a recipe vs a boxed mix; consider number of ingredients needed, such as only water vs needing water, oil, and egg • Premade store-bought batter from a carton • Frozen pancakes • Cooking spray to grease pan
Required actions and timing	• Sit, rather than stand, at stove • Teach one-handed technique to break eggs • Can use a carton holder with handle when pouring liquid eggs from a carton • Keep items in higher shelves of refrigerator and accessible upper cabinets • Rolling cart to move and carry items • Apron with pockets to move and carry small objects	• Use scissors to open package • Sit, rather than stand, to prepare • Keep items in higher shelves of refrigerator and accessible upper cabinets • Rolling cart to move and carry items • Apron with pockets to move and carry small objects	• Can use a suction brush attached to sink to wash fruits • Sit, rather than stand, to prepare • Keep items in higher shelves of refrigerator and accessible upper cabinets • Rolling cart to move and carry items • Apron with pockets to move and carry small objects	• If eggs are needed, teach one-handed technique to break eggs • Sit, rather than stand, to prepare • Keep items in higher shelves of refrigerator and accessible upper cabinets • Rolling cart to move and carry items • Can prepare batter ahead of time • Teach compensatory method to open box of pancake mix • Apron with pockets to move and carry small objects • Can use a carton holder with handle when pouring milk or batter from a carton

Worksheet 5-12: Supported Employment

Resources for goal writing: Gateley & Borcherding, 2012; Morreale & Borcherding, 2013.

Goals need to specify a time frame, measurable criteria, and delineate a desired client behavior relating to function. Goals should reflect what the client needs to achieve, not what the occupational therapy practitioner will do as interventions. Here are some suggested goals for this client. Realize that different settings or practice areas may use slightly different formats or terminology as shown in the various examples that follow. Of course, the actual goals and time frames may be different for a real client.

1. Time management
   - *By the end of 1 month, Joe will demonstrate ability to pack 10 items in a grocery bag within a 2-minute period.*
   - *Joe will adhere to the allotted time for breaks with one verbal cue to set and use a timer within 2 weeks.*

2. Activity transition
    - *After placing a grocery bag in customer's cart, Joe will continue packing remaining groceries without redirection to task within 4 weeks.*
    - *At the end of his allotted break time, client will punch his time card with two verbal cues within 10 days.*
3. Social interaction
    - *With one verbal cue, client will ask customers if they prefer paper or plastic bags, five out of five opportunities, within 2 weeks.*
    - *Joe will greet customers with a smile and say "hello," four of five opportunities, by the end of the month.*
4. Packing groceries
    - *Within 6 weeks, Joe will demonstrate ability to pack cold items together with minimal verbal cues.*
5. Packing groceries
    - *Client will demonstrate ability to place cans/heavier items on bottom of grocery bag with stand-by-assist within 4 weeks.*
6. Packing groceries
    - *Joe will place appropriate number of items to fill bag without risk of bag breaking when carried by handles within 3 months.*

Worksheet 5-13: Additional Interventions: Advocacy, Self-Advocacy, Education, and Training

Suggested resource: AOTA, 2014.

A. Advocacy
B. Self-Advocacy
C. Education
D. Training

1. The practitioner contacts the insurance company to provide rationale for the purchase of a power wheelchair for her client. ___A__
2. The practitioner provides the client's family with information regarding why a power wheelchair is the best choice for him considering the progressive nature of his diagnosis.___C___
3. The client requests contact information about the National Institute of Mental Health to learn more about the programs it provides. ___B___
4. The practitioner sets up a wheelchair obstacle course for the client and works with him until he is able to maneuver safely and independently with a sip-and-puff switch. ___D___
5. The practitioner provides an in-service to the staff of the skilled nursing facility demonstrating the correct way to place a resting pan orthosis on the hand of a client with a flaccid hand. ___D___
6. The practitioner presents a preconference institute at the annual AOTA conference covering the topic of electrical modality application. ___D___
7. The practitioner attends a "Take Back the Night" fundraising event with her client who is the victim of domestic violence. ___A___
8. As part of an intervention session, the practitioner assists the client with an Internet search of organizations that provide services for individuals who have sustained brain injury. ___B___
9. The rural-based practitioner votes for a congressional representative who supports telehealth initiatives. __A__
10. The practitioner reviews the tools and techniques required to don socks using hip precautions. ___D___

Worksheet 5-14: Driving and Community Mobility

Resource: McGuire & Schold-Davis, 2012.

1. T
2. F

Driving and community mobility are areas of IADLs and must be addressed by all OTs. If an OT does not feel competent with complex area of driving modification or teaching community mobility (as in the case of a blind individual), he or she should refer to a specialty practitioner.

3. T
4. T
5. F

An OT should ask a client about his or her ability to drive during an occupational therapy evaluation in a hand therapy setting, but should not assume that clients are unable to drive or require physician approval.

6. T
7. F

Long and costly driving evaluations are not required to identify cognitive or physical deficits that make driving dangerous. A generalist OT can conduct appropriate assessments of various client factors to help a family make an informed decision.

8. T
9. F

Although taking a cab may be a means to maintain independence for some, it may not work for all clients. An assessment of skills and abilities that takes the needs and desires of each client into consideration is the first step in helping that person to maintain or regain appropriate levels of independence.

10. F

Driving and community mobility are important areas of occupation for adolescents as well as adults. Individuals who care for persons with disabilities are also important to assist so that they can safely and effectively transport those they care for.

Chapter 5 References

American Occupational Therapy Association. (2011). The role of occupational therapy in end-of-life care. *American Journal of Occupational Therapy, 65*(Suppl. 6), S66–S75.

American Occupational Therapy Association. (2014). Occupational therapy practice framework: Domain and process (3rd ed.). *American Journal of Occupational Therapy, 68*(Suppl. 1), S1–S48.

Case-Smith, J., & O'Brien, J. (2010). *Occupational therapy for children* (6th ed.). Maryland Heights, MO: Mosby.

Coppard, B. M., Higgins, T., Harvey, K. D., & Padilla, R. (2012). Working with elders who have orthopedic conditions. In R. L. Padilla, S. Byers-Connon, & H. L. Lohman (Eds.), *Occupational therapy with elders: Strategies for the COTA* (3rd ed., pp. 299–311). Maryland Heights, MO: Elsevier Mosby.

Fike, M. L., Pendleton, K., & Hewitt, L. (2015). A telephone repairman with spinal cord injury. In K. Sladyk & S. E. Ryan (Eds.), *Ryan's occupational therapy assistant: Principles, practice issues, and techniques* (5th ed., pp. 268–288). Thorofare, NJ: SLACK Incorporated.

Gateley, C. A., & Borcherding, S. (2012). *Documentation manual for occupational therapy: Writing SOAP notes* (3rd ed.). Thorofare, NJ: SLACK Incorporated.

Gillen, G. (Ed.). (2011). *Stroke rehabilitation: A function-based approach* (3rd ed.). St. Louis: Elsevier Mosby.

Gower, D., & Bowker, M. (2015). A plumber and golfer with total hip arthroplasty. In K. Sladyk & S. E. Ryan (Eds.), *Ryan's occupational therapy assistant: Principles, practice issues, and techniques* (5th ed., pp. 346–357). Thorofare, NJ: SLACK Incorporated.

Logigian, M. (2015). A businessman with a stroke. In K. Sladyk & R. Ryan (Eds.), *Ryan's occupational therapy assistant: Principles, Practice Issues, and Techniques* (5th ed.) (pp. 374-389). Thorofare, NJ: SLACK Incorporated.

Maher, C., & Bear-Lehman, J. (2008). Orthopaedic conditions. In M. V. Radomski & C. A. T. Latham (Eds.), *Occupational therapy for physical dysfunction* (6th ed., pp. 1106–1130). Baltimore: Lippincott, Williams & Wilkins.

McGuire, M. J., & Schold-Davis, E. (2012). *Driving and community mobility.* Bethesda, MD: AOTA Press.

Minor, M. A., & Minor, S. D. (2010). *Patient care skills* (6th ed.). Upper Saddle River, NJ: Pearson Education.

Morawski, D. L., & Padilla, R. (2012) Working with elders who have had cerebrovascular accidents. In R. L. Padilla, S. Byers-Connon, & H. L. Lohman (Eds.), *Occupational therapy with elders: Strategies for the COTA* (3rd ed., pp. 263–274). Maryland Heights, MO: Elsevier Mosby.

Morreale, M. J. (2015). *Developing clinical competence: A workbook for the OTA.* Thorofare, NJ: SLACK Incorporated.

Morreale, M. J., & Borcherding, S. (2013). *The OTA's guide to documentation: Writing SOAP notes* (3rd ed.). Thorofare, NJ: SLACK Incorporated.

Papdapoulos, E., & Deverix, B. (2013). Amputation and prosthetics. In M. B. Early (Ed.), *Physical dysfunction practice skills for the occupational therapy assistant* (3rd ed., pp. 654–675). St. Louis: Mosby.

Peralta, A. M., Powell, S., & Plutschack, D. (2012). Working with elders who have pulmonary conditions. In R. L. Padilla, S. Byers-Connon, & H. L. Lohman (Eds.), *Occupational therapy with elders: Strategies for the COTA* (3rd ed., pp. 323–328). Maryland Heights, MO: Elsevier Mosby.

Schoonover, J., Levan, P., & Argabrite Grove, R. (2006). Occupational therapy and assistive technology in school-based practice: Supporting participation. *OT Practice, 11*(1), CE1–CE8.

Skirven, T., Osterman, A. L., Fedorczyk, J., & Amadio, P. C. (Eds.) (2011). *Rehabilitation of the hand and upper extremity* (6th ed.). Philadelphia: Elsevier.

Spinal Cord Injury Information Pages. (2013). *Spinal cord injury functional goals.* Retrieved from http://www.sci-info-pages.com/function.html

Vacek, K. M. (2015). Upper extremity prosthetics. In B. M. Coppard & H. Lohman (Eds.), *Introduction to orthotics: A clinical reasoning & problem-solving approach* (pp. 424–439). St. Louis: Elsevier Mosby.

Winston, K., & Loukas, K. (2014). Interventions to enhance feeding, eating, and swallowing. In K. Jacobs, N. MacRae, & K. Sladyk (Eds.), *Occupational therapy essentials for clinical competence* (2nd ed., pp. 457–471). Thorofare, NJ: SLACK Incorporated.

Chapter 6

Implementing Preparatory Interventions

Preparatory methods and tasks, such as physical agent modalities (PAMs), orthotic interventions, and therapeutic exercises, are used in occupational therapy to develop or remediate specific client factors (e.g., range of motion [ROM], sensory processing, pain, strength) and manage conditions (e.g., edema, open wounds) with the goal of contributing to the client's occupational performance (American Occupational Therapy Association [AOTA], 2014). Although preparatory interventions can be an important part of a client's intervention plan, these methods and tasks should supplement, but never replace, the use of purposeful activities and occupations (AOTA, 2014). State licensure laws delineate the specific PAMs and other types of interventions that may be used by an occupational therapist (OT) or occupational therapy assistant (OTA) in that state (AOTA, 2012). The worksheets and learning activities presented in this chapter address a variety of preparatory methods and tasks used in occupational therapy for physical conditions. Answers to worksheet exercises are provided at the end of the chapter.

Contents

Morreale, M. J., & Amini, D.
The Occupational Therapist's Workbook for Ensuring Clinical Competence (pp. 205-246).

Worksheet 6-1

Therapeutic Exercises

1. An occupational therapy client is recovering from a shoulder fracture. To achieve independence in home management, the intervention plan includes passive ROM (PROM) to increase the range of motion of the glenohumeral joint. When the OT flexes the client's shoulder to 140°, the client states, "I feel a little stretch." What should the OT do next?
   A. Discontinue PROM to the shoulder for this session
   B. Continue PROM, but only to 130° flexion
   C. Keep joint positioned at 140° flexion for a brief hold time
   D. Notify the referring physician

2. Teaching a client self-ROM is indicated for which of the following conditions?
   A. Flaccid extremity
   B. Frozen shoulder
   C. Extremity with fair minus muscle strength
   D. All of the above

3. To improve ROM for bathing, an OT is performing PROM on a shoulder of a client who has been diagnosed with adhesive capsulitis. The client is positioned in supine with the client's shoulder in 90° abduction. As the OT moves the client's arm into 40° of external rotation, the client reports sharp pain. Which of the following outlines the OT's best course of action for the next session?
   A. Document that the client has a low pain tolerance
   B. Do not attempt any passive external rotation beyond 40°
   C. Attempt passive external rotation with shoulder adducted
   D. Move client to sitting position and attempt passive external rotation with shoulder positioned in 90° abduction

4. An OT has several clients who are interested in improving activities of daily living (ADL) performance. Upper body strength and low endurance are found to be the primary barriers to independence. The clients are instructed in a home exercise program using exercise bands. Which of the following instructions should the OT give to each of the clients for upper extremity strengthening?
   A. Perform each exercise for two sets of 10 repetitions
   B. Perform exercises four times daily
   C. Inspect exercise bands for holes or tears
   D. Perform exercises only every other day

5. When using Thera-Band exercise bands, which of the following would indicate an upgrade of an exercise program or an increase in required effort?
   A. Use the same color exercise band in a shorter length than previously
   B. Use the same color exercise band in a longer length than previously
   C. Change from a red exercise band to a yellow exercise band
   D. Change from a blue exercise band to a green exercise band

Worksheet 6-1

Therapeutic Exercises (continued)

6. A client with rheumatoid arthritis exhibits fair minus muscle strength for right shoulder flexion due to pain and disuse. However, he does not have joint limitations in that shoulder. Muscle strength of his right elbow, wrist, and hand is within functional limits (WFL). Besides incorporating activities and occupations, which of the following would be most appropriate to address this client's shoulder weakness?

   A. Constraint-induced movement therapy (CIMT)

   B. Paraffin and PROM

   C. Bilateral dowel exercises

   D. Using a tabletop exercise skateboard

7. Which of the following activities is an example of a preparatory task to improve a child's finger-to-palm translation for play?

   A. Picking up beads from a table and moving them into palm unilaterally

   B. Stacking 1-inch blocks with index finger and thumb

   C. Flattening clay into a pancake shape using a rolling pin

   D. Using a toy hammer to pop bubble wrap

8. To return to his carpentry job, a client recovering from a Colles fracture is using a 1-pound weight to improve strength for wrist flexion and extension. The muscle contractions used for these exercises are:

   A. Isotonic

   B. Isometric

   C. Isothermal

   D. Isokinetic

9. To regain his ability to play a musical instrument, a client is using an exercise band to improve the strength of the elbow flexors. For the types of biceps contractions used to (1) pull the bands up when the other end is held by the foot and (2) slowly release them, all the following are included except:

   A. Concentric

   B. Eccentric

   C. Isotonic

   D. Isometric

10. An OT is working in a school setting with a child who has cerebral palsy. One of the goals in the child's Individualized Education Program (IEP) is to improve the child's voluntary grasp and release patterns for classroom tasks. During a tabletop activity of putting large pegs in a pegboard, the OT should encourage the child to do which of the following?

    A. Maintain wrist flexion when placing pegs in holes

    B. Abduct shoulder to 90° when placing pegs in holes

    C. Supinate forearm 45° when placing pegs in holes

    D. Maintain wrist extension when placing pegs in holes

Worksheet 6-2

Open and Closed Kinetic Chain Exercises

For each italicized component of the following activities, indicate whether it is an open kinetic chain exercise or closed kinetic chain exercise by putting an "O" or "C" next to each.

1. ____ *Using exercise bands* to improve shoulder strength
2. ____ *Turning a heavy jump rope* with another child holding the other end
3. ____ *Weight-bearing on forearm* while writing with the other hand
4. ____ *Pushing a weighted toy shopping cart* while walking around an obstacle course
5. ____ *Putting cans in upper kitchen cabinets*
6. ____ *Using 1-pound weights* to improve wrist strength
7. ____ *Carrying a lunch tray* in the cafeteria
8. ____ *Sanding* a wooden board using a sanding block
9. ____ *Posing like a bear* with hands and feet on floor
10. ____ *Using a reacher* to remove clothes from dryer
11. ____ *Prone on elbows* while watching a wind-up toy move
12. ____ *Rolling dough into piecrust shape using a rolling pin*
13. ____ *Dynamic standing* when hanging clothes in closet
14. ____ *Hanging clothes in closet* while standing
15. ____ *Pressing and flattening therapy putty with palm* while standing at table
16. ____ *Dynamic standing* while using a hula hoop
17. ____ *Performing pushups against the wall* while standing
18. ____ *Moving rings from one side of an exercise arc to the other side*
19. ____ *Use palm to rub lotion on thigh*
20. ____ *Arm pushups* while seated in preparation for transfers
21. ____ *Cone stacking* to improve grip
22. ____ *Waving a ribbon wand* to music
23. ____ *Scrubbing a floor using a handheld brush*
24. ____ *Painting on an easel* while standing
25. ____ *Sliding board transfer*

Worksheet 6-3

Preparatory Methods and Tasks

1. An OT is working with a client to enable independent self-care by minimizing hand edema and improving ROM of the client's fingers. Which of the following is the least appropriate intervention to address these deficits?
   A. Using a vibrator to improve lymph drainage in the hand
   B. Contrast baths
   C. Retrograde massage
   D. Overhead pumping
2. In occupational therapy, a client recovering from carpal tunnel surgery is putting golf tees in therapy putty. Although an activity or occupation would be more meaningful for the client, this preparatory task was most likely chosen by the OT to address which of the following?
   A. Eye-hand coordination
   B. Tip pinch strength
   C. Pronator teres strength
   D. Hypothenar muscle strength
3. An OT is performing wound care with a client recovering from a finger laceration. In the initial evaluation performed 1 week ago, the OT described the wound as "yellow," and wound size as "9 mm long by 6 mm wide." Which of the following observations made by the OT at this time would indicate that the wound is improving?
   A. Black color
   B. Red color
   C. 1 cm long by .6 cm wide
   D. 8 cm long by 5 cm wide
4. To regain strength to manage clothing fastenings, the OT is instructing an outpatient client in a home program of therapy putty exercises. Which of the following is the least appropriate for the OT to instruct the client to do with the therapy putty at this time?
   A. Squeeze therapy putty into a ball
   B. Roll therapy putty into a log shape on client's thigh
   C. Pinch therapy putty with thumb, index, and long fingers
   D. Squeeze therapy putty between fingers
5. A left-handed 10-year-old child with a traumatic brain injury (TBI) has increased muscle tone in his right upper extremity and fair sitting balance. How should the OT position the child when working on graphomotor skills?
   A. Sitting at desk, feet unsupported, right upper extremity positioned in pronation stabilizing paper on table
   B. Sitting at desk, feet supported, right upper extremity positioned in supination stabilizing paper on table
   C. Sitting at desk, feet supported, right upper extremity holding the pencil, left arm stabilizing paper on table
   D. Sitting at desk, feet supported, right upper extremity positioned in pronation stabilizing paper on table
6. An OT in a rehabilitation hospital is planning a lower body dressing session with a male client recovering from a below-knee amputation (BKA). The OT arrives at the client's room immediately following the client's shower. The client is dressed in a hospital gown, but the long elastic bandage that has been used to shape his residual limb has not been reapplied. What action should the OT take?
   A. Rewrap stump using a circular method to apply the bandage, then work on lower body dressing
   B. Rewrap the stump using a figure-8 method to apply bandage, then work on lower body dressing
   C. Before performing dressing tasks, contact the physical therapist (PT) or physical therapist assistant (PTA) and ask that person to rewrap the stump now
   D. Work on lower body dressing without reapplying bandage

Worksheet 6-3 (continued)

Preparatory Methods and Tasks

7. An OT Level I fieldwork student sees an OT across the room methodically stroking a dry, densely bristled soft brush on a child's arms. The student does not know the child's diagnosis, but also observes that the child eventually begins to engage in a play task of removing beanbags hidden in a bucket of balls. The student should conclude that the outcome the OT is trying to achieve with the brush is most likely which of the following?
   A. Improved wrist extension
   B. Decreased spasticity
   C. Desensitization
   D. Removal of germs for infection control
8. A client post-cerebrovascular accident (CVA) and left hemiparesis is beginning to get some motor return in the affected upper extremity. An OT is using a neurodevelopmental-based technique of upper extremity weight-bearing activities to improve proximal stability. The client is sitting on a mat with his affected arm extended at side and palm on the mat. Which of the following is not correct for the OT to do?
   A. Flatten client's hand completely on the mat
   B. Support client's elbow
   C. Have client shift weight gradually toward affected side
   D. Have client's feet resting on floor
9. An OT is working with a client using an exercise band to improve right shoulder external rotation strength. The OT has tied the exercise band to a doorknob. How should the OT tell the client to position himself?
   A. Stand perpendicular to door with right side of body nearer to doorknob. Use band in right hand and pull across front of body, keeping the weak shoulder adducted.
   B. Stand perpendicular to door with right side of body nearer to doorknob. Use band in right hand and pull away from right side of body, keeping the weak shoulder adducted.
   C. Stand perpendicular to door with left side of body nearer to doorknob. Use band in right hand and pull across front of body with right hand, keeping the weak shoulder adducted.
   D. Stand perpendicular to door with left side of body nearer to doorknob. Use band in right hand and pull away from right side of body, keeping the weak shoulder adducted.
10. When measuring a client for a standard wheelchair, which of the following is correct?
   A. Seat depth should be 1.5 to 2 inches wider than client's hips
   B. Seat back height should be level with superior angle of scapula
   C. Armrest height should be measured with client's elbow placed in approximately 90° of flexion
   D. The front edge of seat should reach to the back of client's knees

Learning Activity 6-1: Client Factors and Motor Skills

For each of the client factors or performance skills in the following table, list two preparatory tasks and two functional activities or occupations that may be used in occupational therapy to improve deficits in those areas. Examples are provided for each category. Also, determine three additional client factors or performance skills to add to this table. Considering each client factor/performance skill category, determine which of the interventions might be more meaningful or effective for a "real" client and the reasons why.

Client Factor/Performance Skill	*Preparatory Task*	*Activities and Occupations*
Shoulder ROM	*Pulleys*	*Put groceries in upper kitchen cabinet*
	1.	1.
	2.	2.
Upper extremity strength	*Exercise bands*	*Carry a laundry basket containing towels or clothes*
	1.	1.
	2.	2.
Cylindrical grip	*Stack cones*	*Use large-handled utensils for feeding*
	1.	1.
	2.	2.
Hand strength	*Squeeze hand gripper*	*Knead bread dough*
	1.	1.
	2.	2.
Standing balance/tolerance	*Stand at table to use shoulder arc*	*Stand at kitchen counter to make a sandwich*
	1.	1.
	2.	2.
Sitting balance/tolerance	*Sit on mat to toss beanbags*	*Sit on tub bench when bathing*
	1.	1.
	2.	2.
Three-point pinch/palmar pinch	*Stack small checkers*	*Put on lipstick*
	1.	1.
	2.	2.
Tip pinch	*Put small pegs in pegboard*	*Put pills in pill organizer (can use beans or small candies to simulate pills)*
	1.	1.
	2.	2.
Lateral pinch	*Pinch therapy putty*	*Hang towels on a clothesline using clothespins*
	1.	1.
	2.	2.
Dexterity/in-hand manipulation	*Pick up foam cubes one at a time and hold in palm*	*Sort a handful of coins into wrappers*
	1.	1.
	2.	2.

Learning Activity 6-1: Client Factors and Motor Skills (continued)

Client Factor/Performance Skill	Preparatory Task	Activities and Occupations
Other:		
	1.	1.
	2.	2.
Other:		
	1.	1.
	2.	2.
Other:		
	1.	1.
	2.	2.

Reprinted with permission from Morreale, M. J. (2015). *Developing clinical competence: A workbook for the OTA*. Thorofare, NJ: SLACK Incorporated.

Learning Activity 6-2: Process Skills

For each of the client factors or performance skills in the following table, list two preparatory tasks and two functional activities or occupations that may be used in occupational therapy to improve deficits in those areas. Examples are provided for each category. Also, determine three additional client factors or performance skills to add to this table. Considering each client factor/performance skill category, determine which of the interventions might be more meaningful or effective for a "real" client and the reasons why.

Client Factor/Performance Skill	***Preparatory Task***	***Activities and Occupations***
Crossing midline	*Moving rings on a shoulder arc from one side to the other*	*Move kitchen utensils from dish drainer to drawer on opposite side*
	1.	1.
	2.	2.
Spatial relations	*Follow a pattern using blocks*	*Place cookie dough evenly spaced on a cookie sheet*
	1.	1.
	2.	2.
Bilateral integration	*Upper extremity pedal exerciser*	*Buttoning a shirt*
	1.	1.
	2.	2.
Short-term memory	*Memory matching game*	*Use calendar to find/schedule appointments*
	1.	1.
	2.	2.
Categorization	*Sort shapes*	*Sort utensils into a divided utensil tray*
	1.	1.
	2.	2.
Sequencing	*Sequencing cards*	*Follow a recipe*
	1.	1.
	2.	2.
Calculation skills	*Math worksheets*	*Use a restaurant menu and calculate cost of a meal including tax and tip*
	1.	1.
	2.	2.
Problem solving	*Logic puzzles*	*Role-play emergency situations*
	1.	1.
	2.	2.
Body scheme	*Orient felt body pieces on a felt board*	*Dressing*
	1.	1.
	2.	2.
Awareness of left visual field	*Pick up beanbags on right side and place in bucket on left side*	*Locate grooming items on left side of counter when brushing teeth*
	1.	1.
	2.	2.

Learning Activity 6-2: Process Skills (continued)

Client Factor/Performance Skill	***Preparatory Task***	***Activities and Occupations***
Other		
	1.	1.
	2.	2.
Other:		
	1.	1.
	2.	2.
Other:		
	1.	1.
	2.	2.

Reprinted with permission from Morreale, M. J. (2015). *Developing clinical competence: A workbook for the OTA*. Thorofare, NJ: SLACK Incorporated.

Worksheet 6-4

Physical Agent Modality Categories

Indicate the pertinent category for each of the following PAMs or devices.

	PAM	Superficial Thermal Agent	Deep Thermal Agent	Electrotherapeutic Agent	Mechanical Device
1.	Fluidotherapy				
2.	Transcutaneous electrical nerve stimulation (TENS)				
3.	Iontophoresis				
4.	Hot pack				
5.	Ultrasound				
6.	Whirlpool				
7.	Vasopneumatic device				
8.	Cryotherapy				
9.	Neuromuscular electrical stimulation (NMES)				
10.	Functional electrical stimulation (FES)				
11.	Continuous passive motion (CPM)				
12.	Paraffin				
13.	High-voltage pulsed current (HVPC)				
14.	Cold pack				
15.	Hydrotherapy				
16.	Phonophoresis				
17.	Short-wave diathermy				
18.	Vapocoolant spray				
19.	Infrared				
20.	Lymphedema pump				

Worksheet 6-5

Selecting Physical Agent Modalities

For each of the client conditions listed, choose an appropriate modality or device from the following list. Only use each modality once.

A. Whirlpool
B. CPM
C. Ultrasound
D. Fluidotherapy
E. Vasopneumatic pump
F. TENS
G. NMES
H. Cold pack
I. Hot pack
J. Paraffin
K. Iontophoresis
L. Biofeedback

1. ___ Acute proximal interphalangeal (PIP) hyperextension injury with pain and edema
2. ___ Shoulder stiffness due to rheumatoid arthritis (RA)
3. ___ Muscle re-education to learn how to minimize involuntary upper trapezius muscle contraction
4. ___ Healed carpal tunnel release with stiffness, fair light touch sensation, intact protective sensation, and scar hypersensitivity
5. ___ Thumb carpometacarpal (CMC) arthritis with pain and stiffness
6. ___ Manage edema following soft tissue trauma
7. ___ Open wound requiring debridement
8. ___ Chronic biceps pain on discharge from occupational therapy
9. ___ Conditions requiring mechanical PROM
10. ___ Lateral epicondylitis requiring topical medication delivery through the skin
11. ___ CVA with hemiparesis and shoulder subluxation
12. ___ PIP joint contracture and scar adhesions following a healed laceration to volar index finger

Reprinted with permission from Morreale, M. J. (2015). *Developing clinical competence: A workbook for the OTA*. Thorofare, NJ: SLACK Incorporated.

Worksheet 6-6

Using Physical Agent Modalities Safely

1. Which of the following conditions would be most appropriate for paraffin?
   A. Wrist fracture resulting in pitting hand edema after cast removal
   B. Crush injury to hand resulting in digital stiffness and poor protective sensation
   C. Healed flexor tendon repair of index and long fingers resulting in tendon tightness
   D. Laceration of thumb with sutures in place and decreased thumb range of motion

2. An outpatient with a shoulder condition requires superficial heat to decrease shoulder stiffness. Before placing a hot pack on the client, the OT should do which of the following?
   A. Ask client to remove watch and rings
   B. Use an antistatic mat under client to prevent electric shocks
   C. Wrap the hot pack with a terry cloth cover and place a plastic bag over it
   D. Check hydrocollator temperature

3. Of the following choices, which primary action should an OT take when a client tells the OT that a hot pack feels too hot?
   A. Lower temperature of hydrocollator
   B. Inform the client that the heat will gradually dissipate
   C. Remove hot pack
   D. Notify the physician

4. Which of the following conditions would be most appropriate for Fluidotherapy?
   A. Rheumatoid arthritis flare-up causing painful hand and swollen joints
   B. Thumb CMC joint stiffness secondary to osteoarthritis
   C. Healed deltoid tendon repair resulting in pain and stiffness, but no sensory loss
   D. Shoulder contracture secondary to complex regional pain syndrome

5. When using a cryotherapy gel pack on a client, the OT should do which of the following?
   A. Place it directly on the affected area without using a cover on gel pack
   B. When done, put the gel pack immediately back in the heating unit so that it stays hot for the next client
   C. Cover it with a towel and then put it over an insensate area
   D. Explain that the client may experience a numb sensation

Worksheet 6-6 (continued)

Using Physical Agent Modalities Safely

6. An inpatient client is morbidly obese and requires a mechanical lift to transfer him out of bed. He rolls side to side using bed rails but cannot roll onto his stomach. The client also has pain in his posterior deltoid for which the doctor ordered occupational therapy, including hot packs. For the past 2 days, to decrease pain and stiffness in preparation for activities of daily living (ADL) performance, the client has received hot packs on his shoulder while sitting in a chair. Today, when the OT arrives with the hot pack, the mechanical lift is not available. What should the OT do?
   A. Place the hot pack underneath the client's shoulder with client supine
   B. Place the hot pack on the client's shoulder with client side-lying
   C. Place the hot pack on the client's shoulder with client prone
   D. Do not use a hot pack at this time

7. When administering a paraffin treatment to a client who has stiffness in digits and intact skin, the OT should do which of the following:
   A. Ask client to perform finger active ROM (AROM) in paraffin bath
   B. Ask client to wash and dry hands before using paraffin
   C. Place a plastic bag over client's hand then dip in paraffin and cover with a towel
   D. Ask client to immerse hand fully to touch bottom of the unit

8. An occupational therapy client with a wrist sprain and resulting stiffness has been receiving hot packs to his wrist followed by ROM and functional activities. When the client arrives, the OT notices the client has bad sunburn on his upper extremities, including his wrist. What primary action should the OT take?
   A. Administer a cold pack, then a hot pack, followed by ROM and functional activities
   B. Defer treatment for today
   C. Defer hot pack and perform functional activities
   D. Call the client's physician

9. An occupational therapy client recently had surgery to remove basal cell carcinoma from his wrist and is currently receiving radiation to eliminate possible remaining malignant cells. The client is having difficulty performing ADLs due to wrist pain and decreased wrist motion. Which of the following modalities would be indicated for this client?
   A. Hot pack
   B. Paraffin
   C. Hot pack and ultrasound
   D. None

10. Which of the following situations is most appropriate for cryotherapy?
   A. Client with an acute wrist sprain and history of a carpal tunnel release 6 months ago with no loss of sensation
   B. Client with Raynaud phenomenon and acute thumb tendonitis
   C. Client with upper extremity peripheral vascular disease and acute finger sprain
   D. Client with an elbow contracture secondary to biceps tendon tightness

Worksheet 6-7

Physical Agent Modality Basics

1. An occupational therapy practitioner is working in a state that does not restrict occupational therapy practitioners from using PAMs. This person is competent in superficial and deep thermal agents and electrotherapeutic modalities. Which of the following intervention plans is not considered occupational therapy?
   A. Hot pack to shoulder, paraffin to hand, contrast baths
   B. PROM, NMES, home management tasks
   C. Hot pack, TENS, home management tasks
   D. Ultrasound, scar massage, ADLs

2. Which of the following PAMs transfer heat strictly by conduction?
   A. Fluidotherapy and hot packs
   B. Ultrasound and paraffin
   C. Paraffin and hot packs
   D. Fluidotherapy and ultrasound

3. Which of the following temperature ranges for paraffin are appropriate for use with a client?
   A. 98°F to 100°F
   B. 134°F to 138°F
   C. 122°F to 124°F
   D. 108°F to 112°F

4. Which of the following is the technique of using therapeutic ultrasound to deliver medication through the skin?
   A. Neuromuscular electrical stimulation
   B. TENS
   C. Iontophoresis
   D. Phonophoresis

5. An OT is working in a state that, regarding PAMs, only allows occupational therapy practitioners to use superficial thermal agents. The client has a diagnosis of carpal tunnel release and the prescription states "Ultrasound, Fluidotherapy, TENS, and ADL retraining." Which of the following should the OT use with the client to decrease pain and improve ROM?
   A. Fluidotherapy and ADL retraining
   B. Fluidotherapy, TENS, and ADL retraining
   C. Fluidotherapy, ultrasound, TENS, and ADL retraining
   D. Only ADL retraining

Worksheet 6-7 (continued)

Physical Agent Modality Basics

6. A client is recovering from a laceration to the hand. Sutures were removed 1 week ago and the wound is healed, but the scar is hypersensitive. The client also has decreased finger ROM and diffuse hand edema. Which of the following PAMs would likely be the most useful?
   A. Fluidotherapy
   B. Paraffin
   C. Hot pack
   D. None of the above

7. An OTA who is competent in administering TENS has moved to a new state that prohibits OTAs from using electrotherapeutic agents. The sole OT at her facility is not competent in administering TENS. However, an occupational therapy client diagnosed with complex regional pain syndrome would really benefit from TENS to manage severe upper extremity pain. The prescription from the doctor says "PAMs PRN." What should the OT do?
   A. Have the OTA administer TENS only under the supervision of a PT
   B. Ask the doctor to write a prescription specifically for TENS for occupational therapy
   C. Have the OT administer TENS with the OTA supervising
   D. Do not use TENS

8. The OT intervention plan for a client with a PIP dislocation injury includes the following PAMs as needed: hot packs, Fluidotherapy, and cold packs. This client has been delegated to the OTA today. At the start of the session, the client tells the OTA that she receives paraffin to her hands when getting manicures at the nail salon and enjoys it very much. The OTA feels that paraffin would be beneficial to decrease the client's finger stiffness today. What should the OTA do during today's session?
   A. Call the client's physician to obtain a prescription for paraffin
   B. Administer paraffin and notify the occupational therapist
   C. Document what the client said and administer paraffin
   D. Administer hot pack or Fluidotherapy

9. A client with thumb tendonitis is at the reconditioning phase in occupational therapy. During an intervention session, which of the following is most likely the proper sequence of interventions for this client?
   A. Hot pack, activities/occupations, paraffin
   B. Hot pack, activities/occupations, cold pack
   C. Paraffin, activities/occupations, hot pack, cold pack
   D. Paraffin, activities/occupations, hot pack

10. Following a client's paraffin treatment, what should the OT do with the used wax?
    A. Put it back in the paraffin unit
    B. Give it to the client to use at home for hand exercises
    C. Throw it away
    D. Put it in a sealed plastic bag with client's name and save it for the client's next paraffin treatment

Worksheet 6-8

Deep Thermal and Electrical Modalities

Occupational therapy practitioners who demonstrate proficiency in their use are able to implement PAMs in preparation for activities and occupations (AOTA, 2012). Accreditation Council for Occupational Therapy Education ({ACOTE}, 2012) Standards call for occupational therapy programs to ensure that students are able to explain the use of deep thermal and electrical modalities. This worksheet is designed to assess your understanding of deep thermal modalities, such as therapeutic ultrasound and a variety of electrical modalities. Practitioners must be sure to check their state licensure laws to determine the specific PAMs that may be used by an OT or OTA in that state (AOTA, 2012).

1. Electrical modalities are successfully used to address many soft tissue problems. Identify the one area that is not addressed through the use of an electrical modality.
   A. Healing of damaged tissue is facilitated
   B. Muscle strength and endurance are enhanced
   C. Pain is modulated
   D. Healing of severed nerves is enhanced

2. Which of the following is not a feature of transcutaneous electrical nerve stimulation (TENS)?
   A. Primarily used for managing chronic pain
   B. Works by blocking the pain signal, and by increasing endorphins in the body
   C. Must be worn all day or will not be effective
   D. Device features include adjustable pulse rate, pulse width, and amplitude (intensity)

3. Which one of the following is a "type" of TENS (based on pulses per second [pps], amplitude, and intensity)?
   A. Massaging TENS
   B. Sundial TENS
   C. Pinprick TENS
   D. Pain threshold TENS

4. Which of the following is a therapeutic effect of NMES/FES?
   A. Stronger than a TENS unit, with a wider pulse width to elicit muscle contraction for a period of time
   B. Prevents disuse atrophy (muscle wasting)
   C. Muscles are contracted and relaxed on and off
   D. Devices have preprogrammed regimens

5. Which of the following is not a diagnosis that may benefit from the use of NMES/FES?
   A. Radial nerve palsy
   B. Weakness due to incomplete spinal cord injury
   C. Shoulder subluxation
   D. Amyotrophic lateral sclerosis (ALS)

Worksheet 6-8 (continued)

Deep Thermal and Electrical Modalities

6. Electrical modalities share many common contraindications. Which one of the following is not a contraindication to the use of electrical stimulation devices?
   A. Use with people fitted with a demand-type heart pacemakers
   B. Use while driving or using machinery
   C. Use over eyes, the heart, or over a pregnant uterus (except during labor)
   D. Use on young children due to active tissue growth

7. Which of the following is not a diagnosis that may respond to iontophoresis using dexamethasone?
   A. Dupuytren disease
   B. De Quervain's stenosing tenosynovitis
   C. Triggering of long finger
   D. Lateral epicondylitis

8. Electromyography (EMG) biofeedback is not a true electrical modality. Which of the following is not true about EMG biofeedback?
   A. It detects electrical responses from muscle tissue
   B. It is painless
   C. It does not provide an electrical charge to the client
   D. It requires the use of a needle electrode for accuracy

9. Microwave and shortwave diathermy are both heat modalities that create heat via ______ and are therefore most similar to __________.
   A. conversion; whirlpool
   B. convection; dry whirlpool
   C. conversion; ultrasound
   D. conduction; ultrasound

10. Interferential current is different from TENS as a method of pain reduction because:
    A. It is delivered via surface electrodes
    B. It penetrates the tissue deeply because of the "interference" created by 2 streams of current
    C. It creates an analgesic effect due to the pain gate mechanism and the release of endogenous opiates
    D. Clients will feel a "pins and needles" sensation during treatment

Worksheet 6-9

Deep Thermal and Electrical Modalities—More Practice

Indicate true (T) or false (F).

1. ________ Ultrasound produces heat within tissue through the process of conduction.
2. ________ Piezoelectric effect occurs when electricity vibrates a crystal.
3. ________ As a deep thermal modality, ultrasound creates frictional heat through the movement of cells created by the sound wave.
4. ________ Electrical modalities, in addition to creating a heat effect, also have a mechanical effect that can be isolated based on direct vs pulsed current.
5. ________ The human body is electrically conductive. Electricity from electrical devices travels through nerves in the skin and muscle to affect nerve endings both motor and sensory.
6. ________ High-voltage electrical stimulation units do not require intact nerves.
7. ________ Dexamethasone is a positively charged medication.
8. ________ Iontophoresis is a drug delivery mechanism used to treat inflammation (e.g., "itis").
9. ________ NMES must be cycled on and off to prevent fatigue of the muscle fibers.
10. ________ High-voltage pulsed galvanic stimulation is a form of electrical stimulation that is primarily used for quickly increasing circulation or reducing edema in a specified area.

Worksheet 6-10

Electrical Modalities

Short answers: Briefly describe the following.

1. Transcutaneous electrical nerve stimulation (TENS) ____________________

2. Neuromuscular electrical stimulation (NMES)/functional electrical stimulation (FES) ____________________

3. Iontophoresis ____________________

4. EMG biofeedback (not a true electrotherapy device) ____________________

5. Voltage ____________________

6. Alternating versus direct current ____________________

7. Waveforms ____________________

8. Pulse rate (pps) ____________________

9. Pulse width (related to pulse rate) ____________________

10. Amplitude (power or intensity) ____________________

11. Polarity ____________________

Learning Activity 6-3: Generating Client Interventions

One of the unique aspects of occupational therapy is the OT practitioner's ability to use everyday objects for therapeutic purposes. In the spaces that follow, list specific ways that a deck of cards might be used to improve the various client factors or performance skills delineated in the *Occupational Therapy Practice Framework* (AOTA, 2014). Examples are provided for each category. Although preparatory methods and tasks can support occupational performance, an OT practitioner should use activities and occupations whenever possible.

Joint, Bone, and Muscle Functions

Example: Improve ROM of the elbow—Deal cards across the table to a partner.

1.

2.

3.

Motor Skills

Example: Improve standing tolerance—Stand at table to play Solitaire for a designated length of time.

1.

2.

3.

Emotional Regulation/Social Interaction Skills

Example: Improve frustration tolerance—Play a card game and wait patiently for one's turn.

1.

2.

3.

Mental Functions/Process Skills

Example: Improve counting and math skills—Count a deck of cards accurately.

1.

2.

3.

4.

5.

6.

Learning Activity 6-4: Generating Client Interventions—More Practice

This exercise will require you to think creatively. One of the unique aspects of occupational therapy is the OT practitioner's ability to use everyday objects for therapeutic purposes. In the box that follows, list specific ways that paper clips might be used to improve the various client factors and performance skills delineated in the *Occupational Therapy Practice Framework* (AOTA, 2014). Examples are provided for each category. Although preparatory methods and tasks can support occupational performance, an OT practitioner should use activities and occupations whenever possible.

Joint, Bone, and Muscle Functions

Example: Improve tip pinch strength—Use index finger and thumb to push paper clips vertically into therapy putty.

1.

2.

3.

Motor Skills

Example: Improve bilateral integration—Stabilize paper on the table while attaching paper clips with the other hand.

1.

2.

3.

Communication/Social Interaction Skills

Example: Improve interpersonal skills—Ask a worker in office supply store where the paper clips are located.

1.

2.

3.

Mental Functions/Process Skills

Example: Safety Awareness—Avoid putting paper clips in mouth while working on a craft project.

1.

2.

3.

4.

5.

6.

Learning Activity 6-5: Generating Creative Interventions

The media used in this exercise will require a bit more thinking "outside of the box." As previously noted, one of the unique aspects of occupational therapy is the OT practitioner's ability to use everyday objects for therapeutic purposes. In the spaces that follow, list specific ways that a container of uncooked rice might be used to improve various client factors, performance skills, and occupations delineated in the *Occupational Therapy Practice Framework* (AOTA, 2014). Examples are provided for each category. Although preparatory methods and tasks can support occupational performance, an occupational therapy practitioner should use activities and occupations whenever possible.

Joint, Bone, and Muscle Functions

Example: Improve upper extremity strength—Carry a 5-pound bag of rice.

1.

2.

3.

Motor Skills

Example: Improve coordination—Move spoonfuls of rice from one container to another without spilling.

1.

2.

3.

Sensory Functions

Example: Reduce tactile hypersensitivity—Locate objects embedded in rice.

1.

2.

3.

Communication/Social Interaction Skills

Example: Express feelings—Discuss significance of rice in one's own culture (e.g., rice and beans, fried rice, rice pudding).

1.

2.

3.

Learning Activity 6-5: Generating Creative Interventions (continued)

Mental Functions/Process Skills

Example: Improve measuring skills—Measure specified amounts of rice accurately.

1.

2.

3.

Occupations (ADL/IADL)

Example: Improve meal preparation skills—Follow a recipe to make rice and beans for lunch.

1.

2.

3.

4.

5.

6.

Occupations (Play):

Example: Improve imaginary play skills—Collaborate with another person and use rice to create a beach scene, decorating with shells, hidden treasure, and dolls suntanning.

1.

2.

3.

Worksheet 6-11

Orthotic Interventions

Match each of these orthotic devices to one of the conditions that follow. Use each only once.

A. Resting hand orthosis
B. Metacarpophalangeal (MP) extension blocking orthosis
C. Airplane orthosis
D. Palm protector
E. Short opponens orthosis
F. Dorsal blocking orthosis
G. Forearm-based thumb spica orthosis
H. Figure-eight finger orthosis
I. Dynamic MP extension orthosis
J. Ulnar deviation orthosis
K. Volar wrist immobilization orthosis
L. Anterior elbow orthosis
M. PIP extension orthosis
N. Forearm-based dorsal extension orthosis
O. Distal interphalangeal (DIP) extension orthosis
P. Ulnar gutter orthosis
Q. Counterforce brace
R. Body-powered prosthesis
S. Composite flexion orthosis
T. Tenodesis orthosis

1. ____ Carpal tunnel syndrome
2. ____ Boutonnière deformity ring finger
3. ____ Upper extremity amputation
4. ____ Small finger metacarpal fracture
5. ____ Dupuytren's release
6. ____ C6–C7 spinal cord injury
7. ____ Flexor tendon repair of digits
8. ____ Brachial plexus injury
9. ____ Swan-neck deformity
10. ____ Mallet finger
11. ____ Low-level ulnar nerve injury
12. ____ Burns to hand/wrist
13. ____ Extrinsic extensor tightness of digits
14. ____ De Quervain's tenosynovitis
15. ____ Elbow flexion contracture
16. ____ MP joints requiring realignment secondary to rheumatoid arthritis (RA)
17. ____ Flexed digits of a client with end-stage dementia causing skin breakdown in hand
18. ____ Low-level median nerve injury
19. ____ Lateral epicondylitis
20. ____ Radial nerve palsy

Worksheet 6-12

Using Orthotic Devices

1. When fabricating a volar wrist extension orthosis for a client with a wrist sprain, an occupational therapy practitioner must mold it carefully to avoid future skin breakdown at which of the following bony prominences?
   A. Radial head
   B. PIP joints
   C. Ulnar styloid
   D. Olecranon

2. A client with an unhealed fracture complains that he is perspiring under his orthotic device. The OT may take the following actions except:
   A. Punch air holes in the splint
   B. Provide washable cotton liners
   C. Discontinue splint
   D. Instruct client how to clean orthotic device

3. When fabricating an orthotic device, the primary reason for making a paper pattern is:
   A. To avoid wasting expensive thermoplastic material
   B. To help ensure proper orthotic size and fit
   C. To keep the pattern in the client's chart
   D. To avoid pen or pencil marks on thermoplastic material

4. After softening thermoplastic material in hot water for orthotic fabrication, what should the OT practitioner do next?
   A. Wait several minutes following removal from hot water, then place on client
   B. Immediately place on client upon removal from hot water
   C. Wait 15 seconds after removal from hot water, then place on client
   D. Cool thermoplastic until comfortable and safe for client to tolerate

5. When fabricating a resting hand orthosis for a client with a flaccid extremity, the thumb should generally be positioned in:
   A. Abduction
   B. Full adduction
   C. 90° interphalangeal (IP) flexion
   D. 70° metacarpophalangeal (MP) flexion

6. When fabricating an index finger mallet orthosis, which of the following is generally not correct?
   A. Conform orthotic device to transverse and longitudinal arches of palm
   B. Allow for full active PIP flexion
   C. Position DIP in extension
   D. Do not incorporate the small finger

Worksheet 6-12

Using Orthotic Devices (continued)

7. When fabricating a forearm-based thumb orthosis for a client with thumb CMC arthritis, which of the following principles does not typically apply?
   A. The orthosis should be half the length of the forearm
   B. Conform to transverse and longitudinal arches
   C. Allow full thumb interphalangeal joint (IP) AROM
   D. Do not immobilize MP joints of other digits

8. A client diagnosed with a right cerebrovascular accident (CVA) exhibits unilateral neglect and poor safety regarding his nonfunctional left hand. The OT fabricated a volar resting hand orthosis to help keep the client's joints in a safe, functional position. The client's wrist spasticity keeps causing the Velcro wrist strap to detach. In addition to possibly fabricating a dorsal wrist orthosis, which of the following is the best course of action for the OT to remedy this problem?
   A. Remold the orthotic device into a flexed wrist position
   B. Discontinue the orthotic device
   C. Instruct the client to refasten the strap
   D. Use a D-ring and longer wrist strap

9. A primary purpose of an outrigger on a dynamic orthosis is:
   A. To ensure proper angle of pull
   B. To conform to the transverse and longitudinal arches
   C. To attach orthotic device to the forearm
   D. To make the orthotic device more durable

10. A child with cerebral palsy was issued a hand-based thumb spica orthosis last week to promote prehension. Today, the child arrives with his mother and tells the OT that the orthotic device is uncomfortable because it is rubbing at the thumb IP joint, and he does not want to wear it. The OT notices that the orthotic edge is rough, causing slight redness at the thumb IP. Which of the following is the OT's best course of action?
    A. Defer treatment and notify the child's physician
    B. Fabricate a new orthotic device
    C. Use a heat gun to smooth rough area
    D. Document that the child is making up excuses to avoid wearing the orthotic device

Worksheet 6-13

Client Education

You have just fabricated and issued an orthotic device for a client who has osteoarthritis of her dominant thumb CMC joint. List at least eight things you need to educate the client about regarding the orthotic device.

1.

2.

3.

4.

5.

6.

7.

8.

Learning Activity 6-6: Custom vs Prefabricated Orthotic Devices

Choose a specific type of orthotic device such as a resting hand orthosis, wrist extension orthosis, elbow extension orthosis, or dynamic MP extension orthosis. Make a list of all the materials and equipment needed to fabricate that device. Use a professional catalogue to calculate the exact cost of materials for making the orthotic device, not including the practitioner's time or standard tools/equipment (e.g., heating unit, scissors). Also, determine whether a similar prefabricated orthotic device is available for purchase. Compare the cost of custom orthotic materials versus the price of the prefabricated device. Which option would you choose for a client? Explain your rationale.

Name of orthotic device ______________________________

List several conditions this orthotic device may be used for:

____

____

Materials Required	***Package Cost and Quantity***	***Unit Cost for One Splint***
Example: *Loop fastener*	*$25 per 25 foot roll*	*24 inches = $2.00*
Equipment Required	***Tools Required***	
Example: *Electric heating pan*	Example: *Scissors*	

Total cost of orthotic device (excluding labor costs): $______________________________

Prefabricated orthotic device cost: $______________________________

Rationale for Using a Custom Orthotic Device	***Rationale for Using a Prefabricated Orthotic Device***

Adapted from Morreale, M. J. (2015). *Developing clinical competence: A workbook for the OTA*. Thorofare, NJ: SLACK Incorporated.

Worksheet 6-14

Upper Extremity Safety

Stella is an 82-year-old client with a diagnosis of right CVA. Her left upper extremity is just beginning to exhibit some limited motor return in her shoulder and elbow, along with some active gross finger flexion. Stella also exhibits poor left upper extremity sensation, homonymous hemianopsia, and moderate left neglect. When Stella sits in the wheelchair, she is unaware that her left arm tends to hang down over the side and get caught in the wheel. List six preparatory or functional interventions that can improve the safety of Stella's upper extremity while she is sitting in her wheelchair. Determine the pros and cons of each method or task.

Intervention	***Pros***	***Cons***
1.		
2.		
3.		
4.		
5.		
6.		

Answers to Chapter 6 Worksheets

OT practitioners must always use clinical judgment when selecting and implementing PAMs, orthotic devices, therapeutic exercises, and other interventions. OTs and OTAs must carefully consider multiple factors, such as the client's medical status and circumstances, precautions, contraindications, evidence-based practice, available methods, and safety. Often, more than one type of physical agent, orthotic device, exercise, or technique is used during a client's intervention program. Functional activities and occupations should always be incorporated into a client's intervention program. Worksheet answers contain general, sound guidelines, but may not be appropriate for all situations.

Worksheet 6-1: Therapeutic Exercises

Resources: Bandy & Sanders, 2008; Fairchild, 2013; Rybski, 2012.

1. C. It will depend on the particular circumstances but, in situations such as the one presented, a report of a minor complaint such as "a little stretch" or "slight pull" is often not cause for major concern. However, if the client had a fragile wound, recent surgery such as a tendon or nerve repair, unstable joints, or reported a more severe complaint during ROM such as "severe pain" or "sharp pain," this would usually require more caution and a different line of thinking. Some other factors to consider are joint end feel and whether a client's pain is new, different, unexpected, or disproportionate to the task at hand. Always keep in mind that pain may signify that something serious is happening, such as an infection, undiagnosed fracture, irritated nerve, or imminent risk of injury. For the situation depicted in this question, *the OT should not aggressively move or force the joint* but might gently try to hold the joint at point of *slight* tension for a brief hold (per client tolerance without creating severe pain) to see whether the muscles relax and further ROM might be obtained. Many clients in occupational therapy have painful conditions that rehabilitation must gradually work through, but clinical judgment is always needed to ascertain what level of pain is or is not acceptable, expected, and safe and the appropriate techniques to apply.
2. D. All answers reflect the inability to actively raise arm fully, which are indicators for self-ROM.
3. C. External rotation with the arm abducted is often a more difficult position for clients with shoulder conditions. The OT can first try an alternate position, with shoulder adducted, to attempt gentle passive external rotation and determine whether this will allow for safer, less painful, and improved ROM. However, caution must be taken with any report of severe or sharp pain. Clinical judgment is always needed to ascertain what level of pain is or is not acceptable, normal, and safe, depending on each client's diagnosis, precautions, and contraindications. Determine if a client's pain is new, different, unexpected, or disproportionate to the task at hand. Pain may signify that something serious is happening, such as an infection, undiagnosed fracture, irritated nerve, or reinjury. *When in doubt, err on the side of caution* and communicate with the referring physician as necessary. In particular situations such as a healing fracture, tendon or nerve repair, or other joint conditions, further communication with the referring physician may also be needed to determine healing status and how hard to "push" the client without risk of injury.
4. C. A tear or hole in an exercise band may cause it to break when it is pulled taut, possibly harming the client. The frequency of exercises and number of repetitions must be individualized for each client.
5. A. A shorter length will create more tension, thus requiring more strength to pull band apart. Thera-Band resistance in order from weaker to stronger is yellow, red, green, blue (Hygenic Corporation, 2008).
6. C. CIMT is not indicated for this client's diagnosis. Although he demonstrates some shoulder weakness, he still has functional use of his right upper extremity and no neurological deficit. He would benefit more from a strengthening program such as active assistive ROM against gravity (answer C) and ADL modification. Functional activities should be incorporated and encouraged. PROM would not be helpful for strengthening because it does not involve active muscle contractions (but can help to maintain joint mobility). Paraffin is not indicated for the shoulder. AROM on the table with a tabletop skateboard is in the gravity-minimized plane (needing only a muscle grade of poor) and would not really facilitate flexion of the shoulder.

7. A. Finger-to-palm translation means manipulating an object to move it from the fingers into the palm. B, C, and D do not do that.
8. A. Isotonic contractions include eccentric and concentric contractions that are occurring in the wrist flexors and extensors.
9. D. The biceps is actively shortening (as the elbow flexes) and lengthening (as the elbow extends) during the task.
10. D. Wrist extension during grasp and release is a typical mature pattern.

Worksheet 6-2: Open and Closed Kinetic Chain Exercises

Closed kinetic chain exercises have a fixed end segment (such as in weight-bearing tasks), whereas open kinetic chain exercises have an end segment that is freely moveable (such as using dumbbells, exercise bands, reaching for objects, or holding items in space; Gillen, 2011b; Wilk & Reinold, 2008). Open kinetic chain exercises may include resistive exercises that facilitate an isotonic, isometric, or isokinetic contraction (Bandy, 2008).

1. O *Using exercise bands* to improve shoulder strength
2. O *Turning a heavy jump rope* with another child holding the other end
3. C *Weight bearing on forearm* while writing with the other hand
4. C *Pushing a weighted toy shopping cart* while walking around an obstacle course
5. O *Putting cans in upper kitchen cabinets*
6. O *Using 1-pound weights* to improve wrist strength
7. O *Carrying a lunch tray* in the cafeteria
8. C *Sanding* a wooden board using a sanding block
9. C *Posing like a bear* with hands and feet on floor
10. O *Using a reacher* to remove clothes from dryer
11. C *Prone on elbows* while watching a wind-up toy move
12. C *Rolling dough into pie crust shape using a rolling pin*
13. C *Dynamic standing* when hanging clothes in closet
14. O *Hanging clothes in closet* while standing
15. C *Pressing and flattening therapy putty with palm* while standing at table
16. C *Dynamic standing* while using a hula hoop
17. C *Performing pushups against the wall* while standing
18. O *Moving rings from one side of an exercise arc to the other side*
19. C *Use palm to rub lotion on thigh*
20. C *Arm push-ups* while seated in preparation for transfers
21. O *Cone stacking* to improve grip
22. O *Waving a ribbon wand* to music
23. C *Scrubbing a floor using a handheld brush*
24. O *Painting on an easel* while standing
25. C *Sliding board transfer*

Worksheet 6-3: Preparatory Methods and Tasks

OT practitioners working in physical rehabilitation settings typically encounter clients who have impairment resulting from neurological conditions such as CVA and traumatic brain injury. Traditional therapeutic approaches to facilitate motor control have included the Bobath method, Brunnstrom movement therapy, the Rood method, and proprioceptive neuromuscular facilitation (PNF) (Radomski & Latham, 2008). However, the evidence supports the use of newer approaches to motor learning such as a task-oriented approach that emphasizes functional interventions

(Gillen, 2011a). Additional techniques, such as edema management or wound care, may be implemented to address other factors. It is important to incorporate the client's affected upper extremity into functional tasks so that it is not just a passive appendage. OT practitioners can use techniques for motor learning, such as CIMT, bilateral activities, mental imagery, and occupation-based activities that facilitate motor skills (Gillen, 2011a, 2011b). While adhering to any precautions and contraindications regarding the client's present situation (such as fracture-healing status and postoperative protocols), OT practitioners should use a function-based approach as much as possible to promote awareness of the involved side, maintain mobility, and improve occupational performance (Gillen, 2011a; Morawski & Padilla, 2012).

1. A. Vibration may be used for scar management or, according to Rood's facilitation principles, the recruitment of muscle fibers (Bentzel, 2008; Rust, 2008). It is not a standard intervention for edema management.
2. B. Eye-hand coordination is not a typical deficit associated with carpal tunnel syndrome or release, although fine-motor skills may be affected due to weakness or sensory deficits (Eaton, n.d.). Median nerve compression may affect strength of the intrinsic muscles in the thenar eminence that control thumb MP flexion, palmar abduction, and opposition, thus affecting tip pinch. The hypothenar muscles (on ulnar side of hand) are intrinsic muscles innervated by the ulnar nerve and involve the small finger. Although pronation is a position that the arm can be placed in during in this task, that particular muscle group is not the focus of this intervention and is not the best answer.
3. B. Wounds are classified as red (healing granulation tissue), yellow (has exudate such as pus or denatured slough), or black (necrotic tissue) (Bracciano, 2008; Skirven, Osterman, Fedorczyk, & Amadio, 2011). Answers C and D actually indicate an increase in wound size.
4. C. Although all of the exercises indicated are appropriate, it is best to avoid using exercise putty directly over clothing because the putty may stick and possibly ruin fabric.
5. D. The child's feet need to be supported for trunk stability. It is not productive for the child to write with the nondominant hand. The affected hand should be positioned with forearm in pronation resting on table for weight bearing to help inhibit tone and provide postural stability (Levit, 2008).
6. B. The OT should have the clinical skill to perform stump wrapping. The appropriate method is a figure 8 diagonal application (Stubblefield & Armstrong, 2008).
7. C. Practitioners specially trained in the Wilbarger protocol use a specific type of brush and special techniques to apply deep pressure and proprioception to a child's limbs and back to help reduce sensory defensiveness (Wilbarger & Wilbarger, 2002). If the arm was simply being cleaned, the OT would be using soap and water.
8. A. Because of its anatomic architecture, the hand should not be completely flattened, and the OT should take care to maintain arches of the hand (Levit, 2008; Morawski & Padilla, 2012). A weak upper extremity may cause the elbow to buckle, which is unsafe. Gradual weight shifting/leaning toward the affected side will help to promote weight bearing through that affected extremity so that it can provide stability during functional tasks. Weight shift toward the unaffected side is also useful to lengthen muscles of weak arm and trunk (Levit, 2008). A function-based approach should be used to incorporate the involved extremity in weight-bearing activities for daily occupations, such as stabilizing objects, wiping a table, or using extremity as a postural support while dressing (Gillen, 2011b).
9. D. The arm must move away from the body to have tension in the exercise band for external rotation. Standing perpendicular to the door with the right side closest to doorknob would not allow for tension in the band.
10. C. A client needing a wheelchair should be assessed to ensure proper fit, adequate support, optimal positioning, and to determine the specific type of seat cushion or adaptations that may be indicated. Seat width (not depth) should provide slight clearance (1.5 to 2 inches) between the client's hips and the side panels of wheelchair to avoid skin breakdown at trochanters. Seat depth should allow for approximately 2 inches of clearance between the edge of seat and popliteal space (back of knees). Armrest height is normally measured with elbow placed at 90°. Wheelchair back height generally should be slightly below inferior angles of scapula, although some clients may need a higher back for greater trunk support or a lower back to allow for greater propulsion (Fairchild, 2013; Minor & Minor, 2010).

Worksheet 6-4: Physical Agent Modalities

Indicate the pertinent category for each of the following PAMs.
Resources: AOTA, 2012; Bracciano, 2008, 2014.

	Physical Agent Modality	Superficial Thermal Agent	Deep Thermal Agent	Electrotherapeutic Agent	Mechanical Device
1.	Fluidotherapy	X			
2.	Transcutaneous electrical nerve stimulation (TENS)			X	
3.	Iontophoresis			X	
4.	Hot pack	X			
5.	Ultrasound		X		
6.	Whirlpool	X			
7.	Vasopneumatic device				X
8.	Cryotherapy	X			
9.	Neuromuscular electrical stimulation (NMES)			X	
10	Functional electrical stimulation (FES)			X	
11.	Continuous passive motion (CPM)				X
12.	Paraffin	X			
13.	High-voltage pulsed current (HVPC)			X	
14.	Cold pack	X			
15.	Hydrotherapy	X			
16.	Phonophoresis		X		
17.	Short-wave diathermy		X		
18.	Vapocoolant spray	X			
19.	Infrared	X			
20.	Lymphedema pump				X

Worksheet 6-5: Selecting Physical Agent Modalities

Resources: Bracciano, 2008, 2014; Cameron, 2009; Knight & Draper, 2013.

1. _H_ Acute PIP hyperextension injury with pain and edema (cold pack)
2. _I_ Shoulder stiffness due to RA (hot pack)
3. _L_ Muscle re-education to learn how to minimize involuntary upper trapezius muscle contraction (biofeedback)
4. _D_ Healed carpal tunnel release with stiffness, fair light touch sensation, intact protective sensation, and scar hypersensitivity (Fluidotherapy)

   The moving particles can be used to reduce hypersensitivity and the modality temperature can be lowered to avoid harm due to client's slightly decreased sensation
5. _J_ Thumb CMC arthritis with pain and stiffness (paraffin)
6. _F_ Manage edema following soft tissue trauma (vasopneumatic pump)
7. _A_ Open wound requiring debridement (whirlpool)

8. F Chronic biceps pain on discharge from occupational therapy (TENS)
9. B Conditions requiring mechanical PROM (CPM)
10. K Lateral epicondylitis requiring topical medication delivery through the skin (iontophoresis)
11. G CVA with hemiparesis and shoulder subluxation (NMES)
12. C PIP joint contracture and scar adhesions following a healed laceration to volar index finger (ultrasound)
Ultrasound can provide thermal and nonthermal effects to promote tissue changes and healing.

Worksheet 6-6: Using Physical Agent Modalities Safely

Resources: Bracciano, 2008, 2014; Cameron, 2009; Knight and Draper, 2013.

1. C. Paraffin is contraindicated for areas containing open wounds, severe edema, or poor sensation. Superficial heat is used to decrease stiffness and facilitate tendon gliding.
2. D. The hot pack is used on the client's shoulder, so there is no need to remove jewelry from wrist and hand. An anti-static mat or plastic bag is not indicated for this modality.
3. C. The client is at risk for a burn, so the hot pack should be removed. It may be appropriate to add extra towel layers if the OT determines that continued use of the hot pack is safe and warranted. The hydrocollator temperature should be checked *before* a hot pack is placed on a client.
4. B. Due to how an extremity must be placed in the Fluidotherapy unit, this modality is not appropriate for shoulder use. Heat should not be applied to a rheumatic joint that is acutely inflamed.
5. D. Cryotherapy is use of a cold thermal agent. A frozen gel pack requires a cover when placed on the skin. It is important to monitor what stage the client is feeling from a gel or ice pack as the client generally experiences a progression of effects. Realize the client is at risk for tissue damage if cold is administered for an extended time or on areas with absent sensation (insensate).
6. B. Care should be taken to protect the client's neck from the hot pack possibly touching it. Clients should not lie directly on a hot pack because pressure on the pack, oozing gel, or excess water may result in a burn.
7. B. Clients should wash and dry hands before a paraffin treatment. A plastic bag is normally placed over the client's hand *after* the hand has been dipped in paraffin. The client's affected hand should typically remain still during paraffin dips to avoid breaking the paraffin "glove," which would allow hot wax to seep underneath and possibly burn the skin. The client should not touch the bottom or sides of the unit as these areas could possibly be very hot, causing a burn.
8. C. It is contraindicated to apply heat to a burn. Most likely, there is no need to contact the client's physician for simple sunburn unless the client is exhibiting other adverse effects such as dehydration, sunstroke, infection, skin rash, or hives. The client should be able to work on other aspects of the intervention plan, such as functional activities.
9. D. Heat modalities and ultrasound are contraindicated for malignant areas. The OT should work on compensatory techniques to enable occupational performance. Fragile tissues may result from the radiation, so the practitioner must use evidence and communicate with the physician to determine any precautions/contraindications regarding wrist ROM.
10. A. Cold is beneficial to reduce acute inflammation but is contraindicated for clients with cold intolerance and poor circulation. Heat, rather than cold, helps to improve soft tissue extensibility. The carpal tunnel release should be well healed by this time and the client has no sensory deficits in the scenario provided.

Worksheet 6-7: Physical Agent Modality Basics

Resources: Bracciano, 2008, 2014; Cameron, 2009; Knight & Draper, 2013.

1. A. The use of PAMs alone is not considered occupational therapy (AOTA, 2012).
2. C
3. C
4. D

5. A. Ultrasound and TENS are not superficial thermal agents, so the OT cannot legally use them in that particular state. The OT should discuss the intervention plan with the referring physician to determine whether a referral to another discipline is warranted for administration of ultrasound and TENS. However, Fluidotherapy, TENS, and ultrasound may not be needed concurrently for this client.
6. A. Fluidotherapy can be used for both desensitization and AROM, and the unit temperature can be lowered to minimize heating effect as necessary so as not to increase edema.
7. D. An OT must have service competency regarding a modality to supervise an OTA administering that modality (AOTA, 2012). If the client needs a modality that the OT is not competent to supervise, the client should be referred to another practitioner. (PRN stands for "as needed.")
8. D. The OTA should only implement the modalities contained in the OT's intervention plan. However, the OTA may document what the client said and then speak to the OT to determine whether the intervention plan should be modified to include paraffin.
9. B. Superficial heat is used to decrease pain, relax muscles, and improve tissue extensibility in preparation for therapeutic exercises/activities. Cold may be used following exercises/activities to prevent flare-up of the condition. It is usually not indicated to implement both hot packs and paraffin to the same area during a single session.
10. C. Used wax should always be discarded to help keep the paraffin unit clean. Paraffin completely hardens, so it will not be useful for exercises at home.

Worksheet 6-8: Deep Thermal and Electrical Modalities

Resources: Bracciano, 2008; Knight & Draper, 2013.

When determining the use of PAMs as part of an intervention plan, the therapist must be proficient in the use of the modality and always carefully consider the client's medical condition and circumstances, any precautions/contraindications, desired functional outcomes, and other pertinent factors.

1. D. Electrical modalities do not affect healing of noncontinuous and nonsutured nerves. Nerves not reconnected after being severed will likely not heal together under any circumstances.
2. C. TENS is intended to be used intermittently throughout the day.
3. A. Massaging TENS is a type of application in which there is a 6-second cycle of concurrent width and pulse rate modulation: Width starts at 200 μS and decreases exponentially to 100 μS in 3 seconds. It then returns back to 200 μS in the next 3 seconds. The rate starts at 100 Hz and decreases exponentially to 65 Hz and then returns to 100 Hz.
4. B. The other responses are properties of the machine but are not therapeutic effects.
5. D. NMES/FES work along intact nerve pathways that are not present in ALS.
6. D. When indicated and under the supervision of a skilled practitioner, electrical modalities can be used safely with children.
7. A. Dexamethasone delivered via iontophoresis is used to decrease inflammation. Dupuytren disease is not the result of inflammation.
8. D. Surface electrodes are used effectively with EMG biofeedback.
9. C. Electromagnetic waves entering the tissue create movement within the cells that produce frictional heat much like the sound waves in ultrasound.
10. B. Unlike TENS, interferential current must have two streams of current to create the desired effect.

Worksheet 6-9: Deep Thermal and Electrical Modalities—More Practice

Resources: Bracciano, 2008, 2014; Knight & Draper, 2013.

1. <u>F</u> Ultrasound produces heat within tissue through the process of conduction.
   Ultrasound works through the process of conversion.
2. <u>T</u> Piezoelectric effect occurs when electricity vibrates a crystal.

3. _T_ As a deep thermal modality, ultrasound creates frictional heat through the movement of cells created by the sound wave.
4. _F_ Electrical modalities, in addition to creating a heat effect, also have a mechanical effect that can be isolated based on direct versus pulsed current.

   Electrical modalities do not create a heat effect but can create a mechanical effect through pulse rate, waveform, voltage, and amplitude. Direct and pulsed current are characteristics of ultrasound.
5. _T_ The human body is electrically conductive. Electricity from electrical devices travels through nerves in the skin and muscle to affect nerve endings both motor and sensory.
6. _F_ High-voltage electrical stimulation units do not require intact nerves.

   Low-voltage units can facilitate contractions of denervated muscle.
7. _F_ Dexamethasone is a positively charged medication.

   Dexamethasone is a negatively charged medication.
8. _T_ Iontophoresis is a drug delivery mechanism used to treat inflammation (e.g., "itis").
9. _T_ NMES must be cycled on and off to prevent fatigue of the muscle fibers.
10. _T_ High-voltage pulsed galvanic stimulation is a form of electrical stimulation that is primarily used for quickly increasing circulation or reducing edema in a specified area.

Worksheet 6-10: Electrical Modalities

Resources: Bracciano, 2008, 2014; Knight & Draper, 2013.

1. Transcutaneous electrical nerve stimulation (TENS) *An electrical modality used primarily to reduce pain*.
2. Neuromuscular electrical stimulation (NMES)/functional electrical stimulation (FES) *An electrical modality used to facilitate contraction of weakened muscles*.
3. Iontophoresis *A drug delivery system using electricity to transport ions of a medicinal substance*.
4. EMG biofeedback (not a true electrotherapy device) *A method of creating a visual or auditory representation of muscle activity to facilitate contraction or relaxation*.
5. Voltage *The amount of potential energy between two points on a circuit. Can be thought of as the pressure or strength of an electrical current. High- and low-voltage electrical stimulation units are capable of affecting muscles differently*.
6. Alternating versus direct current *Alternating current vacillates between positive and negative poles; direct current moves toward one pole only*.
7. Waveforms *The shape of electrical waves forming the electrical current. Shapes of waves can impact the effect of the current in the body. For example, waveforms can be symmetrical or asymmetrical*.
8. Pulse rate (pulses per second [pps]) *The number of separate pulses per second in a current of electricity. Rate of pulses has an impact on the effect of current in the body. For example, a high pulse rate can lead to tetany of a muscle*.
9. Pulse width (related to pulse rate) *Amount of time that a pulse takes to be completed. The greater the width, the fewer pulses are possible within a second*.
10. Amplitude (power or intensity) *The power or intensity of the current. Adjusted for the effect desired in the tissue. For example, high amplitudes may be required to create contraction of weakened muscles when using NMES*.
11. Polarity *Positive or negative charge. Important consideration in iontophoresis in which the charge of the treatment electrode should be the same as the medication to have repulsion of the ions into the skin*.

Worksheet 6-11: Orthotic Interventions

Resources: Coppard & Lohman, 2015; Jacobs & Austin, 2014.

1. _K_ Carpal tunnel syndrome *(volar wrist immobilization orthosis)*
2. _M_ Boutonniere deformity ring finger *(PIP extension orthosis)*
3. _R_ Upper extremity amputation *(body-powered prosthesis)*

4. __P__ Small finger metacarpal fracture (*ulnar gutter orthosis)*
5. __N__ Dupuytren release (*forearm-based dorsal extension orthosis*)
6. __T__ C6–C7 spinal cord injury (*tenodesis orthosis*)
7. __F__ Flexor tendon repair of digits (*dorsal blocking orthosis*)
8. __C__ Brachial plexus injury (*airplane splint [shoulder abduction orthosis]*)
9. __H__ Swan-neck deformity (*figure-8 finger splint [PIP hyperextension block orthosis]*)
10. __O__ Mallet finger *(DIP extension orthosis*)
11. __B__ Low-level ulnar nerve injury (*MP extension blocking orthosis*)
12. __A__ Burns to hand/wrist (*resting hand orthosis*)
13. __S__ Extrinsic extensor tightness of digits (*composite flexion orthosis)*
14. __G__ De Quervain's tenosynovitis (*forearm-based thumb spica splint [long opponens orthosis]*)
15. __L__ Elbow flexion contracture (*anterior elbow orthosis*)
16. __J__ MP joints requiring realignment secondary to RA (*ulnar deviation orthosis*)
17. __D__ Flexed digits of a client with end-stage dementia causing skin breakdown in hand (*palm protector[can also use a soft hand cone]*)
18. __E__ Low-level median nerve injury (*short opponens orthosis*)
19. __Q__ Lateral epicondylitis (*counterforce brace [tennis elbow strap]*)
20. __I__ Radial nerve palsy (*dynamic MP extension orthosis)*

Worksheet 6-12: Using Orthotic Devices

Resources: Coppard & Lohman, 2015; Jacobs & Austin, 2014.

1. C. A volar wrist extension orthosis begins proximal to the MPs and continues two-thirds of the length of the forearm. A potential pressure area is the ulnar styloid.
2. C. The OT should not discontinue the orthotic device without physician approval, particularly for an unhealed fracture.
3. B. While a pattern may be placed in the client's chart for future reference, it is not necessary to do so. Patterns are usually traced onto the thermoplastic material so that process will not avoid marks. Making a pattern does help prevent costly mistakes by not using a trial and error approach. However, the primary purpose of a pattern is to help ensure proper orthosis size and fit, determine best design, and fabricate orthotic device more efficiently.
4. D. Never place softened thermoplastic material from the heating source directly onto the client because the high heat could cause a skin burn. Cooling times vary by type and thickness of material.
5. A. The orthotic device should position the thumb in a functional position
6. A. A mallet finger orthosis typically only immobilizes the DIP joint.
7. A. The orthotic device generally should be two thirds the length of forearm.
8. D. Looping the strap through a D-ring and creating more hook and loop fastener contact will increase stability. This should be considered before fabricating a new orthotic device. However, it is essential to ensure that this new strap configuration does not cause any harmful pressure on the client's wrist. Although answer C would work, it is only a temporary solution and not the best option.
9. A. Orthotic devices with dynamic components require outriggers carefully placed to allow a proper angle of pull (normally 90°) to avoid traction or compression of a joint.
10. C. The OT should be able to easily modify the orthotic device with a heat gun (to smooth the rough edge) for better tolerance by the child. The OT's observation of redness indicates the child is not simply making up an excuse. Education should be provided to the parent and child regarding precautions and monitoring of skin integrity. A follow-up orthotic check should be scheduled. The presence of slight redness in this particular scenario is not an urgent situation that would warrant a call to the child's physician at this time.

Worksheet 6-13: Client Education

1. Purpose of orthotic device
2. Wearing schedule
3. How to don and doff orthotic device
4. Home exercise program to prevent stiffness of immobilized joints
5. Care and cleaning of orthotic device
6. Skin integrity (keeping skin dry, check for pressure areas)
7. Possible problems that may arise (pressure areas, pain, edema, etc.)
8. Protection of orthotic device (keep orthotic device away from heat sources, do not leave in car on hot day)
9. Contact information if problems should arise
10. Follow-up appointment (bring orthotic device)

Worksheet 6-14: Upper Extremity Safety

Although proper body alignment is essential, it is also important to incorporate the client's involved upper extremity into functional tasks as much as possible so that it is not just a passive appendage. For clients who have had a cerebrovascular accident, the OT practitioner can use various techniques (e.g., weight bearing, guiding, bilateral activities, CIMT, task-oriented reaching) incorporated into occupations to facilitate functional motor skills at appropriate stages of recovery (Gillen, 2011a, 2011b). The inclusion of the client's affected extremity in everyday tasks helps to promote awareness of that side, maintain mobility, and improve its function (Gillen, 2011a, 2011b; Morawski & Padilla, 2012). Of course, any precautions or contraindications must always be adhered to (e.g., fracture, fragile wound). OT practitioners must always consider the current evidence, the pros and cons of each intervention method for a specific client, and then choose a method or combination of methods most appropriate for the particular situation.

Intervention	***Pros***	***Cons***
1. Support LUE on a lap tray	• Safer position for left upper extremity (LUE) • Decreased potential for injury • LUE in visual field • May improve trunk upright posture	• May be considered a restraint • Arm may slide off lap tray • Potential for skin breakdown • Passive position
2. Support LUE on an arm trough/arm support	• Safer position for LUE • Decreased potential for injury • LUE may be in visual field • May improve trunk upright posture	• Arm may slide off of arm trough/support • May not be a naturally comfortable position for client's upper extremity • Potential for skin breakdown • Passive position
3. Educate client on proper position of LUE and risk of injury Provide verbal and written reminders Encourage client to self-correct arm position with unaffected hand	• Increases client awareness of problem and self-correction of problem	• Unilateral neglect or cognitive deficits may interfere with carryover • Client may not be able to reach and position extremity with unaffected hand

Intervention	***Pros***	***Cons***
4. Provide sling for LUE	• Keeps arm from getting caught in wheel	• Places arm in a nonfunctional, passive position • May lead to contracture for shoulder adduction and internal rotation • Arm may slide out of sling • May cause pressure around neck • Impedes voluntary motion
5. Have client look in mirror and determine what is problematic with her wheelchair posture	• Increases client awareness of problem and self-correction of problem	• Unilateral neglect or cognitive deficits may interfere with carryover
6. Use bilateral techniques and active involvement of involved arm to incorporate the extremity in functional task performance	• Increases client awareness of extremity • Promotes functional movement patterns and motor learning for occupations • Assists in joint mobility • Helps prevent disuse	• Client may overstretch joints or may drop the arm and cause injury if too aggressive, inattentive, or not careful • Unilateral neglect or cognitive deficits may interfere with carryover
Other:		

Chapter 6 References

Accreditation Council for Occupational Therapy Education. (2012). 2011 Accreditation Council for Occupational Therapy Education (ACOTE™) standards. *American Journal of Occupational Therapy, 66*(Suppl. 6), S6–S74. http://dx.doi.org/10.5014/ajot.2012.66S6

American Occupational Therapy Association. (2012). Physical agent modalities. *American Journal of Occupational Therapy, 66(Suppl. 6),* S78–S80. doi: 10.5014/ajot.2012.66S78

American Occupational Therapy Association. (2014). Occupational therapy practice framework: Domain and process, 3rd edition. *American Journal of Occupational Therapy, 68*(Suppl. 1), S1–S48.

Bandy, W. D. (2008). Open-chain-resistance training. In W. D. Bandy & B. Sanders (Eds.), *Therapeutic exercise for physical therapist assistants: Techniques for intervention* (2nd ed., pp. 103–136). Baltimore: Lippincott, Williams & Wilkins.

Bandy, W. D., & Sanders, B. (2008). *Therapeutic exercise for physical therapist assistants: Techniques for intervention* (2nd ed.). Baltimore: Lippincott, Williams & Wilkins.

Bentzel, K. (2008). Optimizing sensory abilities and capacities. In M. V. Radomski & C.A.T. Latham (Eds.). *Occupational therapy for physical dysfunction* (6th ed., pp. 714–727). Baltimore: Lippincott, Williams & Wilkins.

Bracciano, A. G. (2008). *Physical agent modalities: Theory and application for the occupational therapist* (2nd ed.). Thorofare, NJ: SLACK Incorporated.

Bracciano, A. G. (2014). Physical agent modalities. In K. Jacobs, N. MacRae, & K. Sladyk (Eds.), *Occupational therapy essentials for clinical competence* (2nd ed., pp. 439–456). Thorofare, NJ: SLACK Incorporated.

Cameron, M. H. (2009). *Physical agents in rehabilitation: From research to practice* (3rd ed.). St. Louis: Saunders.

Coppard, B. M., & Lohman, H. (Eds.) (2015). *Introduction to orthotics: A clinical reasoning & problem-solving approach* (4th ed.). St. Louis: Elsevier Mosby.

Eaton, C. (n.d.). The electronic textbook of hand surgery: Carpal tunnel syndrome. Retrieved from http://www.eatonhand.com/hw/hw006.htm

Fairchild, S. L. (2013). *Pierson and Fairchild's principles & techniques of patient care* (5th ed.). St. Louis: Saunders.

Gillen, G. (Ed.). (2011a). *Stroke rehabilitation: A function-based approach* (3rd ed.). St. Louis, MO: Elsevier Mosby.

Gillen, G. (2011b). Upper extremity function and management. In G. Gillen (Ed.), *Stroke rehabilitation: A function-based approach* (3rd ed., pp. 218–279), St. Louis, MO: Elsevier Mosby.

Hygenic Corporation. (2008). Thera-Band® exercise bands. Retrieved from http://www.thera-band.com/store/products.php?ProductID=26

Jacobs, M., & Austin, N. M. (Eds.) (2014). *Orthotic intervention for the hand and upper extremity: Splinting principles and process* (2nd ed.). Baltimore: Lippincott, Williams & Wilkins.

Knight, K. L., & Draper, D. O. (2013). *Therapeutic modalities: the art and science* (2nd ed.). Philadelphia: Lippincott Williams & Wilkins.

Levit, K. (2008). Optimizing motor behavior using the Bobath approach. In M. V. Radomski & C.A.T. Latham (Eds.), *Occupational therapy for physical dysfunction* (6th ed., pp. 642–666). Baltimore: Lippincott, Williams & Wilkins.

Minor, M. A., & Minor, S. D. (2010). *Patient care skills* (6th ed.). Upper Saddle River, NJ: Pearson Education.

Morawski, D. L., & Padilla, R. (2012). Working with elders who have had cerebrovascular accidents. In R. L. Padilla, S. Byers-Connon, & H. L. Lohman (Eds.), *Occupational therapy with elders: Strategies for the COTA* (3rd ed., pp. 263–274). Maryland Heights, MO: Elsevier Mosby.

Morreale, M. J. (2015). *Developing clinical competence: A workbook for the OTA*. Thorofare, NJ: SLACK Incorporated.

Radomski, M. V., & Latham, C.A.T. (Eds.). (2008). *Occupational therapy for physical dysfunction* (6th ed.). Baltimore: Lippincott, Williams & Wilkins.

Rust, K. L. (2008). Managing deficit of first-level motor control capacities using Rood and proprioceptive neuromuscular facilitation techniques. In M. V. Radomski & C.A.T. Latham (Eds.), *Occupational therapy for physical dysfunction* (6th ed., pp. 690–713). Baltimore: Lippincott, Williams & Wilkins.

Rybski, M. F. (2012). *Kinesiology for occupational therapy* (2nd ed.). Thorofare, NJ: SLACK Incorporated.

Skirven, T., Osterman, A. L., Fedorczyk, J., & Amadio, P. C. (Eds.). (2011). *Rehabilitation of the hand and upper extremity* (6th ed.). Philadelphia: Elsevier.

Stubblefield, K., & Armstrong, A. (2008). Amputations and prosthetics. In M. V. Radomski & C.A.T. Latham (Eds.), *Occupational therapy for physical dysfunction* (6th ed., pp. 1264–1294). Baltimore: Lippincott, Williams & Wilkins.

Wilbarger, J., & Wilbarger, P. (2002). The Wilbarger approach to treating sensory defensiveness. In A. C. Bundy, S. L. Lane, & E. A. Murray (Eds.), *Sensory integration theory and practice* (2nd ed.) (pp. 335–338). Philadelphia: F.A. Davis.

Wilk, K. E., & Reinold, M. M. (2008). Closed-kinetic-chain exercise. In W. D. Bandy & B. Sanders (Eds.), *Therapeutic exercise for physical therapist assistants: Techniques for intervention* (2nd ed., pp. 171–188). Baltimore: Lippincott, Williams & Wilkins.

Chapter 7

Evaluating Client Function

A client's level of function and occupational engagement are determined through such various means as skilled observation, formal and informal assessments, and interviews with client or family/significant others. An occupational therapist (OT) is responsible for directing and documenting the initial evaluation and establishing the occupational therapy intervention plan (American Occupational Therapy Association [AOTA], 2010, 2014a). Occupational therapy assistants (OTAs) collaborate with OTs to perform select, delegated responsibilities to help assess and document client function and implement skilled interventions, all in accordance with regulatory guidelines and payer requirements (AOTA, 2010, 2014a). During each intervention session, occupational therapy practitioners use clinical judgment to ascertain safety, changes in the client's situation, areas of progress, and specific factors impeding progress or ability to engage in occupations. This chapter presents worksheets and learning activities to help you identify and document levels of function accurately and measure your ability to implement various assessments correctly. Much of the content and methods referenced in this chapter pertain primarily to adult clients, such as the exercises on manual muscle testing and client factors. However, using clinical judgment, a therapist might determine that some of these tests may be appropriate (or modified) for use with adolescents or younger children in certain situations. Other content in this chapter can more easily be generalized for use with children, such as the exercises regarding assist levels, observation skills, and goal statements. More specific information regarding pediatric practice and the unique needs and occupations of children is presented in Chapter 10. Further information regarding assessments and methods used in mental health practice is presented in Chapter 8. Answers to worksheet exercises are provided at the end of the chapter.

Contents

Morreale, M. J., & Amini, D.
The Occupational Therapist's Workbook for Ensuring Clinical Competence (pp. 247-277).

Worksheet 7-1

Determining Assist Levels

Indicate the specific type of cues or level of assistance (e.g., contact guard, moderate, maximum) you would document for each of the following client scenarios.

1. ______________________ The client donned socks by herself using a sock aid.
2. ______________________ After assessing the resident's transfer skills, the OT determined the resident needs someone next to her for safety in case the resident forgets to lock the wheelchair brakes or moves too quickly.
3. ______________________ The client needed three reminders to look to the left during lunch to find all the food on the plate.
4. ______________________ The client required a hydraulic lift to transfer from bed to wheelchair.
5. ______________________ The resident needed both the OT and PT to help him transfer from the wheelchair to the mat, but was able to bear some weight on his weak leg.
6. ______________________ During a toothbrushing task, the client could not put the paste on or hold and manipulate the brush. She did, however, open her mouth, rinse, and spit on command.
7. ______________________ The OT noted that the resident can feed herself after the containers are opened and food is cut.
8. ______________________ The student zippered her jacket by herself, and the OT told her she did a good job.
9. ______________________ The OT put the crayon in the child's weak hand and helped him hold it. She then guided the child's arm so he could draw a circle.
10. ______________________ The client returned to her room and fed herself after the OT let the client know that the lunch tray was in her room.
11. ______________________ The client needed a little help to bring the shirt around his back and line up the first button when completing upper body dressing.
12. ______________________ During the card-making craft activity, the OT sat next to the client who demonstrated suicidal tendencies.
13. ______________________ During recess, the OT looked out the window periodically to monitor and ensure the child was playing cooperatively with the other children on the playground.
14. ______________________ While the client was standing and cooking at the stove, the OT placed his arm gently on her shoulder in case she became unsteady.
15. ______________________ The client who has chronic obstructive pulmonary disease (COPD) needed several rest breaks to unload the dishwasher.
16. ______________________ Only after the OT put a red line at the left margin could the client with left neglect read the newspaper article.
17. ______________________ During mealtime, the OT had to touch the client's arm a few times to prompt her to bring food to her mouth.
18. ______________________ The child needed help for about half of the shoe-tying task.
19. ______________________ The client would only remember to take her medicine when her cell phone timer buzzed.
20. ______________________ The student demonstrated the ability to use her power wheelchair well, so the OT put a smiley face sticker on the wheelchair.

Worksheet 7-2

Assessing Feeding

Chen, a 75-year-old male from China, sustained a myocardial infarction 4 days ago while visiting his adult children in New York. He has remained hospitalized since that time. Yesterday, the doctor ordered occupational therapy, and Chen was evaluated by the OT. The intervention plan includes goals for increasing Chen's activity tolerance for feeding and grooming while seated in a chair. Today, the OT is working with Chen at breakfast and observes that Chen does not make eye contact, is not picking up the utensils, and is shaking his head "no." What do you think might be a reason for Chen's behavior and refusal to eat? List at least 10 possibilities.

Examples: *Chen may be depressed regarding his recent heart attack.*
Chen may not feel hungry at this time or might have just eaten something else.

1.

2.

3.

4.

5.

6.

7.

8.

9.

10.

Learning Activity 7-1: Client Interview

OT practitioners gather important information by interviewing clients and family/significant others. The focus of an interview and specific questions asked will vary depending on the client's diagnosis and circumstances, the type of practice area, specific services provided, and priorities for care. Besides carefully considering the client's responses, OT practitioners use skilled observations to assess the client's mood, demeanor, social interaction skills, cognitive abilities, and motor skills, among other factors. For example, is the client able to maintain attention for the duration of the interview? Does the client make eye contact? Can the client maintain an upright sitting posture? Are tremors or spasticity exhibited? Does the client have difficulty recalling or understanding information? To practice your interview skills, use the form in Figure 7-1 to interview a family member, classmate, or friend. Although this form may help to determine a client's social history, develop an occupational profile, or screen for problem areas, it may need to be adapted for different populations or situations. Additionally, this form does not include all of the client's demographic data or insurance information that might be present on a "real" form. Be sure to explain the purpose of the interview and let the person you are interviewing know that he or she can choose not to answer any of the questions. It is also important to keep the information confidential, so do not use the person's real name or date of birth on the form. Of course, for an actual client, identifying information would always be included and the OT practitioner would use therapeutic communication techniques to probe further if the client was not forthcoming or particular concerns were noted. Review Chapter 1 for tips regarding active listening and asking open- vs closed-ended questions.

After the interview, elicit feedback about your performance from the person you interviewed. For example, did you speak too quickly or use too much technical jargon? Did you ask questions clearly, confidently, and concisely? Did the interview "flow"? Did the person feel that you appeared interested in his or her responses? Did you spend too much time looking at the form and writing rather than focusing directly on the person? Reflect on any difficulties you may have encountered during this experience. Determine what you might have done better or how you could have worded your questions differently. It is also useful to practice interviewing people from different age groups (e.g., a 10-year-old and an 80-year-old) to compare and contrast factors such as amount of time required, style of questioning, demeanor of the people being interviewed, their life views, and types of responses.

Feedback elicited:

Difficulties encountered:

Changes needed:

Learning Activity 7-1: Client Interview (continued)

Client Interview Form

Client name: ______________________ Date: ______________________
Date of birth: ______________________ Age: ______________________
Gender: ______________________

Diagnosis/medical concerns: ______________________

Marital status: ☐ Married ☐ Widowed ☐ Divorced ☐ Single ☐ Domestic partnership
☐ Other ______________________

Emergency contact: ______________________
Contact phone number: ______________________
Relationship to client: ______________________

Cultural Considerations: ______________________

Communication: ☐ Intact ☐ Impaired ☐ Hard of hearing ☐ Hearing aid ☐ Aphasia
☐ Other ______________________

Level of Education Completed: ______________________
Special training/skills: ______________________
Desired skills or education: ______________________

Work: Type of occupation ______________________
☐ Presently working ☐ Works full-time ☐ Works part-time ☐ Works from home
☐ Works occasionally ☐ Retired ☐ Never worked ☐ Volunteers ______________________
What does client like/dislike about present work? ______________________

Living Situation:
☐ Owns home ☐ Condo/co-op ☐ Apartment ☐ Relative's home ☐ Assisted living facility
☐ Institution ☐ Rents a room ☐ Other ______________________
Children: ☐ Yes ☐ No ______________________
Lives with others: ☐ Yes ☐ No ______________________
Stairs/architectural barriers: ______________________
Pets: ☐ Yes ☐ No ______________________

Emergency Preparedness:
☐ Smoke alarm ☐ CO_2 detector ☐ Flashlight/batteries ☐ Fire extinguisher
☐ Personal emergency response system/panic button ☐ Portable/cell phone ☐ Bottled water
☐ Nonperishable food and manual can opener

BADL/IADL:
Daily living skills that client needs help with: ______________________

Dietary considerations: ______________________

Functional Mobility: Assistance needed ☐ Yes ☐ No
☐ No devices used ☐ Cane ☐ Quad cane ☐ Walker ☐ Rollator ☐ Crutches
☐ Manual wheelchair ☐ Power wheelchair ☐ Power mobility scooter ☐ Other ______________________

Figure 7-1A. Client Interview Form (page 1).

Client Interview Form (continued)

Community Mobility: Transportation adequate for needs: ☐ Yes ☐ No
☐ Drives own car ☐ Relative drives ☐ Friend drives ☐ Walks ☐ Uses a taxi ☐ Bus ☐ Train
☐ County/town transit for elderly/disabled

Rest and Sleep:
Reported stress level (0 to 10 scale) ____________
Hours of sleep per night?____________ Takes naps? ____________
Sleep interrupted by: ☐ Pain ☐ Bathroom needs ☐ Caregiver responsibilities ☐ Anxiety ☐ Noise
☐ Other____________

Play/Leisure:
List three favorite activities and frequency:
1. ____________
2. ____________
3. ____________
Hobbies/special interests or talents:____________
Hours per day watching TV:____________
Does client read: ☐ Books ☐ Newspapers ☐ Magazines
Amount and type of daily/weekly exercise: ____________

Habits Impacting Health:
Tobacco use:____________ Alcohol use: ____________
Other: ____________

Computer Skills:
☐ Excellent ☐ Good ☐ Fair ☐ Poor ☐ Do not use
Hours per day using computer: ☐ Work________ ☐ Leisure ________
Computer or leisure skills desired: ____________

Social Participation:
Clubs, groups, religious organizations:____________
____
Easily engages in activities: ☐ Yes ☐ No
Satisfied with amount of friends: ☐ Yes ☐ No
Prefers: ☐ Individual activities ☐ Group activities ☐ Activities at home ☐ Activities in community
Barriers to leisure or social participation: ____________

Personal Goal: ____________
____
____

OT/OTA signature:____________

Figure 7-1B. Client Interview Form (page 2).

Worksheet 7-3
Assessing Client Factors

1. The OT asked an OTA to use a visual analogue scale with a particular client. This type of scale is used to measure which of the following?
   A. Weight
   B. Oxygen level
   C. Visual acuity
   D. Pain

2. The handle of a Jamar Hydraulic Dynamometer can be adjusted to how many grip positions?
   A. 3
   B. 4
   C. 5
   D. 6

3. When using a Jamar Hydraulic Dynamometer, the OT practitioner should place the client's upper extremity in which of the following positions?
   A. 90° shoulder flexion, adduction, 90° elbow flexion, forearm in neutral position
   B. 0° shoulder flexion, adduction, 90° elbow flexion, forearm in neutral position
   C. 90° shoulder flexion, adduction, 90° elbow flexion, supination
   D. 0° shoulder flexion, 90° abduction, 90° elbow extension, forearm in neutral position

4. When using a manual sphygmomanometer with a client, an OT notices it is not inflating when the device is initially squeezed. Which of the following primary actions should the OT take?
   A. Plug it into a different electrical outlet
   B. Turn the valve in the opposite direction
   C. Change the handle position
   D. Reset the device to zero

5. When using a handheld pinch meter to test lateral pinch, the OT practitioner should place the client's upper extremity in which of the following positions?
   A. 90° shoulder flexion, adduction, 90° elbow flexion, full pronation
   B. 90° shoulder flexion, adduction, 90° elbow flexion, forearm in neutral position
   C. 0° shoulder flexion, adduction, 90° elbow flexion, forearm in neutral position
   D. 0° shoulder flexion, adduction, 90°elbow flexion, full supination

6. To test a client's pinch strength, an OT is using a handheld pinch meter with a manual reset knob. The OT determines that the pinch meter needle is already set at zero. When the client squeezes the device, the OT observes that the needle does not move from the zero position to register pinch strength like the device did earlier in the day. This is the only pinch meter in the clinic. What is the primary action the OT should take?
   A. Turn the pinch meter over and have the client squeeze the device again
   B. Turn the pinch meter knob the opposite way and have the client squeeze the device again
   C. Notify the director of OT that the device is broken
   D. Contact the facility maintenance/engineering department to ascertain if the device can be fixed

Worksheet 7-3 (continued)

Assessing Client Factors

7. When using a volumeter to assess edema, the client should immerse the upper extremity until the plastic stop is between which two digits?
   A. Thumb and index
   B. Ring and small
   C. Index and long
   D. Long and ring

8. During an initial evaluation, the OT assessed a client's right-hand edema using a volumeter containing tap water. The OT documented the results as 550 mL. One week later, the OTA retested the client's same hand and documented the results as 520 mL. However, because there was a problem with the clinic's water supply at that time, the OTA used bottled water to fill the volumeter. The change from 550 to 520 mL is most likely due to:
   A. Decreased edema
   B. Increased edema
   C. OTA tester error
   D. OTA using bottled water rather than tap water

9. A client sustained a dislocation injury to his right index finger proximal interphalangeal (PIP) joint. An OT is taking circumferential measurements of the index finger PIP joint and documents the joint measurement as 6.2 cm. A week earlier the same joint measured 5.7 cm. The client's left index finger PIP joint has a measurement of 5.4 cm. As a result, the OT should document that the client's right PIP joint demonstrates:
   A. Decreased range of motion (ROM)
   B. Decreased edema
   C. Increased edema
   D. An infection

10. An OT is working with a client diagnosed with chronic obstructive pulmonary disease (COPD) who receives oxygen through a nasal cannula. Today, the OT is delegating this client's intervention to an OTA. Because the client has been exhibiting dyspnea on exertion, the OT asked the OTA to assess and document vital signs during the client's self-care routine today. The OTA should interpret this as taking measurements for all of the following except:
    A. Oxygen saturation levels
    B. Heart rate
    C. Systolic pressure
    D. Body temperature

Learning Activity 7-2: Evidence-Based Practice—Grip Strength

With a partner, use a dynamometer that has adjustable grip positions, such as a Jamar Hydraulic Dynamometer. The person being tested should squeeze the dynamometer with the device set at each of the adjustable handle positions. Note grip scores in order, beginning from the narrowest grip position and progressing to the widest handle position. The device should be reset to zero after each squeeze and the person being tested should exert maximum effort for each trial. Plot the measurements on a graph and connect the dots.

1. ______________________ pounds
2. ______________________ pounds
3. ______________________ pounds
4. ______________________ pounds
5. ______________________ pounds

Measure grip strength again with the dynamometer set at each of the handle positions, resetting to zero after each squeeze. This time, however, the person being tested should give less than maximal effort to misrepresent actual strength (as a malingering client might do to avoid showing progress). Note grip scores in order, beginning from the narrowest grip position and progressing to the widest handle position. Plot the measurements on a graph and connect the dots.

1. ______________________ pounds
2. ______________________ pounds
3. ______________________ pounds
4. ______________________ pounds
5. ______________________ pounds

Now compare the two graphs. Are they similar or different in terms of shapes or slopes? Find five evidence-based articles to determine whether graphing the five grip positions is clinically valid when attempting to determine whether a client is actually exerting maximum effort.

Reprinted with permission from Morreale, M. J. (2015). *Developing clinical competence: A workbook for the OTA*. Thorofare, NJ: SLACK Incorporated.

Worksheet 7-4

Assessing Additional Client Factors

1. An OT is assessing static two-point discrimination for a client who has undergone digital nerve repair surgery to his right index finger. When using a Disk-Criminator or aesthesiometer, on the fingertip, which of the following measurements would be considered in the normal range?
   A. 1 cm
   B. 5 cm
   C. 5 mm
   D. 8 mm

2. How much pressure should the occupational therapy practitioner apply when administering a static two-point discrimination test?
   A. Until the filament begins to bend
   B. 5 mm of pressure
   C. Until the client is able to feel the stimulus
   D. Until the skin blanches

3. An OT is using Semmes-Weinstein monofilaments to assess a client's sensation. The progression of colors indicating sensation level in order from better to worse is:
   A. Green, blue, purple, red
   B. Green, yellow, red, blue
   C. Blue, green, purple, red
   D. Blue, purple, red, black

4. A pulse oximeter is used in health care to assess which of the following?
   A. Heart rate
   B. Blood pressure
   C. Oxytocin levels
   D. Blood oxygen saturation levels

5. An OT is assessing a client's right upper extremity passive ROM (PROM). Which of the following observations noted by the therapist would indicate an abnormal end feel?
   A. Shoulder external rotation: Capsular stretch
   B. Wrist flexion: Hard
   C. Elbow flexion: Soft
   D. Elbow extension: Hard

6. An OT is assessing a client's right upper extremity PROM. Which of the following observations noted by the therapist would indicate a normal end feel?
   A. Shoulder flexion: Springy block
   B. Shoulder abduction: Capsular stretch
   C. Thumb MP flexion: Hard
   D. Elbow extension: Soft

Worksheet 7-4 (continued)

Assessing Additional Client Factors

7. An outpatient female client has a diagnosis of adhesive capsulitis. An OT is assessing the client's active ROM (AROM) for right shoulder flexion. The therapist observes that when the client raises the affected arm, the client elevates her right scapula excessively. Which of the following is least appropriate for the therapist to do?
   A. Ask client to perform active shoulder flexion again but tell her to "relax the shoulder"
   B. Document that the client has poor motor planning
   C. Have client perform AROM in front of a mirror
   D. Provide a tactile cue

8. An OT is assessing AROM for a client who has cognitive deficits. When the OT verbally asks the client to follow various upper extremity commands (e.g., "lift your arm up over your head"), the OT observes that the client is attending, but is not performing the motions correctly. What primary action should the OT take?
   A. Write down simple instructions for these motions
   B. Document that the client is noncompliant
   C. Speak in a louder voice
   D. Demonstrate the active motions

9. An OT needs to assess sitting balance for a male client who sustained a cerebrovascular accident (CVA). Of the following choices, which is the most useful method for the OT to assess dynamic sitting balance?
   A. Client sitting on edge of bed and remaining stationary with client's arms folded in lap
   B. Client positioned in Fowler position in bed while self-feeding
   C. Client sitting on the mat and reaching for items on either side
   D. Client sitting in a chair while shaving

10. An OT is assessing a client's muscle tone for the biceps muscle. Which of the following techniques is most appropriate for the OT to use to determine muscle tone?
   A. PROM with a quick stretch
   B. PROM with a slow stretch
   C. Active resisted flexion
   D. Active resisted extension

Assessing Muscle Strength

The questions in Worksheets 7-5 and 7-6 assume that the OT practitioner is performing a *conventional manual muscle test* (MMT), rather than a functional screening, to assess the strength of a muscle or muscle groups for particular joint motions. When administering a MMT, the examiner considers the effects of gravity and places the client in test-specific positions (supine, prone, side-lying, sitting, or standing), according to the motions being tested. Depending on a particular client's situation, such as diagnosis, precautions, contraindications, available time, treatment priorities, and client mobility, an OT practitioner might use clinical judgment to modify standard techniques and perform a functional strength test instead. A functional strength test, rather than a standard MMT, might entail having the client remain lying supine in bed or sitting in a wheelchair for all muscle groups being tested. For example, it may not be contraindicated or not feasible for a client with a recent total hip replacement (THR) or a frail elderly client to assume a prone position. The methods used should be clearly documented in the client's chart. Use Figure 7-2 to help you with the clinical decision-making process for performing a MMT. It is important to realize that, although most sources are generally consistent in defining the muscle grades of Normal (N), Good (G), Fair (F), Poor (P), Trace (T), and Zero (0), differences are evident in the definitions of plus (+) and minus (–) muscle grades (Clarkson, 2013; Flinn, Latham, & Podolski, 2008; Jacobs & Simon, 2015; Latella & Meriano, 2003; Liska & Gonzelez, 2013; Reese, 2012; Rybski, 2012). The muscle grades used in this section delineate Fair– (F–) as incomplete ROM against gravity (greater than 50%) and Poor+ (P+) as incomplete ROM against gravity (less than 50%) (Clarkson, 2013; Reese, 2012). Use the grading system and methods that are standard for your facility.

Some clinical tips when performing a MMT:

- Always adhere to any precautions and contraindications based on the client's condition and situation. Not all clients will require a MMT. Not all clients will be able to assume standard test positions safely.
- Use easy-to-understand instructions instead of technical jargon when asking a client to perform a particular active motion. For example, for shoulder flexion, rather than saying, "*Flex your shoulder,*" you might say, "*Lift your arm up over your head*" or "*Reach up to the ceiling.*" It is helpful to demonstrate the desired motions.
- An easier way to remember and visualize proper client position is to consider that motions against gravity move upward toward the ceiling (e.g., flexion and abduction while seated or standing, horizontal adduction in supine) and the positions minimizing the effects of gravity allow for motions to be performed parallel to the floor (scapula elevation while prone; horizontal abduction while seated; shoulder flexion while side lying).
- If you observe that the client does not exhibit full AROM, do not automatically assume that weakness or joint problems exist. The client will often exhibit more complete motion if you simply provide an additional verbal cue such as, "*Can you lift your arm up any higher than that*?" or "*Can you turn your hand over any further*?"
- A main defining factor and baseline in MMT decision making is determining whether the client can perform full *available* AROM against gravity (at least a muscle grade of Fair). If the client is able to do this, resistance is applied, and the resulting muscle grade can then only be Fair, Fair+, Good, or Normal (some facilities also use G+ and G–). If the client does not meet that baseline, there are two options: (1) the client has already demonstrated the criteria for F– or P+ (depending on amount of motion exhibited) and the test is complete; or (2) based on the criteria, the client must be positioned in a gravity-reduced position to determine a muscle grade of Poor, Trace, or Zero.
- As a means to help with remembering, one of the author's (MJM's) students have dubbed the muscle grade of F+ as "shake and break," meaning that the muscle can sustain a minimal amount of resistance but struggles (shakes) with any greater resistance and lowers downward (breaks).
- A joint limitation or contracture does not necessarily indicate decreased strength. When performing a MMT, if AROM and PROM of a particular joint are equal (client moves through available joint range), then resistance should be applied to determine strength (Reese, 2012). For example, a bodybuilder with pectoralis muscle bulk may demonstrate limited ROM for the antagonist of horizontal abduction. However, this is would not necessarily signify that the bodybuilder has decreased muscle strength for horizontal abduction.

Assessing Muscle Strength (continued)

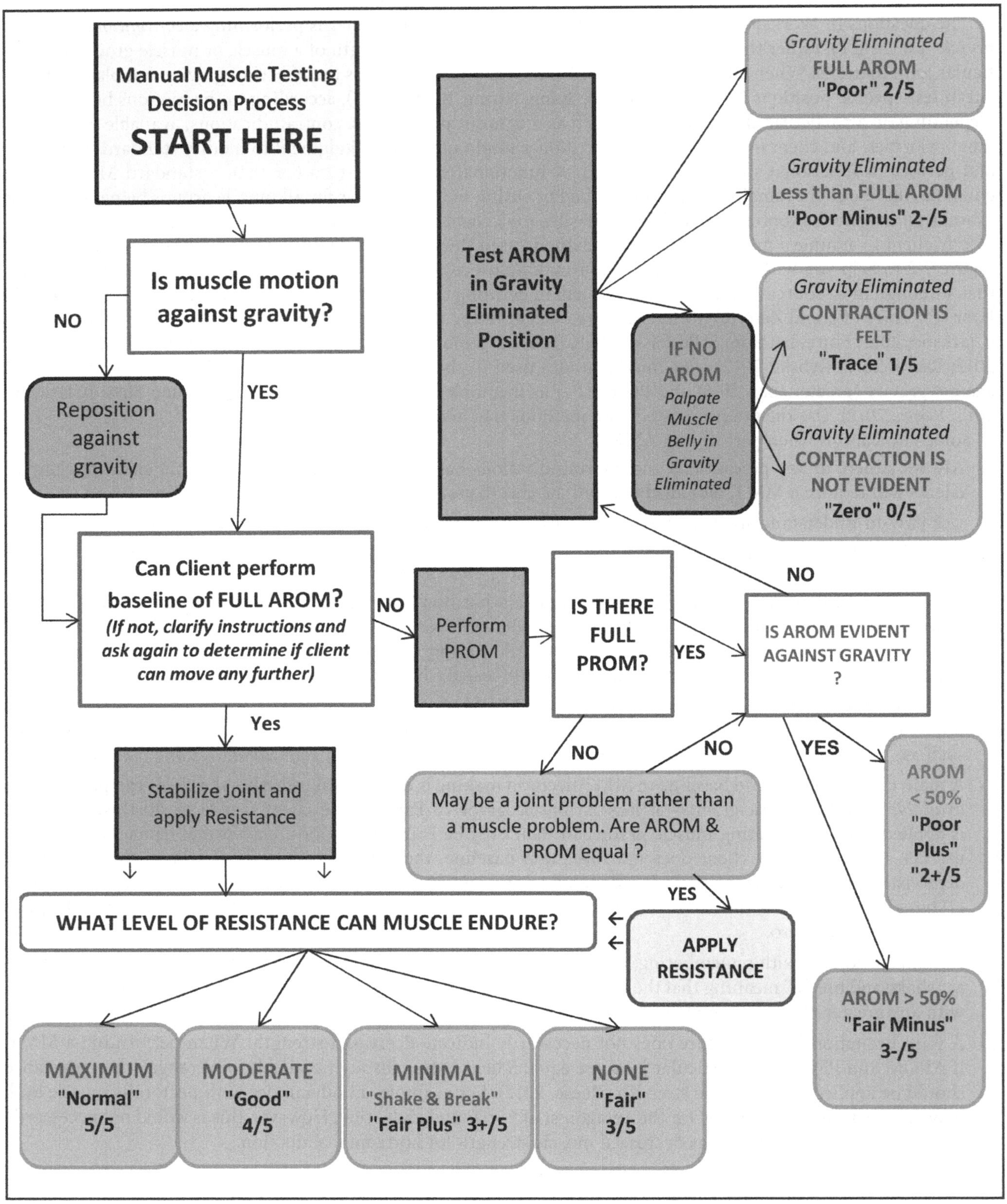

Figure 7-2. Manual muscle test flow chart. (Adapted from Marie Morreale course lecture notes and developed by Elaine Trainor, COTA. Reprinted with permission from Morreale, M. J. [2015]. *Developing clinical competence: A workbook for the OTA*. Thorofare, NJ: SLACK Incorporated.)

Worksheet 7-5

Assessing Muscle Strength

1. An OT is performing a MMT bedside to determine a client's muscle strength for right shoulder flexion. The client, who is seated at the edge of the bed, is unable to initiate lifting his arm into shoulder flexion, but exhibits full PROM. To complete the MMT for shoulder flexion, the OT should place the client in which of the following positions?
   A. Side lying in bed
   B. Supine
   C. Prone with arm hanging off side of bed
   D. Not applicable as the test is now complete

2. An athlete with a shoulder condition is receiving outpatient occupational therapy. When performing a MMT for shoulder external rotation, the OT should initially position the client in which of the following positions?
   A. Sitting in a chair
   B. Side-lying in bed
   C. Supine
   D. Prone

3. When performing a MMT for wrist flexion, on what aspect of the client's extremity should the occupational therapy practitioner apply resistance?
   A. Volar forearm
   B. Volar palm
   C. Volar digits
   D. Dorsal hand

4. While performing a MMT on a 35-year-old client who has good balance and mobility, the OT observes that the client cannot shrug his shoulders while sitting in the chair. For this motion, the next position for the therapist to place the client in is which of the following?
   A. Kneeling on a mat
   B. Sitting on edge of bed
   C. Standing
   D. Prone

5. When assessing muscle strength for wrist extension, a client can perform full AROM with his hand resting sideways on the ulnar side (on a tabletop). However, the client is unable to initiate wrist extension with the palm resting face down on the table. The muscle grade is most likely which of the following?
   A. Fair
   B. Fair –
   C. Poor
   D. Trace

Worksheet 7-5 (continued)

Assessing Muscle Strength

6. A client can perform full active supination against gravity. The next step for the MMT for this motion is:
   A. Nothing as test is completed and muscle grade is fair
   B. Nothing as test is completed and muscle grade is 5/5
   C. Perform PROM to forearm
   D. Apply resistance

7. A client admitted to a skilled nursing facility after a left total knee replacement exhibits both AROM and PROM for right shoulder flexion as 0 to 100°. The OT also observes that the client is unable to sustain any resistance applied to the shoulder flexor muscles. This muscle grade should be documented as:
   A. Poor
   B. Fair
   C. Poor+
   D. Fair+

8. A client exhibits full passive elbow ROM but can only actively flex his elbow three-quarters of the range when seated. This muscle grade should be documented as:
   A. Fair
   B. Fair+
   C. Fair minus
   D. Poor

9. When performing a MMT to test muscle strength for horizontal adduction, the OT should place the client in which start position?
   A. Supine
   B. Sitting
   C. Side-lying
   D. Prone

10. Which of the following clients is likely the most appropriate to place in the standard MMT initial test position to test muscle strength for internal rotation?
    A. A 40-year-old carpenter currently in reconditioning phase of therapy after rotator cuff surgery
    B. A 35-year-old athlete with a shoulder condition who is also 3 weeks status post-open heart surgery
    C. A 70-year-old homemaker 3 days status post-THR who requires upper body strengthening for walker use
    D. A 45-year-old female who underwent surgery for a mastectomy 1 week ago

Worksheet 7-6

Assessing Muscle Strength—More Practice

1. An OT is performing a MMT to test a client's muscle strength for shoulder extension (hyperextension). After completing the initial step, the OT determines the client must be placed in a gravity-reduced position to complete the test, which, for that motion, is which of the following positions?
   A. Sitting
   B. Standing
   C. Side-lying
   D. Prone

2. When performing a MMT to test muscle strength for shoulder abduction, the OT observes that the client exhibits 100° AROM and 160° degrees PROM. The therapist should determine that the muscle grade is which of the following?
   A. Fair
   B. Fair+
   C. Fair–
   D. Undetermined; need to further test in a gravity eliminated position

3. A client can fully flex his biceps muscle against gravity. To complete the MMT for the biceps, the OT should do which of the following?
   A. Nothing; the test is now complete, and muscle grade is 3/5
   B. Nothing; the test is now complete, and muscle grade is 5/5
   C. Place client in gravity minimized position
   D. Apply resistance

4. When performing a MMT to test muscle strength for shoulder internal rotation, the OT should apply resistance to what aspect of the client's upper extremity?
   A. Distal forearm with client prone
   B. Distal forearm with client supine
   C. Distal forearm with client sitting
   D. Distal humerus with client prone

5. An OT is performing a MMT to test a client's muscle strength for MP extension. The therapist should place the client's upper extremity in which start position?
   A. Palm resting face down on table
   B. Hand sideways with ulnar side of hand resting on table
   C. Hand sideways with thumb side of hand resting on table
   D. Hand supported on table with palm facing up

Worksheet 7-6 (continued)

Assessing Muscle Strength—More Practice

6. An OT observes that the client can only touch his thumb to the index and long fingers. Of the following choices, the muscle most likely affected is which of the following?
   A. Flexor digitorum profundus
   B. Opponens pollicis
   C. Abductor digiti minimi
   D. Flexor pollicis longus

7. A client is unable to actively flex his MPs to 70° while simultaneously extending his proximal and distal interphalangeal joints (PIPs and DIPs). PROM is within normal limits. Of the following choices, which muscle is most likely affected?
   A. Lumbricals
   B. Extensor carpi radialis
   C. Flexor digitorum superficialis
   D. Flexor digitorum profundus

8. A client is demonstrating difficulty with tendon gliding after a zone 2 flexor tendon repair. As a result, the OT should primarily work toward facilitating movement of which of the following muscles?
   A. Opponens pollicis and opponens digiti minimi
   B. Extensor pollicis longus and extensor pollicis brevis
   C. Flexor carpi radialis and flexor carpi ulnaris
   D. Flexor digitorum profundus and flexor digitorum superficialis

9. A client diagnosed with carpal tunnel syndrome is exhibiting weakness of his median innervated intrinsic muscles. These would include which of the following muscles?
   A. Adductor pollicis, flexor pollicis brevis, opponens pollicis
   B. Flexor pollicis brevis, opponens pollicis, abductor pollicis longus
   C. Opponens pollicis, adductor pollicis, abductor pollicis brevis
   D. Flexor pollicis brevis, opponens pollicis, abductor pollicis brevis

10. A client has a diagnosis of low-level ulnar nerve lesion. Which of the following observations by an OT would be consistent with that condition?
   A. Inability to perform palmar abduction
   B. Inability to flex thumb metacarpophalangeal (MP)
   C. Inability to flex small finger MP
   D. Inability to flex index finger MP

Learning Activity 7-3: Assessing Pain

As part of a group exercise, participants should create a combined list of situations in which they have experienced (or are currently experiencing) physical pain. Some suggestions are listed below but the group may come up with others. According to each member's comfort level for voluntary disclosure of any personal information, members should describe their personal pain experiences. Consider the particular words needed to specifically describe pain patterns and quantify and qualify pain. For example, was the pain throbbing, burning, knife-like, prickly, or achy? Where exactly did the pain occur? Did the pain travel? Was pain constant, intermittent, or perhaps, only aggravated by specific motions or activities? What methods, if any, helped to reduce the pain? Compare and contrast the description of pain with several members who have experienced the same conditions. Participants might also discuss the personal effects of pain in regards to their occupational performance. Determine what formal or informal pain scales would be useful to assess pain for each participant's condition or situation.

1. Broken bone
2. Sprained ankle
3. Childbirth
4. Kidney stone
5. Exercising/working out at the gym
6. Back injury/sciatica
7. Infection (sinus, ear, wound, urinary tract)
8. Headache/migraine
9. Pneumonia/pleurisy
10. Surgery
11. Toothache
12. Compressed nerve

Specific Condition	***Pain Description***	***Effect on Occupational Performance***	***Formal Pain Scales***	***Informal Pain Scales***

Worksheet 7-7

Improving Observation Skills—Appearance and Hygiene

Clients with conditions such as brain injuries, intellectual disabilities, mental health conditions, or developmental delay require assessment of various factors and skills that reflect mental function, process skills, and ability to interact within social norms. What might you observe and document regarding your client that would indicate a well-groomed appearance vs poor hygiene, health factors, or an unkempt/untidy appearance? In the following chart, list objective factors pertaining to clothing, skin, face, hair, and other features.

Good Hygiene/Well-Groomed Appearance	***Poor Hygiene or Health Factors, Unkempt/Untidy Appearance***

Reprinted with permission from Morreale, M. J. (2015). *Developing clinical competence: A workbook for the OTA*. Thorofare, NJ: SLACK Incorporated.

Worksheet 7-8

Improving Observation Skills—Mood and Behavior

Clients with conditions such as brain injuries, intellectual disabilities, mental health conditions, or developmental delay require assessment of various factors and skills that reflect mental function, process skills, and ability to interact within social norms. Consider what you might observe and document as indicators of the client's present demeanor, mood, or level of thinking. In the following chart, list objective factors, such as types of behavior exhibited and statements expressed.

Behavioral Observations (Give specific examples of what the client actually did)	***Client's Verbalizations (Give specific examples of what the client actually said)***
Example: Arms crossed in front of chest or not	*Example: Client uses courteous words (e.g.,* please, thank you, may I*) or profane words/curses at family, staff, and peers on unit*
Example: Attentive or easily distracted (and by what internal or external factors)	*Example: Verbalizes or does not verbalize understanding of deficits*

Worksheet 7-9

Goal Statements

Indicate which of the statements that follow would be appropriate to use as goals in an occupational therapy intervention plan. For the statements you do not choose, rewrite them to make them appropriate as goals for pretend clients. Keep in mind that for a "real" client, goals must always pertain to the client's specific circumstances, actual needs, wants, and realistic desired outcomes.

1. ______ Client will be able to squeeze therapy putty 10 times with affected hand within 2 weeks.
2. ______ Client will increase right shoulder strength from Fair (F) to Good (G) within 1 month.
3. ______ When dressing, resident will be able to button six half-inch buttons on shirt with modified independence within two intervention sessions.
4. ______ While seated in a chair, client will perform pulley exercises with minimal assistance to increase right shoulder ROM 20° by anticipated discharge on 2/5/2016.
5. ______ Child will demonstrate ability to feed self finger foods independently using right upper extremity within 3 months.
6. ______ To complete school work independently, student will be able to write her name legibly in cursive using a built-up pen 5/5 opportunities by the end of the school year.
7. ______ By the end of 4 weeks, client will demonstrate improved activities of daily living (ADLs) by performing right hand AROM during Fluidotherapy three times a week.
8. ______ To complete bathing routine independently, client will be able to hold a bar of soap in right hand without dropping it within 2 weeks.
9. ______ Veteran will be able to use right three-point pinch to stack five 1-inch cubes 3/3 times.
10. ______ Child will be able to fasten and unfasten a belt buckle with minimal assistance.
11. ______ By the end of next session, client will be able to identify three alternatives to drinking as methods to alleviate stress at work.
12. ______ Client will perform his or her home exercise program daily.
13. ______ Resident will be able to use a right tip pinch to place 10 small pegs in pegboard within 60 seconds.
14. ______ Consumer will demonstrate ability to punch his time card at work with one verbal cue 5/5 opportunities.
15. ______ Client will demonstrate improved dynamic sitting balance while seated on edge of bed within 3 weeks.
16. ______ Client will be issued a left resting hand orthosis within 1 week.
17. ______ When transferring to tub bench, client will remember to lock wheelchair brakes 100% of the time before rising from wheelchair, by expected discharge on 4/16/2016.
18. ______ To perform toileting, client will demonstrate ability to transfer from wheelchair to a commode using a walker with standby assistance within 10 days.
19. ______ To play with mobile, infant will be able to roll from prone to supine with minimal assistance to initiate motion within 1 month.
20. ______ Client will be given a leisure inventory and be asked to complete it within 1 week.

Answers to Chapter 7 Worksheets

Worksheet 7-1: Determining Assist Levels

Resources: Jacobs & Simon, 2015; Logigian, 2015; Morreale & Borcherding, 2013; UB Foundation Activities, Inc., 2002.

Settings may vary in the specific terminology and criteria used to describe levels of function. Always use the terminology and criteria that are standard for your facility, practice setting, and payer requirements. Examples of commonly used terms and definitions are listed in Box 7-1.

1. *Modified independence* The client donned socks by herself using a sock aid.
2. *Standby assist* After assessing the resident's transfer skills, the OT determined the resident needs someone next to her for safety in case the resident forgets to lock the wheelchair brakes or moves too quickly.
3. *Three verbal cues* or *minimal verbal cues* The client needed three reminders to look to the left during lunch to find all the food on the plate.
4. *Dependent* or *total assistance* The client required a hydraulic lift to transfer from bed to wheelchair.
5. *Maximum assistance of two persons (max assist × 2)* The resident needed both the OT and PT to help him transfer from the wheelchair to the mat, but was able to bear some weight on his weak leg.
6. *Maximum assistance* During a toothbrushing task, the client could not put the paste on or hold and manipulate the brush. She did, however, open her mouth, rinse, and spit on command.
7. *Independent with setup* The OT noted that the resident can feed herself after the containers are opened and food is cut.
8. *Independent* The student zippered her jacket by herself, and the OT told her she did a good job.
9. *Hand-over-hand assistance* The OT put the crayon in the child's weak hand and helped him hold it. She then guided the child's arm so he could draw a circle.

Box 7-1.

Levels of Assistance

Total assistance (TOT)	Individual requires 100% assistance to safely complete task. Individual does not assist at all.
Maximum assistance (MAX)	Individual requires 75% of physical/cognitive assistance to safely complete task. Individual assists 25%.
Moderate assistance (MOD)	Individual requires 50% of physical/cognitive assistance to safely complete task. Individual assists 50%.
Minimal assistance (MIN)	Individual needs no more than 25% physical/cognitive assistance. Individual assists 75%.
Standby assistance (SBA)	Supervision or standby assistance for safe, effective task performance.
Set-up assistance	Individual requires set-up of necessary items to perform tasks.
Independent (IND)	No assistance or supervision is required. Able to perform independently. Safety is demonstrated during tasks.

10. *Independent* The client returned to her room and fed herself after the OT let the client know that the lunch tray was in her room.
11. *Minimal assistance* The client needed a little help to bring the shirt around his back and line up the first button when completing upper body dressing.
12. *Supervision within arm's length* or *close supervision* During the card-making craft activity, the OT sat next to the client who demonstrated suicidal tendencies.
13. *Distant supervision* or *supervision within line of sight* During recess, the OT looked out the window periodically to monitor and ensure the child was playing cooperatively with the other children on the playground.
14. *Contact guard assistance* While the client was standing and cooking at the stove, the OT placed his arm gently on her shoulder in case she became unsteady.
15. *Modified independence* The client who has COPD needed several rest breaks to unload the dishwasher.
16. *Visual cue* Only after the OT put a red line at the left margin could the client with left neglect read the newspaper article.
17. *Several tactile cues* or *minimal physical prompting* During mealtime, the OT had to touch the client's arm a few times to prompt the client to bring food to mouth.
18. *Moderate assistance* The child needed help for about half of the shoe-tying task.
19. *Auditory cue* The client would only remember to take her medicine when her cell phone timer buzzed.
20. *Independent* The student demonstrated ability to use her power wheelchair well so the OT put a smiley face sticker on the wheelchair.

Worksheet 7-2: Assessing Feeding

It is important to look at the client holistically, consider all the possibilities, and determine which of the following are applicable to Chen's situation.

1. Chen may be awaiting medical tests for which he is not allowed to eat prior.
2. Chen may not like the food choices because they may be very different from typical food in China.
3. If ethnic food is available, it may be bland or not appealing because of a low-salt or low-fat diet.
4. Chen may normally use chopsticks and may not be comfortable using silverware (Asher, 2006).
5. Food may not conform to the client's values or beliefs (e.g., religious considerations or if Chen is a vegetarian and meat was served).
6. Chen may be embarrassed to have someone helping him or watching him eat, particularly if the person is of a different gender.
7. Chen may have difficulty chewing because of missing teeth or a painful jaw.
8. Chen may have dentures that are not currently in place or are ill fitting and painful.
9. Chen may have nausea, indigestion, or a stomach ache due to constipation or medication.
10. Chen may be very tired or in pain.
11. Chen may have a poor body image or may have an eating disorder.
12. Chen may have underlying cognitive impairment or perceptual problems.
13. Chen may be waiting for his family to arrive before he eats.

Worksheet 7-3: Assessing Client Factors

1. D. This is a simple and common pain scale (Flinn, Latham, & Podolski, 2008).
2. C. (Lafayette Instrument, 2004)
3. B. (Clarkson, 2013; Lafayette Instrument, 2004)
4. B. A sphygmomanometer is a blood pressure device. When using a manual blood pressure device, if the bulb's air valve (knob) is not turned in the proper direction to close it, the cuff will not inflate. This device does not use electricity and automatically starts at zero when the cuff is deflated.

5. C. (Clarkson, 2013; Flinn et al., 2008)
6. B. In this instance, the knob was probably turned the wrong way so that the peak-hold needle (which indicates the measurement) is behind, rather than in front of, the gauge needle, which is supposed to push it.
7. D. (Flinn et al., 2008)
8. A. Bottled vs tap water should not have an effect on test results. Less water was displaced, indicating decreased edema.
9. C. When taking circumferential measurements, an increased number usually indicates increased edema (although girth can also increase due to other factors, such as a nodule, ganglion, or cyst). Although the client could be getting an infection, there are no clinical signs indicated for that, such as increased pain, redness, or increased temperature of digit. ROM measurements are not noted in this example.
10. D. The OT should measure the client's blood pressure, oxygen saturation levels, pulse rate, and note respiration rate/shortness of breath. Although it may be appropriate to assess temperature in certain situations (such as for a suspected fever or joint infection), it is not indicated in this situation.

Worksheet 7-4: Assessing Additional Client Factors

1. C. (Bentzel, 2008)
2. D. (Bentzel, 2008)
3. A. (Bentzel, 2008)
4. D
5. B. (Clarkson, 2013)
6. B. (Clarkson, 2013)
7. B. The client appears to be compensating for weakness in shoulder flexors rather than demonstrating poor motor planning. The OT should try methods to minimize muscle substitution.
8. D. Demonstration would help the client to better process the desired motions. Written instructions could be more confusing, and, unless the client has hearing impairment or is demonstrating poor attention, a louder voice would not help the situation.
9. C. Of the choices provided, sitting unsupported on a mat and weight shifting to either side would best challenge dynamic sitting balance. However, it would be even more challenging if the client were reaching for objects and weight shifting while seated on edge of bed (which is an unstable surface) rather than a static mat surface.
10. A. A quick stretch to a muscle is the traditional evaluation to determine whether resistance occurs as a response to the movement (Gillen, 2011).

Worksheet 7-5: Assessing Muscle Strength

References: Clarkson, 2013; Reese, 2012.

Clinical judgment is needed to determine whether modifications are needed for a particular client. These answers are based on standard MMT procedure.

As previously noted, motions against gravity move upward toward the ceiling (e.g., flexion and abduction while seated/standing, horizontal adduction in supine) and the positions minimizing the effects of gravity allow for motions to be performed parallel to the floor (scapula elevation while prone, horizontal abduction while seated, shoulder flexion while side-lying). Remember, it may not be safe or feasible for some clients to assume a standard test position.

1. A. The OT needs to put the client in a gravity-reduced position, which, in this situation, is side lying. The therapist should support the client's arm or use a powder board.
2. D. The against-gravity start position for external rotation is a prone position. However, this position may be too difficult for elderly clients or contraindicated for some conditions.
3. B. The test begins with client's arm resting on table with palm facing up. The client flexes the wrist and the OT applies pressure on the palm in a downward direction.

4. D. A prone position minimizes the effects of gravity for scapula elevation. Assuming a prone position may be difficult for elderly clients or contraindicated for some conditions.
5. C. The muscle grade is poor as the client is able to perform the motion in a gravity-reduced plane, but cannot move against gravity.
6. D. The test is not yet complete. The OT has determined that the client demonstrates at least a fair muscle grade, but needs to apply resistance to complete the MMT.
7. B. The client's present maximum joint range is 100°. Although the range of motion deficit is documented as a joint contracture, active and passive ranges are equal so the client has at least fair muscle strength. Resistance is then applied to complete the test, which, in this case, the client cannot sustain, so the muscle grade is Fair.
8. C. The client is unable to perform full AROM against gravity, but performs more than 50% of the motion.
9. A. A supine position allows for horizontal adduction to be performed against gravity.
10. A. Resistance is applied to distal forearm with client prone. Resistance and/or a prone position are contraindicated for the other clients because of their medical precautions.

Worksheet 7-6: Assessing Muscle Strength—More Practice

References: Clarkson, 2013; Reese, 2012.

Clinical judgment is needed to determine whether modifications are needed for a particular client. These answers are based on standard MMT procedure.

1. C. The gravity-reduced position for shoulder extension is side lying. The OT should support the client's arm or use a powder board.
2. C. The client demonstrates incomplete AROM against gravity, but more than 50% of available joint range.
3. D. The client demonstrates full AROM against gravity, so the next step is to apply resistance.
4. A. The against-gravity start position for internal rotation is a prone position. This position may not be feasible for frail elderly clients or may be contraindicated for certain conditions (e.g., recent THR).
5. A. The against-gravity start position for MP extension is with the palm facing down.
6. B. The opponens pollicis allows for thumb opposition.
7. A. The motion is performed using the lumbricals.
8. D. A flexor tendon injury in zone 2 affects differential tendon gliding of the flexor digitorum profundus (FDP) and flexor digitorum superficialis (FDS). Of course, other muscles and joints may be affected and require intervention due to secondary complications from the injury or surgery.
9. D. The adductor pollicis is ulnar nerve innervated. The abductor pollicis longus is an extrinsic muscle and is not innervated by the median nerve.
10. C. Inability to perform palmar abduction or MP flexion of thumb may indicate median nerve impairment. Inability to flex finger MPs may indicate weakness of the lumbricals, which are innervated by both the median nerve (index and long fingers) and ulnar nerve (ring and small fingers).

Worksheet 7-7: Improving Observation Skills—Appearance and Hygiene

A client's personal appearance and hygiene could be an indicator of the client's self-image, mood, health, or cognitive status. However, the mere presence of any unkempt/untidy factors listed in the answer table does not necessarily correlate to deficits in mental functions or social skills and does not necessarily need to be documented. For example, a client coming to therapy directly from a landscaping or construction job may be wearing garments with large dirt stains or tears. It is also important not to make value judgments based on one's personal fashion preferences, moral standards, or religious beliefs (Morreale & Borcherding, 2013). The OT practitioner must distinguish between factors such as a client who may have a long beard to meet religious requirements vs a client who has suddenly stopped shaving due to depression, defiance against his parents' wishes, or not understanding a job's dress code. If a client arrives with makeup applied only to one side of face or with lipstick circling her nose, clinical reasoning will ascertain whether these behaviors are influenced by particular deficits, such as left neglect or, perhaps, a psychotic episode. As another example, a teenager wearing flannel pajama pants at a coffee shop may consider himself to be fitting in with peers, whereas an

80-year-old adult would likely consider the teen's fashion choice as inappropriate for outside of the home. However, observations such as a client with disordered clothing, needle track marks, or a skeletal appearance may be quite noteworthy. Clinical judgment is always needed to determine behavior patterns, how your observations may be pertinent or significant to the client's present circumstances, and what should be noted in the client's chart.

Good Hygiene/Well-Groomed Appearance	***Poor Hygiene or Health Factors, Unkempt/Untidy Appearance***
Clean face and skin, no visible dirt or food particles present	Visible dirt or food on face/skin, presence of soap or makeup residue, strong body odor
Hair clean, combed, neatly styled	Hair greasy, dirty, uncombed, matted, presence of lice
Clean teeth, no food particles noted in mouth	Food particles stuck in teeth, gum disease, missing, discolored, or loose teeth
Clothing without wrinkles, neatly pressed, and intact	Clothing wrinkled, torn, number/size of holes, presence of multiple lint balls or large hanging threads, missing buttons
Clothing clean, without stains	Clothing unclean (e.g., has food, grass, or dirt stains, bugs)
Clothing fits properly	Clothing ill fitting (describe such issues as inability to fasten buttons or zipper due to clothing not fitting, clothing several sizes too big, undergarments visible, skirt dragging on floor, etc.)
Buttons lined up properly, fastenings closed, shoelaces tied	Fastenings open or misaligned, shoelaces untied or missing
Clothing right side out	Clothing disordered, inside out or backward
Hat centered on head, socks pulled up	Hat worn backward or falling off, socks down to ankle
Clothing matches and is complete and appropriate for occasion and weather; attention to detail with accessories	Missing an item such as a sock or shoe; clothing does not match or is not appropriate for weather or occasion
Clean shaven, facial hair neatly trimmed	Stubble (e.g., several days facial hair growth), length of beard/mustache, blood present from shaving cuts
Makeup neatly applied	Makeup streaked; lipstick, eyeliner/shadow grossly uneven or beyond typical boundaries
Nails clean, neatly shaped, and polished	Visible dirt beneath nails, length or unevenness of nails, brittleness or fungus present
Smooth, intact skin	Flaky skin, rough/scaly patches, thick callous, open sores, acne, rash, presence of needle track marks, scars from self-mutilation/cutting, nicotine stains
Weight in proportion to height	Weight not in proportion to height (e.g., skeletal, morbidly obese); note specific weight and height
Other:	
Other:	

Reprinted with permission from Morreale, M. J. (2015). *Developing clinical competence: A workbook for the OTA.* Thorofare, NJ: SLACK Incorporated.

Worksheet 7-8: Improving Observation Skills—Mood and Behavior

Avoid judgmental words when describing relevant client actions objectively and use clinical reasoning to determine how those observations are pertinent to the client's condition or situation and what is noteworthy to document (Morreale & Borcherding, 2013). For example, instead of saying, "*Client is paranoid*," a better choice of words might be, "*Client is exhibiting suspicious behavior, such as disassembling his phone and alarm clock several times daily to check if those items are bugged.*" Here are some suggestions of what to look out for, although you may come up with others.

Behavioral Observations (Give specific examples of what the client actually did)	***Client Verbalizations (Give specific examples of what the client actually said)***
Facial expression (e.g., flat affect or smiling, laughing, frowning, tearful/crying)	Identifies mood, such as feelings/thoughts of persecution, depression, happiness, anger, grief, anxiety, guilt, etc.
Eyes open or closed, level of eye contact, looks away	Positive or negative statements about self regarding appearance, abilities, or how others perceive client
Attentiveness, ability to concentrate, easily startled or distracted	Flight of ideas, confusion, lucidity, logical or illogical statements
Head and trunk upright or shoulders hunched, client stooped over	Changes answers/opinions, vacillates, repetitiveness of answers, or replies without thinking
Personal space boundaries	Specific statements that reflect various defense mechanisms (identify with examples)
Arms/legs crossed or open, leans forward or away	Stated opinion regarding future/outlook, past/present rehabilitation, or potential to change
Affectionate behaviors (hugs, kisses), readily shakes hands, or avoids personal contact	Expresses obsessive thoughts, hallucinations, or delusions
Repetitive behavior/rituals or motor activity (e.g., hand wringing, shaking/trembling, tics, nail biting, thumb sucking, rocking, spinning)	Tone and quality of speech, fluency
Client exhibits behaviors such as hitting, kicking, spitting, or hurting others	Client exhibits profane language, yells, screams, or makes other sounds
Threatening approach (points, jabs, is "in one's face")	Client acknowledges or denies problems or deficits
Pacing, timing, and level of energy exhibited (give examples of sedentary, active, manic, impulsive, cautious, reckless, suspicious behavior, etc.)	Client expresses specific realistic or unrealistic fears/anxieties
Alert, awake, energetic vs groggy, sleepy, listless	Client expresses willingness or unwillingness to change thoughts or behavior
Goal-directed behaviors or agitation, restlessness, wandering aimlessly	Client's stated attitude toward completion of task
Sits alone or engages easily with others	Verbalizes understanding of deficits or not
Tantrums or types of acting-out behaviors noted	Length of responses, uncommunicative, rambles, or guarded responses
Handling of objects (rough, destroys or throws items, handles carefully, etc.)	Uses tactful, courteous, respectful words or expresses frustration, is argumentative/tries to pick a fight

Behavioral Observations (Give specific examples of what the client actually did)	***Client Verbalizations (Give specific examples of what the client actually said)***
Avoids or seeks specific sensory stimulation	Stated sleep patterns or changes
Shares items willingly or not (e.g., sitting space, food, cigarettes, craft materials, books/magazines, tools)	Stated changes in weight (time period)
Other:	Asks staff, family, or peers for help when needed
Other:	

Adapted from Morreale, M. J., & Borcherding, S. (2013). *The OTA's guide to documentation: Writing SOAP notes* (3rd ed.). Thorofare, NJ: SLACK Incorporated.

Worksheet 7-9: Goal Statements

Resources: Gateley & Borcherding, 2012; Morreale & Borcherding, 2013; Sames, 2015.

OT goals should be occupation-based, individualized for each client, and contain outcomes that are realistically attainable. Goals must also include measurable criteria, any specific conditions, and delineate a specific time frame for completion. They should reflect functional outcomes that the client is trying to achieve rather what is being done to the client by the therapist. Additionally, goals must meet facility and third-party payer guidelines and any legal requirements.

1. ____ Client will be able to squeeze therapy putty 10 times with affected hand within 2 weeks.

   This is a preparatory intervention, not a goal. This goal needs to include a functional component such as, "Client will be able to squeeze toothpaste onto toothbrush using affected hand, within 2 weeks."

2. ____ Client will increase right shoulder strength from Fair (F) to Good (G) within 1 month.

   This goal needs to include a functional component such as, "To mop kitchen floor independently, client will increase right shoulder strength from Fair to Good within 1 month" or *"Client will increase shoulder strength by one muscle grade in order to wax his car independently within 1 month."*

3. __*__ When dressing, resident will be able to button six half-inch buttons on shirt with modified independence within 2 intervention sessions.

4. ____ While seated in a chair, client will perform pulley exercises with minimal assistance to increase right shoulder ROM 20° by anticipated discharge on 2/5/2016.

   This is a preparatory intervention, not a goal. The goal needs to include a functional component such as "Client will increase right shoulder flexion by 20° to hang clothing in closet with modified independence."

5. __*__ Child will be able to feed self finger foods independently using right upper extremity within 3 months.

6. __*__ To complete school work independently, student will be able to write her name legibly in cursive using a built-up pen 5/5 opportunities by the end of the school year.

7. ____ By the end of 4 weeks, client will demonstrate improved ADLs by performing right hand AROM during Fluidotherapy three times a week.

   This is a preparatory intervention, not a goal. Also, "improved ADLs" is not measurable and needs to specify a level of assistance. The goal should include a specific functional component using right hand such as, "Client will demonstrate ability to use right hand to apply shaving cream to face independently within 2 weeks."

8. __*__ To complete bathing routine independently, client will be able to hold a bar of soap in right hand without dropping it within 2 weeks.

9. ____ Veteran will be able to use right three-point pinch to stack five 1-inch cubes 3/3 times.

   Although this may be a developmental goal for a child and related to play, this task is a preparatory intervention for this adult client, not a goal. It also lacks a time frame. The goal needs to include a functional component such as, "Veteran will be able to don and doff eyeglasses independently using right three-point pinch within 1 month."

10. ____ Child will be able to fasten and unfasten a belt buckle with minimal assistance.

    This goal lacks a time frame for completion and should also indicate the occupation of dressing.

11. __*__ By the end of next session, client will be able to identify three alternatives to drinking as methods to alleviate stress at work.

12. ___ Client will perform his home exercise program daily.

    This goal lacks a time frame for completion and does not indicate occupation. The goal is also unclear and sounds like an intervention. For example, is the intent for the client to "remember" to perform his exercises, to "demonstrate initiative" in performing exercises, or to actually "perform exercises accurately"? Here are some suggestions that incorporate occupation: "Client will go for a daily 15-minute walk 7/7 days to relieve tension within 3 weeks" or "To maintain shoulder AROM needed for IADLS, client will demonstrate ability to perform home exercise program accurately within 1 week."

13. ___ Resident will be able to use a right tip pinch to place 10 small pegs in pegboard within 60 seconds.

    This goal lacks a time frame for completion. It is also not a functional goal for an adult, but rather an intervention or possibly an attempt to measure hand skills. Here is an occupation-based goal that incorporates tip pinch: "Client will demonstrate ability to apply a clear coat of nail polish on left fingernails within 60 seconds using a right tip pinch within 1 month."

14. ___ Consumer will demonstrate ability to punch his time card at work with one verbal cue 5/5 opportunities.

    This goal lacks a time frame for completion. "Within 1 month, consumer will demonstrate ability to punch time card with one verbal cue 5/5 opportunities."

15. ____ Client will demonstrate improved dynamic sitting balance while seated on edge of bed within 3 weeks.

    Goal lacks measurable criteria and a functional component such as, "While donning all upper body garments, client will be able to maintain dynamic sitting balance seated on edge of bed, within 1 month" or *"To perform dressing tasks, client will be able to maintain dynamic sitting balance for 5 minutes while seated on edge of bed, within one month."*

16. ____ Client will be issued a left resting hand orthosis within 1 week.

    This is a planned intervention, not a goal. Here is an example to turn this into a goal: "Client will demonstrate ability to don and doff splint independently within 1 week."

17. __*__ When transferring to tub bench, client will remember to lock wheelchair brakes 100% of the time before rising from wheelchair, by expected discharge on 4/16/2016.

18. __*__ To perform toileting, client will demonstrate ability to transfer from wheelchair to a commode using a walker with standby assistance within 10 days.

19. __*__ To play with mobile, infant will be able to roll from prone to supine with minimal assistance to initiate motion within 1 month.

20. ____ Client will be given a leisure inventory and asked to complete it within 1 week.

    This is a planned intervention, not a goal. Here is an example to turn this into a goal: "By the end of the week, client will complete a leisure checklist and identify three leisure activities that she expresses interest in resuming on discharge from facility."

Chapter 7 References

American Occupational Therapy Association. (2010). Standards of practice for occupational therapy. *American Journal of Occupational Therapy, 64*(Suppl. 6), S106–S111.

American Occupational Therapy Association. (2014a). Guidelines for supervision, roles, and responsibilities during the delivery of occupational therapy services. *American Journal of Occupational Therapy, 68*(Suppl. 3), S16–S22.

American Occupational Therapy Association. (2014b). Occupational therapy practice framework: Domain and process, 3rd edition. *American Journal of Occupational Therapy, 68*(Suppl. 1), S1–S48.

Asher, A. (2006). Asian Americans. In M. Royeen & J. L. Crabtree (Eds.), *Culture in rehabilitation: From competency to proficiency* (pp. 151–180). Upper Saddle River, NJ: Pearson Education.

Bentzel, K. (2008) Assessing abilities and capacities: Sensation. In M. V. Radomski & C. A. T. Latham (Eds.). *Occupational therapy for physical dysfunction* (6th ed., pp. 212–233). Baltimore: Lippincott, Williams & Wilkins.

Clarkson, H. M. (2013). *Musculoskeletal assessment: Joint motion and muscle testing* (3rd ed.). Philadelphia: Lippincott, Williams & Wilkins.

Flinn, N. A., Latham, C. A. T., & Podolski, C. R. (2008). Assessing abilities and capacities: Range of motion, strength, and endurance. In M. V. Radomski & C. A. T. Latham (Eds.). *Occupational therapy for physical dysfunction* (6th ed., pp. 91–185). Baltimore: Lippincott, Williams & Wilkins.

Gateley, C. A., & Borcherding, S. (2012). *Documentation manual for occupational therapy: Writing SOAP notes* (3rd ed.). Thorofare, NJ: SLACK Incorporated.

Gillen, G. (2011). Upper extremity function and management. In G. Gillen (Ed.), *Stroke rehabilitation: A function-based approach* (3rd ed., pp. 218–279). St. Louis: Elsevier Mosby.

Jacobs, K., & Simon, L. (Eds.). (2015). *Quick reference dictionary for occupational therapy* (6th ed.). Thorofare, NJ: SLACK Incorporated

Lafayette Instrument. (2004). Jamar Hydrolic Hand Dynamometer user instructions. Retrieved from http://www.limef.com/downloads/JAMARHandDynamometer.pdf

Latella, D., & Meriano, C. (2003). *Occupational therapy manual for evaluation of range of motion and muscle strength*. Clifton Park, NY: Delmar Learning.

Liska, C., & Gonzelez, T. R. (2013). Assessment of muscle strength. In M. B. Early (Ed.), *Physical dysfunction practice skills for the occupational therapy assistant* (3rd ed., pp. 132–155). St. Louis: Mosby.

Logigian, M. (2015). A businessman with a stroke. In K. Sladyk & R. Ryan (Eds.), *Ryan's occupational therapy assistant: Principles, practice issues, and techniques* (5th ed., pp. 374–389). Thorofare, NJ: SLACK Incorporated.

Morreale, M. J. (2015). *Developing clinical competence: A workbook for the OTA*. Thorofare, NJ: SLACK Incorporated.

Morreale, M. J., & Borcherding, S. (2013). *The OTA's guide to documentation: Writing SOAP Notes* (3rd ed.). Thorofare, NJ: SLACK Incorporated.

Reese, N. B. (2012). *Muscle and sensory testing* (3rd ed.). St. Louis: Elsevier Saunders.

Rybski, M. F. (2012). *Kinesiology for occupational therapy* (2nd ed.). Thorofare, NJ: SLACK Incorporated.

Sames, K. M. (2015). *Documenting occupational therapy practice* (3rd ed.). Upper Saddle River, NJ: Pearson Education.

UB Foundation Activities, Inc. (2002). Description of the levels of function and their scores. In *IRF-PAI training manual* (section III-7). Retrieved from http://www.cms.gov/Medicare/Medicare-Fee-for-Service-Payment/InpatientRehabFacPPS/downloads/irfpai-manualint.pdf

Chapter 8

Applying Knowledge and Skills in Group Leadership and Mental Health Practice

Implementing effective interventions and programs to support a client or population's occupational performance requires that occupational therapists (OTs) in all service delivery areas demonstrate traits such as professionalism, therapeutic use of self, creative problem solving, safety awareness, and good clinical reasoning skills. In the areas of mental health (behavioral health) and other activity programs (such as adult day care or assisted living), an OT must also demonstrate good behavioral observation skills, effective group leadership and mentoring skills, and the ability to select and implement appropriate activities and occupations to meet the clients' therapeutic goals. Review the information in Chapter 1 regarding therapeutic communication techniques. The worksheets and learning activities in this Chapter 8 will help you to identify various mental health settings, understand models of practice, and demonstrate knowledge of mental health interventions, including group leadership skills. Answers to worksheet exercises are provided at the end of the chapter.

Contents

Morreale, M. J., & Amini, D.
The Occupational Therapist's Workbook for Ensuring Clinical Competence (pp. 279-312).

Worksheet 8-1

Assessments for Mental Health Practice

As in all areas of occupational therapy practice, it is important to assess the level of occupational participation experienced by the clients in mental health settings. Assessment tools determine the function of underlying client factors, performance skills and patterns, and the effect of environment and context. Assessment tools assist the therapist, in collaboration with the client, to develop the most appropriate client-centered intervention plan to enhance strengths and minimize the impact of barriers to participation. Tools used by OTs also include outcome measures that determine change from the onset of intervention to treatment discontinuation.

This worksheet will help you to recall the titles of various mental health assessments and outcome measures when given their descriptions.

Write the title of the following measures next to the description (Asher, 2014; Brown & Stoffel, 2011).

- Recovery Enhancing Environment Scale
- Making Decisions Empowerment Scale
- Recovery Self-Assessment
- Hope Scale
- Model of Human Occupation Screening Tool
- Test of Grocery Shopping Skills
- Pediatric Interest Profiles
- Leisure Satisfaction Scales
- Occupational Therapy Quality of Experience and Spirituality Assessment Tool (OT-QUEST)
- Assessment of Motor and Process Skills (AMPS)
- Milwaukee Evaluation of Daily Living Skills (MEDLS)
- Canadian Occupational Performance Measure (COPM)
- Kohlman Evaluation of Living Skills (KELS)
- Bay Area Functional Performance Evaluation (BAFPE)
- Allen Cognitive Level Screen (ACLS-5)
- Allen Diagnostic Module, 2nd edition (ADM-2)
- Mental Health Inventory
- Resiliency Scales for Children and Adolescents
- Independent Living Skills Survey

1. Tool designed to assess executive function and performance within the natural context of a store. ______________________________
2. Measures perceived strength or vulnerability related to psychological resilience to identify adjustment and help determine appropriate interventions.______________________________
3. An occupation-oriented screening tool based on discussion, observation, and record review. It was created for individuals with mental illness who are unable to tolerate lengthy interviews and who demonstrate poor insight and concentration. ______________________________
4. A tool designed to specifically address the issue of spirituality and obtain both qualitative and quantitative information. ______________________________
5. Tool designed to assess areas of mental health through a structured self-report questionnaire. Areas include anxiety, depression, behavioral control, positive affect, and general distress. ______________________________
6. Assesses individual recovery as well as factors in the service environment that are considered to be resilience and recovery enhancing. ______________________________

Worksheet 8-1 (continued)

Assessments for Mental Health Practice

7. Created by an OT, this tool is a brief screening used to estimate a client's cognitive functioning and capacity to learn using a novel leather-lacing task. ______
8. A group of assessments designed to measure interest and involvement in play and leisure occupations. ______
9. Measures the degree to which recovery supporting services are evident to service users. ______
10. A standardized self-report of leisure that measures six subscales, including psychological, educational, social, relaxational, physiological, and aesthetic. ______
11. Standardized craft activities are used to test and treat working memory. ______
12. Tool assesses cognitive, affective, and performance skills in selected daily living tasks and social interactions. Originally created in the late 1970s in the San Francisco area. ______
13. This tool comprises an interview and several interactive tasks resembling typical daily activities. Tool determines the ability of the client to function independently. Created for short-term adolescent and adult inpatient populations. ______
14. A tool recommended for use in mental health settings to measure the level or hope or hopelessness. Can be used with many populations across settings and age span. ______
15. An interview-based tool that determines the level or performance of client-identified areas of occupation and the client's level of satisfaction with that performance. ______
16. Observation-based rating scale used to measure the quality of performance in basic activities of daily living (BADLs) and instrumental activities of daily living (IADLs) and assist in planning intervention. Tool looks at motor, process, and social interaction skills in all populations. ______
17. An outcome measure to determine the extent to which a recovery system transformation was successful for the client (e.g., overcoming stigma, engaging in activities, renewing hope, becoming empowered). ______
18. A comprehensive questionnaire created for persons with serious mental illness. Covers many areas of independent living through either a self-report or informant report version. ______
19. This tool is similar to the KELS, but more comprehensive. Designed to determine baseline functioning in ADL areas before treatment to determine the effectiveness of treatment and assist with planning future living situation. ______
20. Assists in tracking changes in levels of empowerment in persons with mental health challenges. ______

Learning Activity 8-1: Models of Practice for Mental Health

Describe the basic assumptions or tenets, appropriate population, assessments, and interventions used with the following models of practice/frames of reference.

1. Internal Family Systems Model
2. Transactional model
3. Psychobiological attachment theory
4. Sensory integration
5. Consumer-operated services model
6. Model of Human Occupation
7. Canadian Model of Occupational Performance
8. Role acquisition model
9. Occupational adaptation model
10. Recovery model
11. Psychiatric rehabilitation
12. Psychoeducational model
13. Cognitive-behavioral approach
14. Treatment mall approach
15. Clubhouse model
16. Brokerage model
17. Strengths model
18. Assertive community treatment
19. Situated learning theory
20. Wraparound services
21. Transtheoretical model
22. Biopsychosocial model

Worksheet 8-2

Mental Health Settings

For these multiple choice questions, determine the setting where intervention is most likely occurring for the individual in the case study.

1. Consuela is a 2-year-old child with a diagnosis of Down syndrome. Working with the transdisciplinary team, the OT creates an occupational profile to understand the family's experience caring for Consuela. The services of the OT practitioners and other team members are covered under Part C of the Individuals with Disabilities Education Act (IDEA). The type of service setting described is which of the following?

   A. Early Intervention programs/family-centered care setting

   B. Community-based consumer-operated service

   C. Day care program

   D. Forensic setting

2. Kimberly is a 10-year-old child who attends the fourth grade in a local public school. Kimberly rides a bus to school in the morning from her home. In the afternoon, she attends a program at the local YWCA, where she is involved in structured activities to promote socialization and participation in age-appropriate play and leisure activities that encourage physical activity, problem-solving skills, and development of self-efficacy. The setting described is likely which of the following?

   A. Community-based consumer-operated service

   B. After-school program

   C. Forensic setting

   D. Clubhouse

3. Hector is a 39-year-old male with the diagnosis of schizophrenia with negative symptoms. He lives in a group home, where he participates in the required household activities, including cleaning his room, assisting with evening meal preparation and clean up, and washing laundry. During the day, Hector attends a facility-based program with other individuals who have challenges interacting within the community. He is part of the governance board and assists with running the thrift shop that generates revenue to support the program. This program is likely which of the following?

   A. Clubhouse

   B. Community-based case management

   C. Welfare-to-work program

   D. State mental health care facilities (state hospitals)

4. John was found guilty of burglary after an attempt to remove a television from the home of a stranger. He was sentenced to 5 years in a medium-security correctional facility in North Carolina. John is part of an OT life skills and effective communication group that takes place two times per week within the facility. He was selected for this group because of his history of antisocial behavior and lack of completion of secondary education. The OT program is based in which of the following settings?

   A. Community-based consumer-operated service

   B. Partial hospitalization program

   C. Forensic setting

   D. Welfare-to-work program

Worksheet 8-2 (continued)

Mental Health Settings

5. Martha is a 60-year-old female with a long-standing history of major depressive disorder with multiple suicide attempts. Her husband of 41 years, who was her caregiver, passed away recently. The couple had no children and there are no family members to care for Martha. Because of her dependence in ADLs and IADLs, as well as obvious safety concerns, Martha was admitted to an inpatient facility that cares for individuals with significant mental health concerns. The OT, who is part of a team that includes the psychiatrist, nursing staff, and social worker, assessed Martha and initiated a program to maximize her personal care skills for independence while she is living at the facility. This facility is likely which of the following?
   A. Partial hospitalization program
   B. Adult day care program
   C. Community-based case management
   D. State mental health facility (state hospital)

The Occupational Therapy Group Process

Groups in occupational therapy work toward desired outcomes, such as interaction within social norms, expression of feelings, insight into one's actions, improved coping skills and behavior, positive self-image, and the integration of various skills needed for occupational roles. Various leaders in psychology (such as Freud, Skinner, Piaget, and Erikson) and occupational therapy (such as Fidler, Mosey, and Allen) have contributed important theories concerning mental functions and group process that are beyond the scope of this book. The reader is encouraged to review the primary frames of reference and models that have guided occupational therapy mental health practice. Many of these have been clearly summarized by Cole (2012), who describes the following approaches: psychodynamic, developmental, sensorimotor, cognitive-behavioral continuum, Allen's cognitive disabilities, and various approaches that use the Model of Human Occupation. Anne Cronin Mosey has identified five developmental stages for group functioning, each of which addresses acquisition of particular skills: parallel groups, project groups, egocentric-cooperative groups, cooperative groups, and mature groups (Cole, 2012; Early, 2009; Tufano, 2015).

The occupational therapy group leader needs to determine how much direction, structure, and interpersonal reasoning the particular group requires, depending on the activity demands of the particular task, member abilities and limitations, group dynamics, and therapeutic goals (Cole, 2012; Taylor, 2008). Taylor (2008) developed the Intentional Relationship Model, which defines the interpersonal dynamic between the occupational therapist and client (2008). Taylor (2008) describes, at length, six therapeutic communication modes that occupational therapy practitioners use most frequently in therapeutic relationships. These six ways of relating to clients individually and in groups include advocating, collaborating, empathizing, encouraging, instructing, and problem solving (Taylor, 2008).

To lead occupational therapy groups effectively, an OT must demonstrate the ability to design the methods and activities to meet therapeutic goals, encourage and motivate group members, recognize productive and maladaptive group dynamics, manage problem behaviors, set limits, use therapeutic qualities and communication skills (e.g., sensitivity, genuineness, attending, empathy, limited self-disclosure, modeling of appropriate behavior); understand individual and group member roles, and determine capacities and limitations of members (Cole, 2012; Early, 2009; Taylor, 2008; Tufano, 2015). Cole (2012) describes at length seven steps for effective group leadership in occupational therapy that she adapted from Pfeiffer and Jones's *Reference Guide to Handbooks and Annuals* (1977). Cole's Seven-Step Format for Group Leadership, briefly summarized here, is useful for the highest level groups and can also be modified to meet other groups' needs (Cole, 2012).

Cole's Seven-Step Groups (2012)

1. Introduction: The start of a group should include an introduction of the occupational therapy practitioner and participants along with a warm-up to set the mood and encourage attention. The leader explains the group's purpose, outlines the session, and delineates the time frame and expectations.
2. Activity: The leader chooses an activity designed to meet therapeutic goals. The activity is based on multiple factors such as time constraints, the members' mental and physical abilities, and the leader's skill/knowledge. Other considerations for the activity include adaptations needed; amount of intended structure, creativity, or social interaction; and the specific method of instruction to implement the task.
3. Sharing: Group members show their work or explain their feelings. The group leader encourages participation and acknowledges each person verbally or nonverbally.
4. Processing: Group members express their feelings about the group experience and interactions with peers and the leader. The underlying group dynamics may be explored.
5. Generalizing: The leader summarizes the learning aspects and general cognitive principles ascertained through the group process.
6. Application: The identified principles are applied to life situations. Practical methods are discussed and the leader may provide limited self-disclosure to model solutions.
7. Summary: Important aspects of the group are emphasized briefly, such as goals and knowledge achieved. The leader notes changes of behavior and acknowledges and thanks members for their participation.

Learning Activity 8-2: Eating Disorders

Imagine the facility you are working at is starting a new program for young adults with eating disorders. You are developing an ADL group that will be part of this program. Consider occupational therapy discussion topics or activities relating to areas such as dressing, eating, shopping for food or clothing, and health maintenance, among others. Choose a particular self-care ADL or an IADL and use Cole's Seven-Step Format for Group Leadership (2012) to help plan an entire group session for six clients. Determine how much time you will allocate for each stage of this group. Realize that actual activities used in an intervention program will depend on the specific approach or frame of reference that is appropriate for that setting and particular group of clients.

Frame of reference for activity: ____________________

Occupation to be addressed: ____________________

Activity: ____________________

Length of Group: ____________________

1. Introduction. Time allocated: __________ minutes

   What specific words or actions will you use to greet the members and warm-up the group? How will you outline the group's purpose and expectations?

2. Activity. Time allocated: __________ minutes

   What specific activity will the group do? How and where will you set up the activity and position the clients? List the activity demands, such as equipment or supplies needed, specific content of any worksheets/written materials used, method of instruction, and sequence of steps, for example.

3. Sharing. Time allocated: __________ minutes

   What would you like the members to share? What will you ask and do in order to encourage member participation?

4. Processing. Time allocated: __________ minutes
   What will you ask or say in order to encourage member participation? What aspects of the group process will you focus on?

5. Generalizing. Time allocated: __________ minutes
   What concepts do you want the clients to learn?

6. Application. Time allocated: __________ minutes
   How can this experience be applied to other life situations? What limited self-disclosure might you offer?

7. Summary. Time allocated: __________ minutes
   What will you say to summarize and provide a closing for the group?

Adapted from Cole, M. B. (2012). *Group dynamics in occupational therapy: The theoretical basis and practice application of group intervention* (4th ed.). Thorofare, NJ: SLACK Incorporated.

Worksheet 8-3

Social Skills Group—Picnic

Imagine you are leading an occupational therapy social skills group for clients with high cognitive abilities who have been allowed to go on a supervised community outing. The varied diagnoses of the group members include anxiety disorder, mood disorder, obsessive-compulsive disorder, and borderline personality disorder. You have determined that the group should plan and prepare a picnic lunch over the course of several sessions. Food items may be obtained from the facility's food service department (with 24-hour notice), and the facility has a transportation service. Consider some ways in which you can facilitate interaction among the group members for this occupation. For each conversation starter idea you list for this egocentric-cooperative group, indicate a practical method (an activity) for implementing that discussion. Here is an example:

1. Topic:

   Encourage group members to determine a common menu, taking into account likes, dislikes, food allergies, dietary restrictions, and availability of items.

   Possible activity/method:

   a. *Group leader provides each client with a worksheet listing 10 food choices.*

      Clients number them in order of priority from 1 to 10.

      or

   b. *Each client is provided with a list of all available food items to check off or circle one desired item in each category (e.g., beverage, dessert).*

      Worksheet answers can be listed on a white board or flip chart. Group members discuss answers and decide on menu. Consider factors such as decision making, cooperation, and compromise.

2. Topic:

   Activity/Method:

3. Topic:

   Activity/Method:

4. Topic:

   Activity/Method:

5. Topic:

   Activity/Method:

Worksheet 8-3 (continued)

Social Skills Group—Picnic

6. Topic:

   Activity/Method:

7. Topic:

   Activity/Method:

8. Topic:

   Activity/Method:

9. Topic:

   Activity/Method:

10. Topic:

    Activity/Method:

Learning Activity 8-3: Four Current Events Groups

Imagine you are leading four separate occupational therapy current events groups. Choose a recent, interesting article from a newspaper to discuss with the group members. Pick a different article for each group, considering the therapeutic needs of the particular group. For each article, develop eight open-ended questions you might use as conversation starters to facilitate interaction among the group members. Determine the therapeutic purpose for each of the groups and incorporate occupational therapy group process skills. Indicate the lessons that members can learn from discussing the article and application to life situations.

For example, you might ask the group questions such as the following:

- *What is your opinion about that?*
- *What do you think will happen next?*
- *Why do you agree or disagree with that proposed law?*
- *Why is that important?*
- *What are the pros and cons of that?*
- *Can you describe a similar experience you had?*
- *What would you have done in the same situation?*
- *Why do you think that person committed that crime?*
- *Do you think the punishment fits the crime? Why or why not?*

1. **Inpatient Behavioral Health Unit: Substance Use Disorder**

   You are an OT working on an acute inpatient behavioral health unit. The group participants have high cognitive abilities and are diagnosed with substance use disorder (i.e., alcohol, cocaine, opioids).

   Topic of article: ______

   Purpose of group: ______

   General principles to be discussed/applied: ______

   ______

   Conversation starter questions:

   1.
   2.
   3.
   4.
   5.
   6.
   7.
   8.

2. **Senior Citizens Program**

   You are an activity leader for a local senior citizen day program.

   Topic of article: ______

   Purpose of group: ______

   General principles to be discussed/applied: ______

   ______

Conversation starter questions:

1.
2.
3.
4.
5.
6.
7.
8.

3. **Social Day Program: Intellectual Disability**

You are an activity leader working in a social day program for young adults who live with their families. Each of the participants has a developmental condition with mild to moderate intellectual impairment. However, each participant has functional verbal skills.

Topic of article: ____________________

Purpose of group: ____________________

General principles to be discussed/applied: ____________________

____

Conversation starter questions:

1.
2.
3.
4.
5.
6.
7.
8.

4. **School Program: Bullying**

You are an OT working in a school program designed to prevent bullying and are leading a small group of middle-school students.

Topic of article: ____________________

Purpose of group: ____________________

General principles to be discussed/applied: ____________________

____

Conversation starter questions:

1.
2.
3.
4.
5.
6.
7.
8.

Worksheet 8-4
Social Skills Group—Collage Craft

Imagine you are leading an occupational therapy social skills group for clients who have high cognitive abilities and various mental health conditions, such as mood disorders, anxiety, and substance use disorder. You have determined that the group members should work together to make one big collage. List 10 possible ways to facilitate interaction among group members as they are making the collage.

Here is an example:

Group participants must decide on a common theme, such as "happiness" or "family."

1.

2.

3.

4.

5.

6.

7.

8.

9.

10.

Learning Activity 8-4: Interventions in Mental Health—Frames of Reference

For each of the following occupational therapy groups, list the frame of reference you will use and three therapeutic activities appropriate for adult clients with depression.

Activity Group

Frame of reference: ______________________________

List three craft projects that the clients can choose from and explain why you chose each craft. For example, is the craft a quick-success project, or does it allow the client to express emotions? You will also need to decide whether tasks will be performed individually or as a collaborative effort.

1.

2.

3.

According to the frame of reference, this particular activity was chosen because ______________________________

____

Expressive Group

Frame of reference: ______________________________

List three discussion topics or activities for this group and explain why you chose each of them. For example, does the activity facilitate interpersonal skills or exploration of feelings?

1.

2.

3.

According to the frame of reference, this particular activity was chosen because ______________________________

____

IADL Group

Frame of reference: ______________________________

List three possible IADL activities for this group and explain why you chose each of them. For example, does the activity facilitate role performance or promote healthy habits?

1.

2.

3.

According to the frame of reference, this particular activity was chosen because ______________________________

____

Learning Activity 8-5: More Interventions in Mental Health

For each of the following occupational therapy groups, list three therapeutic activities appropriate for young adults diagnosed with substance use disorder. You will also need to decide if tasks will be performed individually or as a collaborative effort.

Activity Group

Frame of reference: ______________________________

List three craft projects that the client can choose from and explain why you chose each craft. For example, is the craft a quick success project, or does it allow the client to express emotions?

1.

2.

3.

According to the frame of reference, this particular activity was chosen because ______________________________

____

Expressive Group

Frame of reference: ______________________________

List three discussion topics or activities for this group and explain why you chose each of them. For example, does the activity encourage the client to express emotions or teach coping strategies?

1.

2.

3.

According to the frame of reference, this particular activity was chosen because ______________________________

____

Leisure Group

Frame of reference: ______________________________

List three possible activities for this group and explain why you chose each of them. For example, does the activity develop leisure skills or help alleviate stress?

1.

2.

3.

According to the frame of reference, this particular activity was chosen because ______________________________

____

Five-Stage Group Format Designed by Ross

Ross (1997) designed a Five-Stage Group format, based on neurophysiological principles, for clients who have low cognitive or social abilities, developmental disability, nonverbal/limited communication, or behavioral problems (e.g., hostility, acting out). Ross advocates a structured progression of sensory stimulation as a means to motivate the group, improve behavior and social skills, and help members process and organize information. Desired responses are elicited through sensory activities (e.g., vestibular, tactile, proprioceptive, visual) and the activities' effect on the central nervous system (Ross, 1997). Ross's five stages are briefly summarized as follows (Ross, 1997):

1. Orientation—Introductions and a simple 1-minute activity (e.g., handle simple instruments, pass around items, use scents, noisemakers) to increase alertness, facilitate calmness and relaxation, and provide sensory stimulation.
2. Movement—This stage consists of motor activities, such as reaching, walking, hopping, dance, or activities using props such as a parachute, ball, ribbon wand, scarves, and hoops.
3. Visual-motor perceptual activities—Consists of more challenging tasks, such as puzzles, activities addressing body parts (e.g., Simon Says), eye-hand coordination (e.g., golf putting, plastic bowling).
4. Cognitive stimulation and function—Activities such as stories, short poems, discussions, and memory and guessing games are used to increase communication and help organize thoughts and behavior.
5. Closing the session—A brief, familiar routine is used to signal the end of the session and provide positivity (e.g., a song, snack, hold hands).

Reprinted with permission from Morreale, M. J. (2015). *Developing clinical competence: A workbook for the OTA*. Thorofare, NJ: SLACK Incorporated.

Learning Activity 8-6: Assisted Living Facility

Imagine you are an activity leader for the Alzheimer's unit in an assisted living facility. You would like to provide the residents with meaningful opportunities to reminisce, handle objects, engage in familiar activities, and socialize. Use Ross's Five-Stage Group Format (1997) to design a group session. Create an activity box, relating to a familiar occupation, and plan the group around this theme. Keep in mind any safety concerns or dietary restrictions. An example of an activity box and relevant group activities for a session are provided.

Occupation	*IADL: Baking*	
Activity box contents	*Egg beater, wooden spoon, spatula, small muffin tin, sifter, plastic measuring cups, measuring spoons, small rolling pin, cookie cutters*	
Stage 1	*Greeting and introduction* *Smell spices used in baking (e.g., vanilla, cinnamon, ginger)*	
Stage 2	*Roll out prepared sugar cookie dough with a rolling pin*	
Stage 3	*Cut out cookies with a cookie cutter and place on a cookie sheet*	
Stage 4	*Each group member selects a kitchen item to handle and name* *Reminisce about baking, favorite desserts*	
Stage 5	*Closing remarks, provide a snack that clients are allowed to eat (e.g., cookies)*	

Reprinted with permission from Morreale, M. J. (2015). *Developing clinical competence: A workbook for the OTA*. Thorofare, NJ: SLACK Incorporated.

Worksheet 8-5

Mental Health Situations

1. A client with severe violent tendencies needs a one-on-one session to review a leisure checklist. When delegated this task, an OT should take which of the following actions:
   A. Keep the door closed for privacy
   B. Refuse to treat the client
   C. Ask a staff member to remain in vicinity
   D. Review the leisure checklist during an OT leisure group

2. An OT is working with a client who is hostile and attending an anger management program. Which of the following interventions would probably be least appropriate for the therapist to implement at this time to help reduce this client's tension?
   A. Sweeping the floor
   B. Wiping tables
   C. A 15-minute walk
   D. Sanding a small wood project

3. An OT brings a client with an eating disorder over to the craft supply closet. The therapist asks the client to choose a craft project from among the items on the shelves. The client is passive, insecure, and says repeatedly, "I don't know what I should do" and "I can't decide." What primary action should the therapist take?
   A. Use a timer to facilitate decision making
   B. Give the client a choice of two craft projects
   C. Have another client choose a project for this client
   D. Have the OT choose a project for this client

4. An OT in a mental health setting is leading a sensorimotor group for clients with chronic schizophrenia. Which of the following activities is most appropriate as the primary activity for this group?
   A. Writing down feelings with lively music playing in background
   B. Talking about bright colors of the rainbow
   C. Tossing and hitting a beach ball
   D. Lying on yoga mats and listening to music

5. A client in a group the OT is leading is becoming aggressive, out of control, and appears ready to hit someone. Of the following choices, the last course of action the therapist should consider taking is which of the following?
   A. Try to physically restrain the client
   B. Ask another client to go get help
   C. Talk to the client in a calm voice
   D. Remove other clients from the area

Worksheet 8-5 (continued)

Mental Health Situations

6. An OT and OTA are working on an acute psychiatric unit. They are collaborating to develop a policy and procedure manual for all the occupational therapy groups to ensure safety and meet therapeutic goals. Which of the following craft group procedures is least appropriate for inclusion in the manual?
   A. Hand out sharps individually to clients needing them for the activity
   B. Count the number of scissors before and after the group
   C. Avoid using permanent markers and oil-based stains
   D. Give clients the autonomy to retrieve craft supplies, scissors, yarn, and other supplies from the OT supply closet

7. A client with schizophrenia has been attending a community mental health program but has not shown up for the past week. Today the client arrives and begins talking about how her neighbors are watching her through the TV. She also states that they come in her apartment at night and move her belongings, even though her doors have a deadbolt lock. Which of the following is most likely the best activity for the OT to choose for this client?
   A. Writing in a journal
   B. Peeling potatoes in an IADL group
   C. Painting a picture in a crafts group
   D. Discussing feelings in an expressive group

8. During an occupational therapy craft group, a client keeps picking lint off his clothing. He also keeps trying to pick lint off the other clients' clothing, despite the OT asking him repeatedly to stop this behavior. The other clients are becoming irritated at being touched. The therapist should document the lint-picking behavior in the client's chart and describe it using which of the following terms?
   A. Obsessive behavior
   B. IADL retraining
   C. Compulsive behavior
   D. Attention to detail

9. A client attending a partial hospitalization program has a diagnosis of anxiety disorder. The client is exhibiting a panic attack and is trembling, crying, and stating that she is going to die. Which primary action should the OT take?
   A. Encourage the client to take slow, deep breaths
   B. Call an ambulance
   C. Call the client's doctor
   D. Go get the OT's supervisor

10. An OT is leading a group for clients on an acute psychiatric unit who are diagnosed with depression. The group members are making items to decorate their individual hospital rooms. Of the following choices, which would likely be the most appropriate?
    A. A painted ceramic piggy bank
    B. A decorative wreath made with artificial flowers glued to a wire hanger
    C. A painted picture made with the use of stencils
    D. A colorful macramé wall hanging

Worksheet 8-6

Therapeutic Responses

Provide the therapeutic response indicated to the client comments that follow.

1. "I am so confused by all of the rules and regulations surrounding Medicare reimbursement, I may just scream."
   Reflective listening response ______________________________

2. "I just completed a 5K marathon in 6 hours."
   Affirmation ______________________________

3. "I am looking forward to graduation."
   Open-ended question to gain specific information. ______________________________

4. "I had a couple of drinks last night, but I deserve it since I had not had one for 2 weeks."
   Therapeutic paradox ______________________________

5. "I am sure you have never seen anyone with a stroke as bad as the one I have had. I will never do anything again."
   Normalizing statement ______________________________

Worksheet 8-7

Mental Health Intervention Techniques

This worksheet is based on communication techniques and interventions used by OTs in mental health practice (Davis, 2011). Models to consider include the Kawa model (Iwama, 2006), Positive Psychology (Snyder, Lopez, & Pedrotti, 2011), Motivational Interviewing (Rollnick, Miller, & Butler, 2008), Dialectical Behavioral Therapy (DBT; Linehan, 2015), and the Wellness Recovery and Action Plan (WRAP) (Copeland, 2011). For the following multiple-choice questions, chose the answer that best describes what you would first say or do when assisting the client to regain occupational participation.

1. A client who has severe and persistent mental illness in the area of depression is seen by the OT for an initial evaluation. The therapist learns that the client is motivated to take control of her own life and wants to enhance her level of participation in things that she had previously found enjoyable. One of her concerns is that she never knows when a bout of depressive anxiety will hit. She also constantly worries about how others will treat her and if they will have her wishes in mind if things go badly. What technique may the OT use to help this patient become more empowered to take control over her mental health concerns?
   A. Ask the client to create the metaphor described in the Kawa model
   B. Assist the client in seeing her ambivalence through motivational interviewing
   C. Assist the client in the creation of a notebook that contains her medications, triggers, and advanced directives and describes her typical behaviors as she is entering a crisis
   D. Use a dialectical behavior approach to prevent her from committing suicide

2. You are interviewing a client as a part of information gathering for the occupational profile. During the interview, the client states that he was a firefighter in New York City on 9/11 and that he helped to rescue several first responders who were in the area of Building 2. What is the most appropriate statement that you may make upon hearing that news while using your best "therapeutic use of self"?
   A. "WOW, can we talk about that for a minute? That must have been an amazing day!"
   B. "My ... I can't even imagine what that must have been like."
   C. "OK. How are you doing with your self-care activities?"
   D. "Wow.... That is cool, you are a real hero."

3. Your client experiences persecutory delusions and sometimes becomes defensive when personal questions are asked. You are interested in knowing more about his childhood, with regard to how many brothers and sisters he has and his experience growing up in a large family. How could you best ask this question to gain insight into his childhood experiences?
   A. "Good morning, George. Today I want to start with asking you about your childhood. How many brothers and sisters do you have?"
   B. "Hi George. I hope that you had a good breakfast. I am wondering if we can chat today about your thoughts on global warming?"
   C. "I enjoyed talking to you about your time in the service, George. I found it very interesting that your brothers also served in the army. I am wondering if you have any other siblings?"
   D. "Hi, George. I was just talking to some of the staff in the break room—they said you have eight brothers and sisters. What was it like growing up in that huge family?"

Worksheet 8-7 (continued)

Mental Health Intervention Techniques

4. Stefanie is a second-semester high school senior who is struggling with school. She has a high rate of absenteeism and spends her time walking in her backyard or watching cooking shows on television; she has few friends. Stefanie has been referred to occupational therapy by her primary care physician; today is your first visit. From a positive psychology perspective, understanding that teenagers who do not like school and do not have extracurricular activities that provide successful skill development can become depressed, what might your OT intervention plan include?
   A. Asking her if she would like to explore some culinary classes at the community college
   B. A referral to a personal trainer so that she can learn to exercise daily
   C. Asking Stefanie's mom if it would be ok to purchase her a puppy for companionship
   D. Bringing a knitting kit to your first session and teaching Stefanie how to knit a sweater

5. Amaya is a 55-year-old female from Cambodia who immigrated to the United States after the recent death of her husband. Amaya has been despondent for the past 3 months and will not participate in self-care or IADLs. Amaya has been admitted to the acute behavioral health unit of the medical center where you work, after her son brought her to the emergency department. She is diagnosed with major depressive disorder and has been referred to occupational therapy for an evaluation and intervention. Unfortunately, you are finding it difficult to communicate with Amaya regarding her thoughts about her occupational performance and interest in regaining her independence. Which one of the following activities and associated model of intervention may be beneficial to you as you begin building the occupational profile of Amaya?
   A. Filling out a Venn diagram indicating interested in occupation as a technique from the Person–Environment–Occupation–Performance (PEOP) model
   B. Have Amaya draw a river that depicts her life and obstacles to her full participation as described in the Kawa model
   C. Conduct the Occupational Performance History Interview—II (OPHI-II) based on the Model of Human Occupation
   D. Ask Amaya to create diary cards that describe therapy interfering behaviors that she may display, a Dialectical Behavioral Therapy technique.

Learning Activity 8-7: Therapeutic Interaction

Imagine a client who is diagnosed with a particular substance use disorder (i.e., alcohol, opioids, cocaine, etc.). In the box next to each area of communication, write a statement that you may say to the client during your first treatment encounter and their response back. Share your thoughts with an occupational therapy classmate and reflect on the accuracy of the script that you have created.

Area	*Reflection*
1. Greeting client	You say: The client says:
2. Explaining purpose of visit	You say: The client says:
3. Ask an appropriate "open-ended question" to seek information	You say: The client says:
4. Ask follow-up questions to explore relevant areas mentioned in response to question 3	You say: The client says:
5. Ask a closed-ended question	You say: The client says:
6. Reflective listening—restatement of responses	You say: The client says:
7. What might you say to demonstrate active listening?	While the client is speaking, you may say:
8. Describe your posture during this interaction	What is an appropriate posture? What are you doing with your arms and face?
9. Describe your position relative to client	
10. What is an affirmation that you may give to your client based on a statement that he or she makes?	The client says: You say:
11. Can you identify a "direction" to the interview?	

Worksheet 8-8

Behavioral Observation Skills in Mental Health

For each of the following categories, list specific behaviors that an occupational therapy practitioner might expect to see in a client who is depressed and how those behaviors might interfere with occupational performance.

Occupations:

ADLs:

Rest and Sleep:

Leisure:

Work/Education:

Social Participation (include the following areas):

Intrapersonal factors:

Interpersonal behaviors:

Task behaviors:

After you have completed your list of behaviors, review the following case study. On the basis of the client information provided, look at each of your listed behaviors and circle only the ones in the list you created that are *actually observed* for Laurie while she is on the unit. Then complete Learning Activity 8-8 to develop an intervention plan for Laurie.

Laurie, a 38-year-old bank teller, was admitted to an acute psychiatric unit with a diagnosis of depression. After her spouse's cancer death 3 months ago, Laurie states that she has stopped attending her weekly college business class and her daily routine of going to the gym. She reports having frequent headaches and muscle tension in her upper back for the past 4 weeks. For the 2 weeks before admission, Laurie has stayed in bed all day in her pajamas, missed work, lost weight due to decreased appetite, and not answered phone calls, text messages, or e-mail. She states that she is "not good enough" to return to work. When asked if she has contacted her college or job to discuss a medical leave, Laurie replied, "Why bother?" She denies suicidal ideation at this time. Laurie does not have any children. She has one sister who lives in the next town, and her parents live in a retirement community 1,000 miles away.

Learning Activity 8-8: Intervention Planning

Review the case study presented in Worksheet 8-8.
Do you think the client Laurie will be able to return home? Why or why not? ____________________

____

____

Considering the categories in the *Occupational Therapy Practice Framework* (AOTA, 2014), fill in the boxes below to develop an intervention plan for the client, Laurie.

Problem Area	*Client Behavior Exhibited That Hinders Her Occupational Performance*	*Develop One Long-Term Goal for Each Category Listed in the First Column*	*Develop Two Short-Term Goals for Each Long-Term Goal You Listed*	*OT Interventions (Indicate whether these are preparatory, activities, occupations, education, advocacy, or groups)*
ADLs **1.** **2.** **3.**				
IADLs **1.** **2.** **3.**				
Work				
Leisure/play **1.** **2.** **3.**				
Education				
Social Participation				
Rest/sleep				
Performance Skills **1.** **2.** **3.**				
Performance Patterns **1.** **2.** **3.**				
Client factors **1.** **2.** **3.**				
Contexts and Environments **1.** **2.**				

List at least three follow-up recommendations or community supports that are likely indicated for this client upon her discharge from the facility.

1. ______________________________
2. ______________________________
3. ______________________________

Answers to Chapter 8 Worksheets

Worksheet 8-1: Assessments for Mental Health Practice

References: Asher, 2014; Brown & Stoffel, 2011.

1. Test of Grocery Shopping Skills
2. Resiliency Scales for Children and Adolescents
3. Model of Human Occupation Screening Tool
4. Occupational Therapy Quality of Experience and Spirituality Tool
5. Mental Health Inventory
6. Recovery Enhancing Environment Measure Scale
7. Allen Cognitive Level Screen
8. Pediatric Interest Profiles
9. Recovery Self-Assessment
10. Leisure Satisfaction Scale
11. Allen Diagnostic Module
12. Bay Area Functional Performance Evaluation
13. Kohlman Evaluation of Living Skills
14. Hope Scale
15. Canadian Occupational Performance Measure
16. Assessment of Motor and Process Skills
17. Recovery Self-Assessment
18. Independent Living Skills Survey
19. Milwaukee Evaluation of Daily Living Skills
20. Making Decisions Empowerment Scale

Worksheet 8-2: Mental Health Settings

1. A
2. B
3. A
4. C
5. D

Worksheet 8-3: Social Skills Group—Picnic

In general, the OT should facilitate positive interaction among group members; provide necessary feedback regarding appropriate and inappropriate language and behavior exhibited; and provide opportunities for socialization, leisure, and learning, such as application of the group experience to life and strategies (Cole, 2012). Here are some practical suggestions to facilitate interaction among group members for this picnic task. Realize these are only suggestions, which may not be appropriate for each group of clients. Actual implementation and choice of a particular method or activity will depend on the specific approach or frame of reference that the OT (and team) determines is appropriate for a particular group of clients:

1. Topic:

   Encourage group members to determine a common menu, taking into account likes, dislikes, food allergies, dietary restrictions, and availability of items.

   Possible activity/method:

   a. *Group leader provides each client with a worksheet listing 10 food choices.*

      Clients number them in order of priority from 1 to 10.

      -or-

   b. *Each client is provided with a list of all available food items to check off or circle one desired item in each category (e.g., beverage, dessert).*

      Worksheet answers can be listed on a white board or flip chart. Group members discuss answers and decide on menu. Consider factors such as decision making, cooperation, and compromise.

2. Topic:

   Group members can discuss feeling/attitudes toward picnics or going outdoors, considering past experiences and anticipation of task.

   Possible activity/method: *Have client anonymously write a word or phrase on an index card describing his or her feelings toward the upcoming picnic activity (such as* fun, anxious, relaxing, boring*) and place it in a basket for discussion.*

   or

   Worksheet: Each client circles or checks off from a list describing how the client is feeling regarding the upcoming picnic and then discusses this.

3. Topic:

   Once menu has been decided, group members must come up with a list of all items needed for the picnic.

   Possible activity/method:

   Group leader (or member) writes down member suggestions on a large flip chart or white board. Can list by categories (e.g., specific food items/condiments, eating and serving equipment, recreational items).

4. Topic:

   Group members must determine time frames for preparatory tasks (e.g., order food 2 days before, bake cupcakes 1 day before, make sandwiches morning of the picnic).

   Possible activity/method:

   Group leader (or member) writes down list of steps and member suggestions on a large flip chart or white board. Discuss factors such as organization and time management.

5. Topic:

   Group members must decide on a picnic location within a certain radius.

   Possible activity/method:

   Group leader provides each client with a worksheet listing five choices of locations. Clients are asked to number them in order of priority from 1 to 5, then to discuss and decide on location. The pros and cons can be written on a flip chart or white board.

6. Topic:

   Group members should discuss alternatives if it rains.

   Possible activity/method:

   Worksheet: Clients write down two alternative solutions or can choose from a list of possible alternatives. Member suggestions can be written on a flip chart or whiteboard for discussion.

7. Topic:

   Group members can plan for other recreational activities at picnic site, such as sedentary or active leisure tasks.

   Possible method/activity:

   Each member fills out leisure inventory/checklist. Clients choose two items to suggest to the rest of group or can write them on index cards and place in a basket for discussion. Consider factors of cooperation and compromise.

8. Topic:

   Group members must plan how food items will be prepared (e.g., Will the dietary department provide premade sandwiches? Will each person prepare his or her own sandwich? Will each member prepare a component of the meal for everyone? Will the group bake a batch of cookies together?).

   Possible method/activity:

   List options on flip chart or white board, discuss, and decide. Consider factors such as food safety, decision making, and cooperation.

9. Topic:

   Cooperation/compromise

   Possible method/activity:

   Perform a meal preparation task (such as baking cookies or preparing a salad) for which group members must work cooperatively and actually have to share such items as kitchen tools, spices, plastic wrap.

10. Topic:

    Favorite recipes (their own or someone else's)

    Possible method/activity:

    Members can look up recipes for various picnic foods or bring a familiar recipe to share with the group. Group members can discuss or teach their own method/recipe for the meal components, such as a favorite recipe for cookies or potato salad.

    or

    Members can use a worksheet to list one or more favorite homemade foods and answer such questions as whether this food is healthy/unhealthy, a special treat, a childhood favorite, holiday-related, and how often it was available, for example.

11. Topic:

    Group members must decide how food will be packed (e.g., individual boxed lunches or shared platters of food).

    Possible method/activity:

    List options on flip chart or white board and discuss. Consider factors such as food safety, decision making, and cooperation.

12. Topic:

    Group members can discuss and critique the prepared food, picnic outing experience, and interaction with peers.

    Possible method/activity:

    Have each client anonymously write a word or phrase on an index card describing his or her feelings/attitude toward the picnic activity (such as fun, anxious, relaxing, stupid*) and place in a basket for discussion.*

    or

    Worksheet: Each client circles or checks off from a list describing how the client felt regarding the picnic, then discusses it.

    or

    Worksheet: Rate each category (e.g., food, location, overall experience) on a scale from 0 to 10 and then discuss.

13. Topic:

    Group members can discuss feelings and attitudes toward food (e.g., emotional eating, comfort foods, healthy/unhealthy foods).

    Possible activity/method:

    Worksheet: Have clients write down specific foods that they usually eat in various designated situations, such as when feeling stressed, watching TV, needing energy, and as a reward or treat.

Worksheet 8-4: Social Skills Group—Collage Craft

The OT should encourage positive interaction among group members and provide feedback regarding appropriate and inappropriate language and behavior exhibited. Here are some suggestions to facilitate interaction among group members as they are making the collage.

1. *Group participants must decide on a common theme such as "happiness" or "family." They may be provided with a list to choose from if more structure is needed.*
2. *Ask a group member who has made a collage before to teach others how to do the craft.*
3. *Limit materials so that clients will have to share (e.g., only 1 bottle of glue).*
4. *Ask group members to divide up the activity demands and decide who will do which aspects of the project (e.g., one person has to find magazines on the unit, another person has to clear and set up the work surface with newspapers).*
5. *Ask group members to explain why they chose the pictures they did.*
6. *Ask group members to comment on others' pictures.*
7. *Group members can be asked to collaboratively decide on picture placement.*
8. *Ask group members to decide on other possible art materials to decorate the collage (e.g., glitter, foam letters).*
9. *Ask group members to discuss or critique the finished product.*
10. *Create some situations to address frustration tolerance or facilitate problem-solving or decision-making skills, such as creating time constraints, running out of some materials, establishing additional criteria (e.g., cannot use a picture of a person or all words must have red letters).*
11. *Ask group members to discuss their feelings regarding participation in this activity.*
12. *Ask group members to decide where to place the finished collage.*

Worksheet 8-5: Mental Health Situations

1. C. For safety reasons, the OT should keep the door open and ensure that a staff member is in the vicinity in case the client becomes aggressive.
2. A. A client can use a mop or broom as a weapon (Early, 2009).
3. B. Although a timer could possibly work, it is not the best option because it could create more stress for the client and lessen feelings of self-control. A full closet of craft options may be too overwhelming for this client, so minimizing the choices to two options would be appropriate to facilitate decision making. Having others choose the project would not allow for the client to experience any self-control or decision making.
4. C. The only choice consisting of a gross motor activity is the beach ball activity.
5. A. If a client is becoming out of control, it is best for the OT to call for help, talk in a calm voice, and remove other clients from the area. Physically restraining a client should be avoided and used only as a last resort (Early, 2009).
6. D. To help ensure safety, an occupational therapy practitioner must carefully keep track of sharps and other hazardous objects such as string and yarn. Items with fumes (e.g., stains, dyes) can also be dangerous (Early, 2009).
7. B. A client experiencing hallucinations would benefit from activities that are structured, familiar tasks to help the client to maintain appropriate focus (Early, 2009).
8. C. The client is acting on his obsessive thoughts and demonstrating compulsive behavior.

9. A. An OT should always use clinical judgment to distinguish between a true medical emergency vs the client's pattern of panic attacks and take action accordingly. For a panic attack, generally the first course of action is to encourage the client to take slow, deep breaths to help the anxiety to pass.
10. C. A wire hanger, glass, and cords can be used by a client to harm self or others (Early, 2009).

Worksheet 8-6: Therapeutic Responses

References: Rollnick, Miller, & Butler, 2008.

1. "I hear you saying the Medicare rules and regulations are difficult to keep straight and it affects your ability to do your job."
2. "I can see how proud you are of your accomplishment. It is great that you were able to complete your very first attempt at a 5K."
3. "Please tell me more about the aspect of graduation that you are looking forward to the most."
4. "I think it is time for you to consider managing your alcoholism on your own. You do not seem ready to take help from anyone else."
5. "I know that things seem very difficult now, but I have worked with people who have also had significant strokes who have been able to return to many of their activities."

Worksheet 8-7: Mental Health Intervention Techniques

References: Copeland, 2011; Davis, 2011; Iwama, 2006; Kielhofner, 2008; Law et al., 1996; Linehan, 2015; Rollnick, Miller, & Butler, 2008; Snyder, Lopez, & Pedrotti, 2011.

1. _C_ A WRAP notebook will empower the client to take control of her own care plan in the event that symptoms become severe. Although the Kawa river activity in Answer A is helpful in identifying barriers to occupational participation, it is not a strategy to ensure future resilience. Answer B is not correct because the client is not ambivalent; she understands what concerns her and is taking steps to improve her response. The client is not described as being suicidal in the case study, therefore DBT (Answer D) is not appropriate at this time.
2. _B_ You are providing an empathetic response, yet not dwelling on the topic. Choice A, although seemingly supportive, is an overly enthusiastic response to your client's comment during the initial interview. It will be distracting and may not be what the client was hoping to focus upon. For choice C, not addressing the client's comment is not appropriate because the client did find it important enough to mention this significant event to you. Choice D is not the best response because first responders and others in jobs where saving lives is part of their daily duty do not consider themselves heroes. Saying that being present at ground zero is "cool" may be interpreted as a disrespectful response that does not indicate understanding of the gravity of the experience.
3. _C_ This is the correct answer because George was speaking to you openly about his brother in the army; you are showing interest in a topic that he has discussed. Choice A is not the best answer because you have not established enough trust with George to ask a question that he may consider very personal. Controversial topics that could have political overtones (choice B) should be avoided, especially when you have not yet established rapport with the client. For choice D, it is not appropriate to discuss staff conversations with a client. In this case, it is particularly concerning to mention to George that others were talking about him because this knowledge will support his persecutory delusions.
4. _A_ The case mentions that Stefanie has an interest in cooking shows, which may indicate an interest in the culinary arts. Taking part in courses that interest her may lead to a higher level of self-efficacy and, ultimately, success in life. Choice B is not the best answer because there is no reason to believe that Stefanie is not physically fit and that she requires or would be interested in the use of a trainer to teach her how to exercise. For choice C, animals do provide companionship, but having a puppy may not lead to enhanced self-efficacy and may not provide her with the incentive to try new educational activities or develop new human friendships. Choice D, knitting, could lead to a successful outcome and improve self-efficacy, but it is a solitary activity that has not been described in the case study as an interest of Stefanie's.

5. _B_ The Kawa (river) model uses the metaphor of the river to assist clients in thinking about their life to identify barriers to occupational performance. The metaphor and associated activity is useful across many cultures. Choice A, filling out a Venn diagram, is not a treatment or assessment technique. Choice C, the OPHI-II, would not be your first choice because the interview format requiring extensive dialogue with Amaya, who is not communicative at this time. Choice D, "diary cards," are indicated for individuals who have difficulty complying with a therapy program. According to the information provided, there is no reason to suspect that Amaya has had, or will have, a difficult time with treatment compliance on the mental health care unit.

Worksheet 8-8: Behavioral Observation Skills in Mental Health

Each client is different, but some suggestions are presented here as possible symptoms of depression that an occupational therapy practitioner might observe. Tufano (2003) urges caution when depressed clients show sudden peacefulness and behavioral changes along with sudden declaration that depression is resolved. This new vigor, for some clients, could be an indicator of suicidality (Tufano, 2003). The giving away of items can also be a warning sign. Only the items below in bold are those that are **actually observed** with Laurie on the unit, based on the information provided. She may exhibit other behaviors during her hospitalization or during group activities, but these are not noted in the case study.

ADL

- Change in appetite (note specific amount eaten and/or types of foods). *Laurie has lost weight before admission due to decreased appetite. It is not noted whether Laurie's eating patterns have changed since she was admitted.*
- **Specific weight loss or gain.** *Laurie has lost weight recently due to decreased appetite. although exact amount is not noted. This will need to be monitored on unit.*
- Lacks initiation to get out of bed (note amount of cueing/assistance needed). *Prior to admission, Laurie had stayed in bed all day. However, it is not noted whether she is continuing this pattern of behavior on the unit.*
- Lacks initiation to get dressed or shower (note amount of cueing/assistance needed). *Before admission, Laurie had stayed in bed all day in her pajamas. However, it is not noted whether she is currently getting dressed on the unit.*
- Inattention to grooming and hygiene (describe). *Not noted at present time.*

Rest and Sleep

- Atypical amount of time sleeping or inability to sleep (note sleep patterns). *Not noted at present time.*
- Reports poor sleep quality. *Not noted.*

Leisure

- **Withdraws from regular leisure routine.** *Laurie reports she has stopped her daily routine of going to the gym.*
- Does not express interest in resuming leisure activities. *Not noted currently.*
- Refuses or demonstrates limited participation in leisure activities on unit (specific tasks, length of time, level of participation). *Not noted.*
- Expresses unwillingness to resume her exercise regimen or go for a 15-minute walk with staff. *Not noted.*

Work/Education

- **Misses work or school.** *Laurie reports she has stopped attending her weekly college business class and, for the past 2 weeks, has also missed work.*
- Expresses lack of desire to return to work and/or school. *Expresses inability.*
- **Difficulty with initiating contact with employer or teachers for a plan to return to work, complete studies, or arrange for a medical leave.** *She states, "Why bother?"*

Social Participation

Intrapersonal factors

- **Expresses feelings of hopelessness**, sadness, depression, or suicidal ideation (note specific statements). *States "not good enough" to return to work and "why bother?" Denies suicidal ideation.*

- **Verbalizes negative attributes about self** (note specific statements). *States "not good enough" to return to work.*
- **Expresses negative outlook regarding future or ability to cope** (note specific statements). *Regarding contacting her boss and college, Laurie states, "Why bother?"*
- Crying exhibited. *Not noted.*
- **Somatic complaints.** *Reports frequent headaches and muscle tension in her upper back.*
- Inability to identify coping mechanisms for dealing with a depressed mood (e.g., does not identify people client can contact to discuss feelings, expresses unwillingness to exercise/go for a 15-minute walk). *Not noted.*

Interpersonal behaviors

- Lack of eye contact (describe situation). *Not noted.*
- Flat affect/does not smile. *Not noted*
- Does not initiate conversation. *Not noted*
- **Uncommunicative or minimal level of engagement in conversation (note length and type of responses).** *Does not answer phone calls, respond to text messages or e-mail.*

Task behaviors *(The following behaviors are not noted in case study)*

- Refuses or minimally participates in group activities (note how often and for how long).
- Poor task initiation.
- Poor decision making (Describe what happens when presented with choosing an activity/craft project or components such as colors or materials).
- Does not complete project/gives up.
- Poor attention to detail/does not recognize or correct errors (describe/give examples).
- Low frustration tolerance (describe the situation and behavior).

Chapter 8 References

American Occupational Therapy Association. (2014). Occupational therapy practice framework: Domain and process, 3rd edition. *American Journal of Occupational Therapy, 68*(Suppl. 1), S1–S48.

Asher, I. (Ed.). (2014). *Asher's occupational therapy assessment tools: An annotated index* (4th ed.). Bethesda, MD: AOTA Press.

Brown, C., & Stoffel, V. (Eds.). (2011). *Occupational therapy in mental health: A vision for participation.* Philadelphia: F. A. Davis.

Cole, M. B. (2012). *Group dynamics in occupational therapy: The theoretical basis and practice application of group intervention* (4th ed.). Thorofare, NJ: SLACK Incorporated.

Copeland, M. E. (2011). *Wellness recovery action plan* (5th ed.). San Francisco: Peach Pit Press.

Davis, C. (2011). *Patient practitioner interaction: An experiential manual for developing the art of heath care* (5th ed.). Thorofare, NJ: Slack Incorporated.

Early, M. B. (2009) *Mental health concepts and techniques for the occupational therapy assistant* (4th ed.). Baltimore: Lippincott Williams & Wilkins.

Iwama, M. (2006). *The Kawa Model: Culturally relevant occupational therapy.* Philadelphia: Churchill Livingstone.

Morreale, M. J. (2015). *Developing clinical competence: A workbook for the OTA.* Thorofare, NJ: SLACK Incorporated.

Kielhofner, G. (2008). *Model of human occupation: Theory and application* (4th ed.). Philadelphia: Lippincott, Williams & Wilkins.

Law, M., Cooper, B., Strong, S. S., Rigby, P., & Letts, L. (1996). The person–environment–occupation model: A transactive approach to occupational performance. *Canadian Journal Occupational Therapy, 63*(1) 9–23.

Linehan, M. (2015). *DBT® skills training manual* (2nd ed.). New York: Guilford Press.

Pfeiffer, J., & Jones, J. (1977). *Reference guide to handbooks and annals* (2nd ed.). La Jolla, CA: University Associates.

Rollnick, S., Miller, W., & Butler, C. (2008). *Motivational interviewing in health care: Helping patients change behavior.* New York: Guilford Press.

Ross, M. (1997). *Integrative group therapy: Mobilizing coping abilities with the five-stage group.* Bethesda, MD: American Occupational Therapy Association.

Snyder, C. R., Lopez, S., & Pedrotti, J. (2011). *Positive psychology: The scientific and practical explorations of human strengths* (2nd ed.). Thousand Oaks, CA: Sage.

Taylor, R. (2008). *The intentional relationship: Occupational therapy and use of self.* Philadelphia: F.A. Davis.

Tufano, T. (2003). Mental health occupational therapy (Suicidality: section 6-31). In K. Sladyk (Ed.), *OT study cards in a box.* Thorofare, NJ: SLACK Incorporated.

Tufano, R. (2015). Group intervention. In K. Sladyk & R. Ryan (Eds.), *Ryan's occupational therapy assistant: Principles, practice issues, and techniques* (5th ed., pp. 444–462). Thorofare, NJ: SLACK Incorporated.

Chapter 9

Demonstrating Knowledge and Skills in Adult Rehabilitation and Geriatrics

Occupational therapy practitioners working in settings such as home care, hospitals, nursing homes, inpatient and outpatient rehabilitation centers, and specialty areas of practice (e.g., low vision, hand therapy, eating and swallowing, etc.) require specialized knowledge and skills unique to those practice areas. Occupational therapists (OTs) and occupational therapy assistants (OTAs) implement skilled interventions that focus primarily on safety, improving client factors/skills, and various methods to support health and engagement in areas such as activities of daily living (ADLs), instrumental ADLs (IADLs), and work. The worksheets and learning activities in this chapter will assess your understanding of the needs of adult and elderly clients who have physical conditions. It is imperative that OTs demonstrate understanding of common medications, medical devices, and procedures; adhere to protocols regarding precautions and contraindications for various medical conditions and circumstances; make good clinical decisions; develop appropriate intervention plans; and implement skilled interventions effectively.

Note that space limitations in this chapter allow for only select initial evaluation data to be presented for case studies. A "real" evaluation would include more complete information, such as the specific aspects of occupations needing assistance and the various factors, contexts, or performance skills hindering or supporting occupational participation. Answers to worksheet exercises are provided at the end of the chapter.

Contents

Morreale, M. J., & Amini, D.
The Occupational Therapist's Workbook for Ensuring Clinical Competence (pp. 313-356).

Worksheet 9-1

Diseases and Conditions

List another common name for the diseases and conditions listed below.

1. Colles fracture ______
2. Complex regional pain syndrome ______
3. Lou Gehrig disease ______
4. Herpes zoster ______
5. Golfer's elbow ______
6. Degenerative joint disease ______
7. Adhesive capsulitis ______
8. Tennis elbow ______
9. Gamekeeper's thumb ______
10. Epstein-Barr virus ______
11. Ewing sarcoma ______
12. Barlow syndrome ______
13. Varicella ______
14. Decubitus ulcer ______
15. Hypoglycemia ______
16. Myocardial infarction ______
17. Hypertension ______
18. Hyperemesis ______
19. Trisomy 21 ______
20. Hyperlipidemia ______
21. Thrombus ______
22. Osteogenesis imperfecta ______
23. Diplopia ______
24. Ecchymosis ______
25. Hematuria ______

Worksheet 9-2

Common Medications

Match each of the conditions in the following chart to one of the generic or brand name medications listed. Although some medications may be used to treat multiple problems, list each of the conditions below only once.

Multiple sclerosis	Infection	Pain	Angina
Osteoarthritis	Hypertension	Schizophrenia	Diabetes
Osteoporosis	Parkinson's disease	Asthma	Shingles
Atrial fibrillation	Cancer	Depression	Dementia
Iron deficiency	Anxiety	Attention-deficit disorder	Seizure

1. Warfarin __________
2. Nitroglycerin __________
3. Naproxen __________
4. Aricept __________
5. Risperdal __________
6. Atenolol __________
7. Diazepam __________
8. Boniva __________
9. Levodopa __________
10. Topamax __________
11. Demerol __________
12. Methotrexate __________
13. Adderall __________
14. Lexapro __________
15. Proventil __________
16. Augmentin __________
17. Avonex __________
18. Acyclovir __________
19. Humulin R __________
20. Slow FE __________

Worksheet 9-3

Generic Medications

Match the brand name medications in the following chart to the generic equivalent listed.

Neurontin	Aleve	Tenormin	Valium
Advil	Xanax	Lipitor	Tylenol
Tums	Coumadin	Cymbalta	Cardizem
Vasotec	Humulin R	Prozac	Klonopin
Prilosec	Ventolin	Vicodin	Paxil

1. warfarin ______________________
2. omeprazole ______________________
3. ibuprofen ______________________
4. diazepam ______________________
5. naproxen sodium ______________________
6. hydrocodone bitartrate ______________________
7. albuterol ______________________
8. gabapentin ______________________
9. atorvastatin calcium______________________
10. clonazepam ______________________
11. enalapril maleate ______________________
12. alprazolam ______________________
13. insulin ______________________
14. fluoxetine hydrochloride ______________________
15. diltiazem ______________________
16. acetaminophen ______________________
17. paroxetine ______________________
18. duloxetine hydrochloride ______________________
19. calcium carbonate ______________________
20. atenolol ______________________

Reprinted with permission from Morreale, M. J. (2015). *Developing clinical competence: A workbook for the OTA*. Thorofare, NJ: SLACK Incorporated.

Worksheet 9-4

Rehabilitation Hospital—Total Hip Replacement Goals

Mary, a 70-year-old retired secretary, had left hip replacement surgery (posterolateral approach) 5 days ago due to a hip fracture sustained in a fall on an icy sidewalk. Her current weight-bearing status for the left lower extremity is partial weight bearing. Mary's medical history includes hypertension, coronary artery disease, and hyperlipidemia. She was transferred to a rehabilitation hospital yesterday, with expected discharge to home in 10 days. Here is some additional information taken from Mary's occupational therapy evaluation report:

Living situation: Widowed and lives alone in a third-floor condominium, with elevator access, in an adult retirement community. There is a shower stall in one bathroom and shower/tub in a second bathroom. Client's daughter works full time, has two children in elementary school, and lives in the next town. Her son also works full time and lives approximately 100 miles away.

Prior level of function: Before her fall, client was independent in all ADLs and IADLs. She volunteers 1 day a week at a food pantry and is active in several church groups (choir and Bible study). Client uses the town's senior citizen bus service for transportation.

ADLs: Currently unable to perform lower body dressing and bathing due to total hip precautions. Client needs moderate assistance for transfers using a rolling walker.

IADLs: Dependent in household chores at this time

Cognition: No functional deficits noted

Upper extremity strength and range of motion (ROM): Within functional limits (WFL)

Use a professional format to list four *functional* occupational therapy goals for Mary.

1.

2.

3.

4.

Worksheet 9-5

Home Care

1. An OT arrives at a client's home for a scheduled occupational therapy visit. The therapist rings the doorbell several times but no one answers. The therapist should perform which primary action?
   A. Use a cell phone to call 911
   B. Use a cell phone to call the rehabilitation director
   C. Use a cell phone to call the client
   D. Leave and document that no one answered the door

2. An OT arrives at an 80-year-old female client's home for a scheduled occupational therapy visit. A person answers the door and introduces herself as the client's niece, who is visiting from out of town. She tells the therapist that the client is upstairs napping. The niece asks why her aunt was hospitalized recently and what her aunt needs to work on in therapy. The therapist should perform which primary action?
   A. Help the client's niece to understand the client's condition and intervention plan
   B. Wake the client up and ask for permission to talk to her niece
   C. Reschedule therapy to another day
   D. Call the nurse case manager

3. For clients with Medicare who require that occupational therapy services be provided at their residence, the guidelines for home care must be followed except if the client is living in which of the following settings?
   A. A relative's home
   B. An assisted living facility
   C. A skilled nursing facility
   D. A subsidized apartment in a senior housing complex

4. An OT is providing services to a client who resides in a continuing care retirement community. The client is diagnosed with a shoulder fracture, hypertension, and diabetes. Today the client expresses that he is thirsty, nauseous, and the therapist observes that the client has labored breathing with a fruity breath odor. The therapist should conclude that the client is most likely at risk for which of the following?
   A. Hypoglycemia
   B. Ketoacidosis
   C. Insulin shock
   D. Orthostatic hypotension

5. A client in home care is diagnosed with chronic obstructive pulmonary disease (COPD). He exhibits deficits in endurance, which limit his ability to perform IADLs such as meal preparation and laundry. The client tells the OT he has been driving to a local restaurant for dinner most nights and to a dry cleaning establishment occasionally to get his laundry done. What is the therapist's best course of action
   A. Work on other community mobility activities in collaboration with the physical therapist (PT)
   B. Do not document that the client is driving because Medicare will deny home-care services
   C. Document that the client no longer needs OT services
   D. Recommend outpatient OT services

Worksheet 9-5 (continued)

Home Care

6. For adult clients with Medicare or Medicaid receiving skilled home care services, which of the following outcome measures is required?
   A. OASIS
   B. DASH
   C. Minimum Data Set
   D. FIM

7. According to Medicare guidelines, when a physician approves the plan of care, which of the following conditions must be met in order for an OTA to provide home care services?
   A. The OT is present during the OTA's session
   B. The physician also signs the OTA's treatment notes
   C. The OT has established the plan and provides supervision
   D. The OTA cannot provide home care for clients with Medicare

8. A client receiving home care services is recovering from bilateral lower extremity fractures. He requires assistance from his wife to use his wheelchair. When teaching wheelchair mobility in an area that lacks curb cuts, the OT should instruct the client's wife to use which of the following methods with the wheelchair to descend a curb from the sidewalk?
   A. Approach curb with the wheelchair facing curb and tilted backward, castor wheels off the ground, and bring large wheels over the curb
   B. Approach curb with the wheelchair facing curb, lift large wheels off the ground and bring castor wheels gently over the curb
   C. Approach curb with the wheelchair backward, ease large wheels over the curb and tilt wheelchair backward to lift castor wheels over curb
   D. Approach curb with the wheelchair backward, tilt wheelchair forward to lift the large wheels and ease castor wheels gently over the edge of curb

9. An OT is working with a client in home care who has a neurological condition. As the therapist begins today's session, the client begins to exhibit a seizure. Besides obtaining medical assistance, the therapist should perform which primary action?
   A. Try to restrain the client to minimize convulsions
   B. Adjust clothing around the client's neck to loosen it
   C. Place a washcloth or wallet in client's mouth to prevent him from biting his tongue
   D. Use smelling salts and place a cool washcloth on the client's forehead

10. Which of the following statement is accurate regarding hospice services?
    A. Palliative care is provided
    B. Medicare will not reimburse for OT and PT because the client is not expected to have improved health or functional gains
    C. A physician must always certify that the client is within 1 month of death
    D. Most third-party payers will only provide reimbursement for hospice services if the diagnosis is cancer

Worksheet 9-6

Acute Care

1. A client in acute care has a Foley catheter in place. The collection bag is filled halfway with urine. When transporting the client in a wheelchair to the OT department, what should the therapist do with the catheter bag?
   A. Disconnect it
   B. Place it in the client's lap
   C. Attach it to the top of the wheelchair back support
   D. Attach it below the seat

2. An occupational therapy client contracted a nosocomial infection. This is normally classified as which of the following?
   A. An infection that causes a coma
   B. A hospital-acquired infection
   C. An infection of the nasal cavity
   D. Nonmalignant sarcoma

3. A client recovering from congestive heart failure has an intravenous line placed in his left antecubital vein. When taking this client's vital signs, where should the OT should place the blood pressure cuff?
   A. On the client's right upper arm
   B. On the client's right forearm
   C. On the client's left upper arm
   D. On the client's left forearm

4. An OT is working with a client who has hemiparesis and a nasogastric tube in place. Which of the following activities will most likely create the greatest risk for dislodging the tube?
   A. Active ROM (AROM) of the affected upper extremity
   B. Donning and doffing a turtleneck sweater
   C. Using a transfer belt around the client's waist
   D. Retrograde massage to the affected arm

5. When preparing to transfer a client from a hospital bed to a wheelchair using the bed rail for support, the OT should do which of the following?
   A. Move intravenous pole to maintain tension at infusion site
   B. Raise the hospital bed
   C. Swing away wheelchair footrests
   D. Lower the bed rail

6. In acute care, when does discharge planning begin for most clients?
   A. After an OT evaluation is complete
   B. Upon admission
   C. After all goals are met
   D. The day before discharge

Worksheet 9-6 (continued)

Acute Care

7. During which of the following tasks is a client more likely to experience orthostatic hypotension?
   A. Elevating the foot of the bed
   B. Bilateral dowel exercises to increase shoulder ROM
   C. Transferring sit to stand
   D. Exercising with weights

8. A client confined to bed requires maximum assistance of two people for bed mobility. Which of the following methods is likely the most useful for the OT and nurse to use together when attempting to position the client closer to the head of the bed?
   A. Use a trapeze
   B. Lift the patient up by holding under his arms and legs
   C. Hold onto a sturdy cloth beneath the client
   D. Have client pull on the bed rails

9. Which of the following isolation conditions require droplet precautions?
   A. *Clostridium difficile*
   B. Tuberculosis
   C. Scabies
   D. *Streptococcus A*

10. A 50-year-old client was admitted to the intensive care unit and is unable to communicate. The client's nephew has presented documentation to the hospital staff that indicates that he is the client's health care agent. The kind of documentation the nephew presented is most likely which of the following?
    A. Insurance card
    B. Living will
    C. Do not resuscitate form
    D. Health care proxy

Learning Activity 9-1: Medical Devices

Clients with acute or chronic medical conditions may undergo special procedures or require temporary or long-term use of various medical devices. It is essential that occupational therapy practitioners working with those clients have knowledge of the particular devices and procedures used which can impact occupational therapy intervention and client recovery. Define the medical terms in the table below and list several conditions which would necessitate their use. For each device/condition listed, indicate any precautions impacting occupational therapy intervention and possible effect on a client's ADL performance (e.g., mobility, dressing, sexual activity, etc.).

Medical Devices and Procedures	*Definition*	*Possible Conditions Requiring Use*	*Precautions*	*Effect on Occupational Performance*
Left ventricular assist device (LVAD)				
Suprapubic catheter				
Foley catheter				
Central venous catheter/central line				
Peripherally inserted central catheter (PICC line)				
Implanted venous access port				
Tunneled central venous catheter				
Nasogastric tube (NG-tube)				
Percutaneous endoscopic gastrostomy (PEG)				
Gastric feeding tube (G-tube)				
Nasal cannula				
Percutaneous pinning				
External fixation device				
Tracheostomy				
Sequential compression device				
Neurostimulator/drug pump				
Halo				

Learning Activity 9-2: Medical Devices and Procedures Terminology

Define the following medical terms:

Incentive spirometer:

Nebulizer:

Hyperbaric oxygen therapy:

Bag-valve mask:

Peak flow meter:

Pulse oximeter:

Endoscopy:

Gastrostomy:

Jejunostomy:

Enteral nutrition:

Gavage:

Lavage:

Stent:

Glucometer:

Insulin pen:

Insulin pump:

Sphygmomanometer:

Define stoma/stomata (surgical) and list five examples:

1.
2.
3.
4.
5.

Indicate several situations in which a client may be required to use a condom catheter instead of an indwelling catheter and the challenges associated with the use of that device.

1.
2.
3.

Worksheet 9-7

Cardiac Care—Ventricular Assist Device

Advances in medicine have resulted in the use of ventricular assist devices (VAD) to prolong life for certain clients diagnosed with heart failure. These devices, implanted via a sternotomy, consist of a mechanical pump connected to the heart and a driveline, which connects externally to a controller and power source (Wells, 2013; Wilson, Givertz, Stewart, & Mudge, 2009). OTs working with clients who have undergone this procedure should have special training regarding this specialized device.

Indicate if the following statements are true (T) or false (F).

1. ______ A ventricular assist device is used only with clients who are candidates for a heart transplant.
2. ______ Surgeons will not implant a left ventricular assist device (LVAD) in children under age 12.
3. ______ Health team goals include teaching the client and caregiver aseptic technique for changing bandages around the driveline exit site.
4. ______ The occupational therapy intervention plan should include teaching the client how to change the power source from alternating current (AC) to a battery and vice versa.
5. ______ When the client is medically allowed to take a shower, the OT should instruct the client to place a plastic grocery bag over the device to keep it dry.
6. ______ For a client with a VAD who is deconditioned but allowed to sit up in a chair, initial interventions for transfer training should include wheelchair pushup exercises
7. ______ A client with a LVAD and good recovery can generally resume taking a bath at approximately 8 to 10 weeks.
8. ______ Clients with an implanted nonpulsatile VAD may not have a palpable pulse.
9. ______ The OT should instruct the client to wear elastic waist pants over the driveline.
10. ______ For a client with a VAD, a noncontact sport such as swimming is generally recommended to help with reconditioning.
11. ______ The traditional method of assessing blood pressure may not be reliable with a client with a VAD.
12. ______ Clients with a VAD and/or their caregivers must be able to distinguish between several types of alarms associated with the particular device.
13. ______ For a client with a LVAD, it is preferable that the client have a posterior pelvic tilt when in a seated position.
14. ______ To better accommodate the VAD driveline, the OT might recommend the use of button-down shirts when dressing.
15. ______ Clients whose lives were saved with a VAD are not considered at risk for anxiety or depression because they are generally happy to be alive.

Worksheet 9-8

Skilled Nursing Facility

1. Which of the following ADL impairments is typically one of the earliest symptoms an individual may exhibit as an early sign of Alzheimer's disease?
   A. Incontinence
   B. Forgetting how to shave or brush teeth
   C. Forgetting how to operate a car
   D. Difficulty with remembering names or appointments

2. An OT is working with a client, Stella, diagnosed with Alzheimer's disease and functioning at Allen Cognitive Level 3. The client is recovering from a thoracic compression fracture and appears to have back pain. Stella requires assistance for all ADLs and often asks when her mother, who is deceased, will be coming to visit. When assisting the client with upper and lower body dressing, which of the following methods is probably the least useful for this client?
   A. Teaching use of a sock assist to don socks
   B. Using validation technique
   C. Using chaining technique to don a shirt
   D. Using task breakdown

3. Mary, a client with dementia, cannot remember to ask staff for assistance when she wants to get out of her wheelchair. She is at risk for falls due to poor balance and inability to remember to use her walker. Mary also has poor fine motor skills. Which primary intervention should an OT suggest as an alternative to a restraint while Mary sits in her wheelchair?
   A. Seat belt with buckle
   B. Vest restraint
   C. Seat alarm
   D. Lap board

4. An OT in a skilled nursing facility (SNF) is working with a client who exhibits left neglect. Which of the following activities is least appropriate for the therapist to do?
   A. Implement a symmetrical bilateral activity
   B. Implement an asymmetrical bilateral activity
   C. Apply lotion to the client's left arm
   D. When leaving, the OT should state that the call bell is on the client's left side

5. An OT is working with a client with dementia functioning at Allen Cognitive Level 2. During an intervention session, the client is exhibiting agitation and keeps asking when her husband will arrive. The therapist knows that the client's spouse has been deceased for 10 years. Which of the following methods would probably be the least effective in regard to this situation?
   A. Reality orientation
   B. Therapeutic fib
   C. Redirect attention
   D. Validation

Worksheet 9-8 (continued)

Skilled Nursing Facility

6. Lydia, an 80-year-old client with congestive heart failure (CHF), has been admitted to a SNF for short-term rehabilitation. When the OT session has ended, the therapist brings Lydia back to her hospital room and transfers her into a chair per her request. A cup of hot herbal tea and a snack have just been delivered by the dietary department. Lydia states that she is a bit sleepy but happy to see her hot beverage. Because the therapist has a busy schedule and cannot stay with Lydia while she drinks her hot tea, which action is best for the therapist to take?
   A. Quickly make sure that the cup of tea has not become cold
   B. Place the tea and snack in Lydia's hands while she sits in the chair so that she does not need to walk to the bedside table to get them
   C. Tell Lydia that you are not comfortable with letting her drink her tea because she is sleepy
   D. Place the tea on the over-bed table, move it close to Lydia, and alert the nurse's aide that the client is sleepy and drinking hot tea.

7. An OT working in an SNF is assessing a 75-year-old client's cognitive abilities following a brain aneurysm sustained 2 weeks ago. The client emigrated from Russia to the United States 20 years ago, is fluent in English, and was transferred from an acute care hospital yesterday. The client correctly states his first and last name and the name of the facility. However, although today is December 30, the client states that today's date is "29th of December." The therapist asks the client to state the major holiday that is coming up in January and the client's response is "*Christmas.*" The client's daughter is in the room and quietly states, "*My Dad is Russian Orthodox—he follows the old calendar.*" The OT should conclude which of the following? (Note: Judith Wolansky contributed to this question.)
   A. The client is oriented to person, place, and time
   B. The client is oriented to person and place but not time
   C. The client is hard of hearing
   D. The client is confused

8. Saul, a 78-year-old male with COPD, was diagnosed with pancreatic cancer last month, which necessitated surgery. After surgery, Saul experienced an exacerbation of his COPD. As soon as he was medically stable, he was transferred to an SNF for 3 weeks of rehabilitation and was then discharged to his home. A few days later, the OT who had worked with Saul daily in the SNF went out to dinner with a friend and happened to see Saul eating in the same restaurant and sitting with three other people. Saul was one of her favorite clients. What should the therapist do?
   A. Go over to Saul and ask how he is doing in remission
   B. Wait for Saul to acknowledge the OT first
   C. Get Saul's attention, wave "hello" and tell his companions he has done remarkably well recovering from cancer surgery
   D. Pretend she does not see him and mention to her friend that Saul was one of her favorite nursing home clients

Worksheet 9-8 (continued)

Skilled Nursing Facility

9. An OT is using the constraint induced movement therapy approach with a client who is diagnosed with a right CVA and left side weakness. Which of the following is considered a primary intervention for that approach?
   A. Use a transfer belt during functional mobility and transfers
   B. Put a sling on the client's right arm during selected functional tasks
   C. Put a sling on the client's left arm during selected functional tasks
   D. Use a seat belt to prevent falls

10. For clients with Medicare or Medicaid in a skilled nursing facility, which of the following is part of the Resident Assessment Instrument?
   A. Outcome Assessment Information Set
   B. Functional Independence Measure
   C. Canadian Occupational Performance Measure
   D. Minimum Data Set

Worksheet 9-9

Speech and Language

Indicate which of the following terms are typically used in documentation to describe speech and/or language.

1. ____ dysarthria
2. ____ dysphagia
3. ____ dystonia
4. ____ dysphonia
5. ____ cadence
6. ____ dysrhythmia
7. ____ aspiration
8. ____ intelligibility
9. ____ shuttering
10. ____ intonation
11. ____ apraxia of speech
12. ____ hemianopsia
13. ____ aphasia
14. ____ dysphasia
15. ____ fluency
16. ____ articulation
17. ____ dysthymia
18. ____ anomia
19. ____ dysesthesia
20. ____ pitch

Worksheet 9-10

Wheeled Mobility

1. Leona, a 58-year-old female with a chronic neurological disease, was referred to OT for a wheelchair assessment. Because of the progressive nature of her condition, Leona has been nonambulatory for the past 6 months and requires moderate assistance to transfer. Her husband is the one who generally pushes her standard adult wheelchair. The OT notes that Leona weighs 200 pounds and determines that Leona has moderate impairment in upper extremity function requiring use of a joystick for wheeled mobility independence. Leona would like to resume her part-time work as a greeter at a large discount store, and she desires to volunteer 1 day a week reading to a kindergarten class. The town she lives in provides door-to-door transit service for wheelchair users. Which of the following options is most appropriate for the therapist to recommend?
   A. Standard wheelchair with a Roho seat cushion
   B. Sip-and-puff wheelchair with a gel seat cushion
   C. Heavy duty adult wheelchair with a Roho seat cushion
   D. Tilt in space power wheelchair with a gel seat cushion

2. Tyler, a 18-year-old male weighing 180 pounds, has a diagnosis of paraplegia due to a random drive-by shooting through his kitchen window. Before his injury he was planning to attend college to study accounting and was admitted on a basketball scholarship. He is currently using a lightweight manual wheelchair independently. Of the following choices, which is the most appropriate for an OT to recommend at this time?
   A. Power wheelchair
   B. Heavy-duty adult wheelchair
   C. Sports wheelchair
   D. Power mobility scooter

3. Marisa, a 45-year-old female diagnosed with multiple sclerosis (MS), lives with her spouse in a wheelchair-accessible apartment. She is able to transfer independently but cannot stand for more than a few minutes or ambulate long distances safely. Because of her MS and a chronic right shoulder condition, she fatigues easily when self-propelling her standard wheelchair. Marisa desires to continue working as a college professor and maintain independence in IADLs, such as shopping and driving. Which of the following options is most appropriate for an OT to recommend at this time?
   A. Power mobility scooter
   B. One arm drive wheelchair with adjustable reclining seat
   C. Tilt-in-space power wheelchair
   D. Sip-and-puff wheelchair

4. Massimo, a 67-year-old male, 5' 6" and weighing 148 pounds, has a diagnosis of right cerebrovascular accident (CVA) resulting in left hemiplegia. He was recently admitted to a rehabilitation hospital with the goal for him to return home in several weeks. Massimo does not have any functional cognitive deficits. A goal in the occupational therapy intervention plan is for the client to attain independence in wheeled mobility because it is not likely Massimo will be able to ambulate independently on discharge. Which of the following options is most appropriate for the therapist to recommend at this time?
   A. Adult bariatric wheelchair
   B. One-arm drive wheelchair
   C. Power wheelchair
   D. Ultralight wheelchair

Worksheet 9-10 (continued)

Wheeled Mobility

5. An "amputee" wheelchair for a client with bilateral lower extremity amputations is different from a standard wheelchair in which of the following ways?
   A. The rear wheel axles are in a more posterior position
   B. The rear wheel axles are in a more anterior position
   C. It has four anti-tippers attached
   D. The caster wheels are larger than the rear wheels

6. Which of the following would least likely be part of a fall injury prevention program for wheelchair users in an SNF?
   A. Merry Walker
   B. Hipster
   C. Toggle lock extension
   D. Chest harness

7. Saul is a 40-year-old male carpenter who sustained an incomplete lumbar level spinal cord injury due to a recent fall from a deck that he was building. The OT determined that the safest way for Saul to transfer is for him to use a sliding board. When ordering Saul's wheelchair for home use, which of the following wheelchair options would likely be least useful?
   A. Removable front rigging
   B. Removable arm rests
   C. Scissors lock
   D. Toggle lock

8. Abdoul is an 82-year-old male admitted to a rehabilitation hospital with a diagnosis of Guillain-Barré syndrome. He is beginning to regain gross motor function in his upper extremities. However, because of poor trunk control, he tends to slide forward while seated in his wheelchair and is at risk for falling. A wheelchair lap belt with an attached buckle would be considered a restraint because Abdoul cannot yet manage unfastening it. Which of the following choices should the OT try next to keep him seated safely in the wheelchair?
   A. Wheelchair seat alarm
   B. Abduction wedge
   C. Lap belt with a loop Velcro closure
   D. Lap tray

Worksheet 9-10 (continued)

Wheeled Mobility

9. Which of the following statements is incorrect?
   A. The larger outer rim on a one-arm drive chair propels the near drive wheel
   B. A reclining wheelchair usually has a longer back than a standard wheelchair
   C. Releasing the locking mechanism allows the front rigging to move outward
   D. Pneumatic caster tires tend to provide a smoother ride and function better on rougher surfaces than rubber tires

10. When instructing a client in performing a standing pivot transfer from the wheelchair to a bed, the OT should instruct the client to do which of the following for safety?
    A. Lock the front rigging in place
    B. Engage the toggle mechanism
    C. Elevate the footrests
    D. All of the above

Worksheet 9-11

Amputation Levels

Occupational therapy practitioners may work with individuals who have experienced either a lower extremity or upper extremity amputation. Typically, when working with an individual with a lower extremity amputation, the OT and OTA will address functional mobility/transfers, and self-care ADLs including dressing and prosthetic donning and doffing. Upper extremity prosthetics require instruction in the use of the device and well as facilitating return to participation in desired occupations using the device.

Match the levels of upper and lower extremity amputations with their descriptions (Murphy, 2014).

	Transfemoral amputation (above-knee amputation; AKA)	A	Intact forearm supination and pronation and flexion and extension of the wrist
	Chopart amputation	B	Removal of entire leg
	Transcarpal amputation	C	Removal of navicular, cuboid, cuneiforms, metatarsals, and phalanges
	Pirogoff amputation	D	Removal of entire arm and scapula
	Partial hand amputation	E	Between tibia and calcaneous
	Transhumeral amputation	F	Comprises 85% of all lower extremity amputations; desirable when below-knee amputation (BKA) will not heal
	Transradial amputation	G	Fingers and or part of the thumb
	Scapulothoracic amputation	H	Best results when the deltoid insertion is maintained
	Hip disarticulation	I	Best lever arm when radial length is no shorter than 2 centimeters above the wrist

Worksheet 9-12

Prosthetic Devices

Indicate whether the statement about prosthetic devices and occupational therapy interventions for individuals with upper extremity or lower extremity prosthetics is true (T) or false (F).

1. ______ Clients with bilateral lower extremity amputations will require an amputee axle plate to ensure that the center of gravity is repositioned.
2. ______ Anti-tippers are also a solution for the change in center of gravity in a wheelchair for an individual with amputation of bilateral lower extremities, but these can create difficulties with maneuvering the chair on uneven surfaces.
3. ______ Three types of hand prosthesis include the robotic mini, the functional mind control, and passive prosthesis devices.
4. ______ Transfer training should include transfers onto the floor and instruction in moving along the floor for individual with lower extremities amputations.
5. ______ Maintaining the knee in extension by artificial means (splinting) immediately following a below-knee amputation in not required as the quadriceps will keep the knee joint in extension automatically.
6. ______ Ideally, a hand prosthesis will allow for only a gross grasp, a lateral pinch, and three-jaw chuck grasp.
7. ______ Commercial shrinkers for lower extremity amputations are preferred over ace wrap wrappings, especially for those who have poor hand dexterity.
8. ______ Phantom limb pain occurs in approximately 85% of those with amputations. Many report that the sensation is similar to a tickling sensation or very itchy.
9. ______ It is very important for a client with an amputation to make regular inspections of his or her skin to ensure that skin breakdown of the stump does not occur.
10. ______ A passive nonfunctional prosthesis may be desired by an individual who wants a device that looks more lifelike.
11. ______ Terminal hand devices, such as a hook, are typically driven by motion of the scapula and glenohumeral joint.
12. ______ Externally powered devices that are activated by impulses from muscles are expensive and reserved for individuals who have a mature stump.

Worksheet 9-13

Dysphagia

Occupational therapists work with individuals who have feeding, eating, and swallowing difficulties that can result from central nervous system damage caused by stroke or traumatic brain injury, acquired conditions such as amyotrophic lateral sclerosis, or as the result of developmental disabilities such as cerebral palsy. The National Dysphagia Diet (NDD) was created by the National Dysphagia Diet Task Force of the American Dietetic Association (2002). This diet establishes standard terminology along with guidelines for dietary texture modification to assist practitioners and clients in the management of dysphagia (National Dysphagia Diet Task Force, 2002; AOTA, 2007).

For this worksheet, fill in the criteria for each level identified by the NDD including the name of the level, and at least two examples of the type of food for each level (except level III) including the levels of liquid viscosity.

National Dysphagia Diet Level I:

Dysphagia

"____________________________"

1.
2.
3.

National Dysphagia Diet Level II:

Dysphagia

"____________________________"

1.
2.
3.

National Dysphagia Diet Level III:

Dysphagia

"____________________________"

1.

Regular:

No Dysphagia

Proposed levels of liquid viscosity:

Thin ____________________________

1.
2.
3.

Nectar-like ____________________________

1.
2.
3.

Honey-like ____________________________

1.
2.
3.

Spoon-thick ____________________________

1.
2.
3.

Worksheet 9-14

Feeding and Eating Terms

Fill in the following chart. Either define the term listed or identify the definition listed.

1.	Adaptive feeding equipment	
2.		The prevention of accidental introduction of liquids, food, or medications into the trachea during eating or drinking (AOTA, 2007).
3.	Aspiration	
4.	Bolus	
5.		Tube feedings where nutrients are placed in and absorbed in the intestinal tract (AOTA, 2007).
6.		Swallowing phase where the bolus of food travels along the esophagus and into the stomach (AOTA, 2007).
7.	Mendelsohn maneuver	
8.	Oral phase	
9.		Swallowing phase where the bolus of food is chewed and manipulated by the lips, cheek, and tongue to create the bolus that is the correct texture for swallowing (AOTA, 2007).
10.	Oral stage function	
11.	Pharyngeal phase	
12.	Pocketing	
13.		A U.S. Food and Drug Administration–cleared method to of neuromuscular electrical stimulation that promotes swallowing by strengthening and reeducating muscles (AOTA, 2007)
14.	Upper aerodigestive tract	
15.		The provision of nutrients through an intravenous tube (AOTA, 2007).
16.	Therapeutic feedings	
17.		"A swallowing technique used for airway protection where the client is told to take a breath and hold it while swallowing and then coughs after the swallow; results in the voluntary closure of the vocal folds before, during, and after the swallow" (AOTA, 2007, p. 696).
18.		The leakage of food into the lungs without overt coughing or choking; may indicate a motor or sensory deficit (AOTA, 2007).
19.		The ability of the individual to set up food and bring to mouth without assistance (AOTA, 2007).
20.	Secretion management	
21.	Preoral phase	
22.		Two or more attempts are used to swallow food (AOTA, 2007).

Worksheet 9-15

Low Vision Rehabilitation

Visual difficulties are a major factor in occupational disruption, particularly for the older adult. Occupational therapy practitioners provide low-vision rehabilitation services to facilitate the ability of those with low vision to participate in desired activities. Worksheet 9-15 and Worksheet 9-16 check your knowledge of low vision, the conditions that lead to it, how to assess for visual loss and how to facilitate participation.

1. Which of the following is *not* true about Certified Orientation Mobility Specialists (COMS)?
   A. They provide instruction to individuals with visual impairments to assist them in using their remaining senses to know their position in the environment and move around with it.
   B. They provide services to all age groups.
   C. Occupational therapists can become COMS through participation in a training session.
   D. COMS teach compensatory techniques and the use of adaptive equipment.

2. Which of the following is not a component of vision?
   A. Visual acuity
   B. Visual resonance
   C. Visual field
   D. Contrast sensitivity

3. Optical devices used to overcome low-vision deficits have both advantages and disadvantages. Which one of the following is a disadvantage of using a handheld magnifier?
   A. Client more likely to accept because of familiarity
   B. Illumination is available for low-light environments
   C. Client moves device in and out to find desired level of magnification
   D. Lower cost when compared with many higher tech options

4. Appropriate visual function measures help ensure that rehabilitation is comprehensive to ensure dramatic results and improved functional abilities. Which of the following lists of functional vision components do OTs assess most often?
   A. Visual acuity, glare, light adaptations
   B. Reading acuity, visual acuity, preferred retinal locus (PRL)
   C. Color vision, glare, visual acuity
   D. Preferred retinal locus, visual acuity, depth perception

5. Which one of the following areas of low-vision intervention is beyond the scope of practice of a generalist OT (refer the client to a Certified Orientation Mobility Specialist)?
   A. Safety issues regarding tub, shower, and rugs
   B. Locating appliances within the home
   C. Locating light switches within the home
   D. Bus or subway travel

Worksheet 9-16

Low Vision Basics

True (T) or false (F):

1. _______ Low vision visual impairments are correctable with the appropriate surgical intervention.
2. _______ Low vision is not the same as blindness. Low vision allows for the visualization of light; blindness does not.
3. _______ Occupational therapists have been providing services for low vision since the 1940s.
4. _______ Medicare has covered the cost of low vision services provided by occupational therapists since the 1960s.
5. _______ Low vision positively correlates with the incidence of clinical depression in older adults.
6. _______ Vision comprises five separate components.
7. _______ Diabetes can lead to scattered spotty areas of vision loss called *scotomas*.
8. _______ A cataract is an area of blindness located in the center of the visual field.
9. _______ Autoimmune deficiency disorder (AIDS) can lead to blindness due to the cytomegalovirus.
10. _______ An optical device such as a magnifier will provide clear vision for someone with a low-vision deficit.
11. _______ The role of an OT providing low vision interventions is not to know how optical devices work; that is the role of the optometrist.
12. _______ In addition to performing specialized assessments to determine the visual abilities of a client, it is important to ask the client how their vision is specifically affecting his or her overall occupational participation.
13. _______ When using an eye chart, such as the Bailey-Lovie Chart or the Lea Acuity chart to measure visual acuity, the lighting of the chart is crucial.
14. _______ An occupational therapist can recommend adapted keyboards, such as those with high contrast or large letters, to assist a person with low vision in typing
15. _______ Voice-activated and audio-output devices should only be recommended to a client by a Certified Orientation Mobility Specialist.

Learning Activity 9-3: Spinal Cord Injury Interventions

Individuals diagnosed with spinal cord injuries (SCI) do not necessarily have predictable and absolute outcomes because injuries sustained often are incomplete, rather than complete, lesions. Persons with incomplete lesions may vary greatly regarding specific viable client factors, present functional abilities, and ultimate outcomes for occupational participation. For this exercise, imagine three persons who are diagnosed with complete spinal cord lesions, each at one of the three levels designated in the following chart. Choose one of the 10 activities/occupations listed and compare and contrast occupational therapy interventions for each of the three clients. Consider whether the client will likely achieve independence in this occupation or if the assistance of another person is needed to complete this task. Using activity analysis, consider how the client will perform each step. Determine the compensatory methods, equipment, or occupational adaptations that would be helpful and any caregiver education required.

<u>Activity/Occupation List</u>

1. Bowel and bladder management (including feminine hygiene)
2. Grooming (shaving face/legs, applying makeup, brushing teeth)
3. Lower body dressing (donning/doffing underwear, pants, socks, shoes)
4. Upper body dressing (donning/doffing button-down shirt, tie, bra, polo shirt, undershirt)
5. Upper and lower body bathing
6. Hair care (shampoo and style)
7. Feeding (managing finger foods, utensils, knife, cup)
8. Medication management (include oral medication and diabetic care)
9. Driving
10. Preparing lunch (frozen pizza and salad)

Occupation Requiring Intervention:	***Client With Complete C-5 Lesion***	***Client With Complete C7-C8 Lesion***	***Client With Complete T-6 Lesion***
Attainable assistance level desired outcome (e.g., modified independence, mod, max assist, etc.)			
Client position and where the intervention will take place (e.g., sitting upright in bed, sitting in wheelchair at sink, table)			
Mobility devices indicated			
Aspects of task requiring setup/ assistance			
Compensatory methods, orthotics, and/or adaptive equipment/durable medical equipment indicated			
Sequence of steps and instructional methods			
Caregiver education required for this task			

Learning Activity 9-4: Cognitive Levels

The Rancho Los Amigos Coma Scale, also known as the Levels of Cognitive Functioning, was developed at the Rancho Los Amigos Hospital in Downey, California, in 1972. The authors of the scale were Chris Hagen, Danese Malkmus, and Patricia Durham, members of the head injury treatment staff (Whyte, 2011). The purpose of this tool is to assist the intervention team in determining the client's state of consciousness, the extent of the brain injury, and the prognosis. The scale also assists health care workers in understanding and evaluating the client's behaviors as he or she progresses through the 8 levels (Whyte, 2011). Occupational therapists find the scale helpful in intervention planning by providing an outline of what functional abilities and behaviors are expected at various levels.

The following learning activity provides you an opportunity to recall the eight levels of the Rancho Los Amigos scale, including the names and description of the client at each level. In addition, the activity provides you with an opportunity to consider various techniques, tasks, activities, and occupations that may be appropriate as occupational therapy interventions at various levels. Information for Level I has been provided as an example.

Level of Cognitive Functioning	***Name of Level***	***Type of Response at Level***	***Activities (one preparatory task or technique and, if indicated, one activity or occupation)***
Level I	*No response*	*Patient appears to be in deep sleep and is completely unresponsive*	*Coma stimulation techniques*
Level II			
Level III			
Level IV			
Level V			
Level VI			
Level VII			
Level VIII			

Learning Activity 9-5: Cognitive Interventions

OTs work with clients who have various conditions that affect functional cognition. One model used in occupational therapy practice to aid therapists in evaluation and intervention planning is the Cognitive Disabilities Model developed by Claudia Allen (1985). Allen delineates global characteristics for six distinct levels of cognitive function (1985). Current information about the specific assessments used with this model can be found at www.allen-cognitive-network.org. For the following exercise, imagine three adults with no physical limitations but who are diagnosed with schizophrenia, each currently at one of the three levels designated in the chart below. The clients have been referred for an occupational therapy consultation to assess existing functional abilities, safety, and to provide caregiver education. Choose one of the 12 activities/occupations listed and compare and contrast occupational therapy interventions for each of the three clients. Consider whether the client will likely achieve independence in this occupation or if the assistance of another person is needed to complete this task. Using activity analysis, consider how the client will perform each step and any safety concerns. Determine the compensatory methods, equipment, or occupational adaptations that would be helpful; specific types of cues indicated (tactile, visual, verbal, etc.); and any caregiver education required.

<u>Activity/Occupation List</u>

1. Bowel and bladder management
2. Grooming (shaving, applying makeup, brushing teeth, nail care)
3. Dressing
4. Bathing
5. Using a telephone (include situations such as social calls, contacting service providers, dealing with telemarketers)
6. Feeding (managing finger foods, utensils, knife, cup)
7. Hearing aid management
8. Hair care (wash, cut, style)
9. Banking and paying bills
10. Care of a pet
11. Preparing breakfast (tea and toast)
12. Preparing lunch (soup and salad)

Occupation Requiring Intervention	***Client With Schizophrenia: Allen Level 2***	***Client With Schizophrenia: Allen Level 4***	***Client With Schizophrenia: Allen Level 5***
Attainable assist level/desired outcome (e.g., modified independence, mod, max assist, etc.)			
Likely setting where the client resides and where the intervention will take place			
Safety concerns for task			
Aspects of task likely requiring setup/assistance			
Compensatory methods, adaptive equipment and/or durable medical equipment indicated			
Sequence of steps and instructional methods			
Caregiver education required for this task			

Learning Activity 9-6: Intervention Planning—Upper Extremity Conditions

In this activity you will find information about two individuals who have sustained injuries to their upper extremities. Read the cases and complete a plan of care as instructed for each of the clients. Compare and contrast your two plans of care. For additional practice, complete Learning Activity 9-7.

1. Determine three or four assessments that you may find appropriate to determine the client's occupational status and the status of skills or client factors.
2. Once you have determined the areas of occupation that are affected, create three long-term goals and a minimum of two short-term goals for each. Use a professional format to formulate proper goals that are occupation-based and measurable. A useful goal format that contains all the necessary elements is the COAST method, which stands for client, occupation, assist level, specific conditions, timeline (Gateley & Borcherding, 2012; Morreale & Borcherding, 2013).
3. Finally, list several activities that you will do to facilitate the client's return to occupational participation. Identify the type of interventions that you chose, keeping in mind that any preparatory methods and tasks selected must be used in preparation for activities and occupation-based engagements.
4. When you are done creating your plan, share it with a fellow occupational therapy student and discuss your ideas using the following questions:
   - Are the assessment tools appropriate for your client's age, diagnosis, and your hypothesis regarding areas of challenge?
   - Is your plan relevant for the context and environment in which this client lives and works?
   - Are your goals measurable and occupation-based?
   - Do your goals contain all components identified in a method such as COAST?
   - Which frame of reference or practice model is your intervention plan based on?
   - How are the activities, tasks, and techniques that you have chosen going to work to realization of the goals?
   - Are the activities appropriate for the context, environment, and interests of the client and the diagnosis?
   - Are you aware of evidence to support your treatment activity choices? Where would you locate this evidence?
   - Note that there are many similarities in case study 1-A and 1-B. To what do you attribute differences in the intervention plans that you created for these very similar client injuries?

<u>Case 1-A</u>

Mrs. P is a 63-year-old married female. She does not work outside of the home, but is very involved in civic organizations such as the Junior League and the local garden club. She and her husband, who recently retired as the vice president of an electronics firm, purchased a large historical home in the downtown area of their city. Because swimming is an important leisure and health pursuit of Mrs. P, the couple installed a large swimming pool almost immediately.

Approximately 3 weeks ago, while walking her dog poolside, Mrs. P slipped and sustained a fracture to the olecranon of her dominant right elbow. As a result, she underwent an open reduction and internal fixation (ORIF) procedure with Kirshner wire to secure the bone fragments for healing. At this time, the sutures have been removed and the wound is healing well. Mrs. P is currently keeping occupied by having multiple friends visit throughout the day. They spend many hours poolside discussing world events. Her husband transports Mrs. P to all of her doctor appointments and assists her with some activities, such as grocery shopping.

Mrs. P has her first occupational therapy visit today and is to begin active mobilization of the elbow joint and to address occupational concerns. The cast provided by the physician immobilizes her elbow in 60° of flexion and does not include her wrist. Although initially circumferential, the cast was cut in half and is now applied with an ace wrap. It is effective in immobilizing and protecting the joint while Mrs. P attempts to complete all desired activities. However, she reports the following difficulties:

- Dependency in application of splint (Ace wrap)
- Limited wrist mobility due to length of splint/cast

Learning Activity 9-6: Intervention Planning—Upper Extremity Conditions (continued)

- Bulkiness of splint/cast creating difficulty with dressing into long sleeve shirts and jackets
- Heaviness of splint/cast, leading to shoulder soreness
- General dependency for all self-care and transportation
- Unable to attend garden club activities
- Unable to attend and participate in Junior League activities

Case 1-B

Mrs. M is a 64-year-old single female who currently works outside of the home as an electronic assembler in a local emergency lighting plant. She has a 12-year history of type II diabetes and has early signs and symptoms of COPD due to chronic bronchitis. She attends church on a regular basis and occasionally volunteers with church-related activities. Mrs. M lives in a 2-bedroom apartment with her 32-year-old son and his 25-year-old girlfriend, neither of whom is employed. Her home is several miles from the nearest store and her work is a 20-minute drive.

Approximately 3 weeks ago, Mrs. M sustained a fracture to her dominant right elbow following a fall down the stairs of her apartment. She underwent an open reduction and internal fixation procedure (ORIF) with Kirshner wire to secure the bone fragments for healing. A cast was provided by the physician that immobilizes her elbow in 55° of flexion and leaves the wrist free. At this time, Mrs. M is occupying herself by watching television and searching the Internet for jobs that may suit her son and his girlfriend.

Today Mrs. M has her first occupational therapy visit to begin active mobilization of the elbow joint and to address occupational concerns. Her neighbor has brought her to therapy. The therapist observes that the circumferential cast has been cut in half and is now applied as a splint with an Ace wrap. The wound and bone are healing well. Mrs. M reports the following difficulties to the therapist during her initial evaluation:

- General dependency for all self-care and transportation
- Unable to work
- Unable to cook for son and girlfriend or do their laundry
- Dependency in application of splint (Ace wrap)
- Limited wrist mobility due to length of splint/cast
- Bulkiness of splint/cast creating difficulty with dressing into long sleeve shirts and jackets
- Heaviness of splint/cast, leading to shoulder soreness

Plan of Care

Assessment tools: ____________________

____

____

Functional problem 1 ____________________

Occupation-based long-term goal 1 ____________________

Short-term goal 1a ____________________

Short-term goal 1b ____________________

Functional problem 2 ____________________

Long-term goal 2 ____________________

Learning Activity 9-6: Intervention Planning—Upper Extremity Conditions (continued)

Short-term goal 2a ____________________

Short-term goal 2b ____________________

Functional problem 3 ____________________

Long-term goal 3 ____________________

Short-term goal 3a ____________________

Short-term goal 3b ____________________

Activity 1 (based on short-term goal ____________)

Activity 2 (based on short-term goal ____________)

Activity 3 (based on short-term goal ____________)

Learning Activity 9-7: Intervention Planning—More Practice

In this activity, you will find information about two other individuals who have sustained injuries to their upper extremities with many similarities. Read the cases and complete a plan of care as instructed for each of the clients. Compare and contrast your two plans of care with each other and with the plans you created in Learning Activity 9-6.

1. Determine three or four assessments that you may find appropriate to determine the client's occupational status and the status of skills or client factors.
2. Once you determine the areas of occupation affected, create three long-term goals and a minimum of two short-term goals for each. Use a format, such as COAST, to formulate proper goals that are occupation-based and measurable.
3. Finally, list several activities that you will do to facilitate the client's return to occupational participation. Identify the type of interventions that you chose, keeping in mind that any preparatory methods and tasks selected must be used in preparation for activities and occupation-based engagements.
4. When you are done creating your plan, share it with a fellow occupational therapy student and discuss your ideas using the following questions:
    - Are the assessment tools appropriate for your client's age, diagnosis, and your hypothesis regarding areas of challenge?
    - Is your plan relevant for the context and environment in which this client lives and works?
    - Are your goals measurable and occupation-based?
    - Do your goals contain all components identified in a method such as COAST?
    - On which frame of reference or practice model is your intervention plan based?
    - How are the activities, tasks, and techniques that you have chosen going to work to realization of the goals?
    - Are the activities appropriate for the context, environment, and interests of the client and the diagnosis?
    - Are you aware of evidence to support your treatment activity choices? Where would you locate this evidence?
    - Note that there are many similarities in Case Study 2-A and 2-B. To what do you attribute differences in the intervention plans that you created for these very similar client injuries?

<u>Case 2-A</u>

Julia is a 54-year-old divorced female who works as an assistant manager at a local branch of a large national discount store. One week ago, Julia lacerated her dominant right wrist at work when a bottle of tequila that she was shelving broke in her hand. She sustained a laceration of her ulnar nerve, flexor digitorum superficialis and profundus to the ring and small fingers, and to the ulnar artery. All structures were surgically repaired and Julia was referred to occupational therapy for treatment of her nerve and tendon injuries. At this time, the therapist observes that Julia's wounds are healing well, no infection is present and her hand is protected in a postsurgical half cast securing her wrist and digits in moderate flexion.

In addition to issues surrounding her injury, Julia is showing signs of significant stress that she attributes to work-related concerns. Her boss has refused to allow her access to the broken liquor bottle that she needs as evidence to seek damages from the manufacturer of the faulty glass. She was also to receive a promotion to manager within weeks of this accident and was told by her employer that they will not promote someone who is injured. Despite 25 years of dedicated service, she will be put back on the list and may have to wait many months or years before another position becomes open. These work-related issues are causing Julia a great deal of emotional stress. She is beginning to show signs of complex regional pain syndrome (CRPS) and posttraumatic stress disorder (PTSD).

While creating the occupational profile, the occupational therapist asked Julia about her home life, her support system, and her interests other than work. He found that Julia lives in her own home with her adult daughter and enjoys home decorating, craft activities, and cooking. At this time, Julia is not working and is unable to care for her home or engage in leisure activities. She is able to prepare light meals for herself and to dress and bathe with increased time required. Her daughter works full time and must adjust her schedule to help her mother with transportation and home tasks.

Case 2-B

Ralph is a 54-year-old married male who works as an assistant manager at a local branch of a large national discount store. Two days ago, Ralph lacerated his nondominant right wrist at work when a bottle of tequila that he was shelving broke in his hand. He sustained a laceration of his ulnar nerve, flexor digitorum superficialis and profundus to the ring and small fingers, and to the ulnar artery. All structures were surgically repaired, and Ralph was referred to occupational therapy for treatment of his nerve and tendon injuries.

In addition to issues surrounding his injury, Ralph is showing signs of significant stress that he attributes to issues related to work and his fear of not being able to provide for his family. Ralph's boss has refused to allow him access to the broken liquor bottle that he will need as evidence to seek damages from the manufacturer of the faulty glass. He was also to receive a promotion to manager within weeks of this accident and has been told by his employer that they will not promote someone who is injured. Despite 25 years of dedicated service, he will be put back on the list and may have to wait many months or even years before another position becomes open. These work-related issues are causing Ralph a great deal of emotional stress. He is beginning to show signs of CRPS and PTSD.

While creating the occupational profile, the occupational therapist asked Ralph about his home life, his support system, and his interests other than work. He found that Ralph lives in his own home with his wife and adult daughter and enjoys home maintenance, lawn care, and working on his 1964 Corvair. At this time, Ralph is not able to complete any home maintenance or engage in leisure activities. He is not working and spends his time watching television and occasionally reading a how-to book or magazine about cars. His wife is responsible for driving him to all appointments and caring for the basic household needs. She readily assists Ralph with any self-care concerns and is a good listener, according to him.

Plan of Care

Assessment tools: ______________________________

____

____

Functional problem 1 ______________________________

Occupation-based long-term goal 1 ______________________________

Short-term goal 1a ______________________________

Short-term goal 1b ______________________________

Functional problem 2 ______________________________

Long-term goal 2 ______________________________

Short-term goal 2a ______________________________

Short-term goal 2b ______________________________

Functional problem 3 ______________________________

Long-term goal 3 ______________________________

Short-term goal 3a ______________________________

Short-term goal 3b ______________________________

Activity 1 (based on short-term goal ____________)

Activity 2 (based on short-term goal ____________)

Activity 3 (based on short-term goal ____________)

Answers to Chapter 9 Worksheets

Worksheet 9-1: Diseases and Conditions

1. Colles fracture—*Distal radius fracture*
2. Complex regional pain syndrome—*Reflex sympathetic dystrophy*
3. Lou Gehrig disease—*Amyotrophic lateral sclerosis*
4. Herpes zoster—*Shingles*
5. Golfer's elbow—*Medial epicondylitis*
6. Degenerative joint disease—*Osteoarthritis*
7. Adhesive capsulitis—*Frozen shoulder*
8. Tennis elbow—*Lateral epicondylitis*
9. Gamekeeper's thumb—*Ulnar collateral ligament injury*
10. Epstein-Barr virus—*Mononucleosis*
11. Ewing sarcoma—*Bone cancer*
12. Barlow syndrome—*Mitral valve prolapse*
13. Varicella—*Chickenpox*
14. Decubitus ulcer—*Pressure sore/bed sore*
15. Hypoglycemia—*Low blood sugar*
16. Myocardial infarction—*Heart attack*
17. Hypertension—*High blood pressure*
18. Hyperemesis—*Vomiting excessively*
19. Trisomy 21—*Down syndrome*
20. Hyperlipidemia—*Elevated lipid levels/High cholesterol*
21. Thrombus—*Blood clot*
22. Osteogenesis imperfecta —*Brittle bone disease*
23. Diplopia—*Double vision*
24. Ecchymosis—*Bruise*
25. Hematuria—*Blood present in urine*

Worksheet 9-2: Common Medications

Resource: Wilson, Shannon, & Shields, 2014.

1. Warfarin *Atrial fibrillation*
2. Nitroglycerin *Angina*
3. Naproxen *Osteoarthritis*
4. Aricept *Dementia*
5. Risperdal *Schizophrenia*
6. Atenolol *Hypertension*
7. Diazepam *Anxiety*
8. Boniva *Osteoporosis*
9. Levodopa *Parkinson's disease*
10. Topamax *Seizure*
11. Demerol *Pain*

12. Methotrexate *Cancer*
13. Adderall *Attention-deficit disorder*
14. Lexapro *Depression*
15. Proventil *Asthma*
16. Augmentin *Infection*
17. Avonex *Multiple sclerosis*
18. Acyclovir *Shingles*
19. Humulin R *Diabetes*
20. Slow-FE *Iron deficiency*

Worksheet 9-3: Generic Medications

Resource: Wilson et al., 2014.

1. Warfarin *Coumadin*
2. Omeprazole *Prilosec*
3. Ibuprofen *Advil*
4. Diazepam *Valium*
5. Naproxen sodium *Aleve*
6. Hydrocodone Bitartrate *Vicodin*
7. Albuterol *Ventolin*
8. Gabapentin *Neurontin*
9. Atorvastatin calcium *Lipitor*
10. Clonazepam *Klonopin*
11. Enalapril Maleate *Vasotec*
12. Alprazolam *Xanax*
13. Insulin *Humulin R*
14. Fluoxetine hydrochloride *Prozac*
15. Diltiazem *Cardizem*
16. Acetaminophen *Tylenol*
17. Paroxetine *Paxil*
18. Duloxetine hydrochloride *Cymbalta*
19. Calcium carbonate *Tums*
20. Atenolol *Tenormin*

Worksheet 9-4: Intervention Planning—Total Hip Replacement

Resources for goal writing: Gateley & Borcherding, 2012; Morreale & Borcherding, 2013.

Goals need to specify a time frame, measurable criteria, and delineate a desired client outcome relating to occupational participation. Goals should reflect what the client needs to achieve, not what the occupational therapy practitioner will do as interventions. Here are some examples of possible goals for this client. Realize that different settings or practice areas may use slightly different formats or terminology as shown in the various examples below. Of course, the actual goals and time frames may be different for a real client.

1. *Client will complete dressing routine with modified independence and adhering to all total hip precautions by expected discharge in 10 days.*

   or

   Client will complete lower body dressing with modified independence and adhering to all total hip precautions by 3/26/2016 discharge date.

or

By expected discharge on 3/26/2016, client will don lower body garments independently using adaptive equipment and adhering to hip precautions.

2. *While seated at sink, client will perform morning grooming routine with modified independence by expected discharge on 3/26/2016.*

   or

   Client will manage grooming tasks independently, demonstrating ability to stand at sink for 8 minutes using rolling walker, within 10 days.

3. *While seated on tub bench, client will complete bathing routine with modified independence and adhering to all total hip precautions by expected discharge in 10 days.*

   or

   While seated on tub bench and adhering to hip precautions, client will be able to bathe upper and lower body independently using a long-handled sponge by expected discharge in 10 days.

   or

   Client will perform lower body bathing with modified independence and adhering to all total hip precautions by expected discharge date of 3/26/2016.

4. *By expected discharge in 10 days, client will demonstrate ability to prepare a frozen microwave meal with modified independence while adhering to all total hip precautions and using wheeled walker.*

   or

   Client will demonstrate ability to prepare a simple stovetop meal (e.g., eggs, soup) while standing at stove with walker and contact guard assistance within 10 days.

5. *Client will complete toilet transfers with modified independence (using wheeled walker, elevated seat, and grab bar) and adhering to all total hip precautions by expected discharge in 10 days.*

Worksheet 9-5: Home Care

1. C. The client may be in the bathroom or might not have heard the doorbell so the primary course of action would be try and reach him by phone. If there is still no answer, the OT should follow agency policy, such as contacting a supervisor or nurse case manager and document the situation.
2. B. An OT must always adhere to HIPAA (Health Insurance Portability and Accountability Act) guidelines. Because the therapist must wake up the client for therapy, she should ask the client for permission to discuss the client's medical information with her niece. The client may or may not want it disclosed.
3. C. According to Centers for Medicare and Medicaid Services (CMS) guidelines, A, B, and D may be considered as the client's residence (CMS, 2003b). If a client is in a skilled nursing facility, regulations for that setting would apply instead.
4. B. These may be symptoms of hyperglycemia, which can cause ketoacidosis (diabetic coma), a serious condition (George, 2013; Oakes, 2014).
5. D. If the client is able to drive around the community independently, he may no longer ethically meet the Medicare criteria for being homebound, and this should be discussed with the health team (CMS, 2003a). The client may still benefit from therapy to address his ADL deficits and can be referred to an outpatient clinic.
6. A. The Outcome Assessment Information Set (OASIS) is required (CMS, 2012), although the health practitioner may choose to use any additional assessments, such as the Disability of Arm, Shoulder, and Hand (DASH) and Functional Independence Measure (FIM). The Minimum Data Set (MDS) is used in skilled nursing facilities.
7. C. Medicare guidelines for occupational therapy (CMS, 2011) require that an OT perform the assessment and establish, manage, and supervise the plan of care. The OT must also perform client reassessments at specified intervals. An OT does not have to be physically present when an OTA implements a delegated intervention session between those intervals. Although the physician must certify changes in the plan of care, there is no requirement that the physician sign treatment notes.
8. C. (Fairchild, 2013)

9. B. During a seizure, do not restrain the client or place objects in client's mouth. Adjust clothing around neck to help keep the client from having a restricted airway and call for medical help (George, 2013; Oakes, 2014).
10. A. Typically, a client must be terminally ill with a prognosis of 6 months or less to receive hospice care, which a physician must certify. In addition to cancer diagnoses, benefits are provided for other terminal conditions, such as congestive heart failure, non-Alzheimer's dementia, failure to thrive, and chronic kidney disease (CMS, 2013).

Worksheet 9-6: Acute Care

1. D. The urine collection bag should be below the bladder level to avoid backflow (Fairchild, 2013; George, 2013).
2. B. A nosocomial infection is a generic term for a hospital-acquired infection, which can include hepatitis B, *Clostridium difficile*, and other conditions. The more recent term, *health care–associated infections*, is now being used to reflect all areas of health practice (Siegel, Rhinehart, Jackson, Chiarello, & the Healthcare Infection Control Practices Advisory Committee, 2007).
3. A. Avoid placing the cuff above the intravenous insertion site (Fairchild, 2013).
4. B. The tube is inserted through the nose. Care must be taken so that donning and doffing an overhead sweater does not tug or pull at the tube.
5. C. The IV line should not be taut. The bed should be lowered so that the client's feet can reach the floor when seated on the edge of bed for safety. Wheelchair footrests should be in the swing away position or removed. If a client is using bed rails to aid in transfers, the rails should be locked in the up position.
6. B. Length of stay in acute care is often very short. As soon as the client is admitted, the team members consider whether the client will be returning home, will need continued rehabilitation at another facility (e.g., skilled nursing facility, rehabilitation hospital), or will be transfered to a different setting (e.g., relative's home). This will help give the discharge planner time to coordinate the transfer or any discharge recommendations. In acute care, not all clients will need or receive occupational therapy.
7. C. Sudden postural changes, for some clients, may cause the client's blood pressure to drop significantly and may cause lightheadedness or fainting.
8. C. A draw sheet under the client makes it easier for staff to move and position a client in bed who requires much assistance. Lifting a client up by the arms and legs poses greater risk for injury to both the client and health workers. Although the client can attempt to assist by pulling up using a trapeze or bed rails, they are not the best option in this situation.
9. D. In terms of isolation procedures, *Streptococcus* A requires droplet precautions, tuberculosis requires airborne precautions, and scabies and *Clostridium difficile* require contact precautions (Siegel et al., 2007).
10. D. A health care proxy designates an individual who can make health care decisions on one's behalf in case of incapacitation.

Worksheet 9-7: Cardiac Care—Ventricular Assist Device

Indicate whether the following statements are true (T) or false (F).

1. _F_ A ventricular assist device is used only with clients who are candidates for a heart transplant. *Devices may be used as destination therapy for patients who are not appropriate for a heart transplant* (Padmanabhan & Thankachan, 2011; Wells, 2013; Wilson et al., 2009).
2. _F_ Surgeons will not implant a left ventricular assist device (LVAD) in children under age 12. *These devices are used even with infants* (McIntyre, 2007).
3. _T_ Health team goals include teaching the client and caregiver aseptic technique for changing bandages around the driveline exit site. *It is extremely important that procedures are in place to prevent infection* (Padmanabhan & Thankachan, 2011; Wilson et al., 2009).
4. _T_ The OT intervention plan should include teaching the client how to change the power source from alternating current (AC) to a battery and vice versa. *This is especially important during shower training* (Abramson, Harvey, Greenfield, Lauman, & Metzler, 2012; Padmanabhan & Thankachan, 2011).

5. _F_ When the client is medically allowed to take a shower, the OT should instruct the client to place a plastic grocery bag over the equipment to keep it dry. *A specialized manufactured waterproof bag/shower kit is used* (Abramson et al., 2012; Padmanabhan & Thankachan, 2011).
6. _F_ For a client with a VAD who is deconditioned but allowed to sit up in a chair, initial interventions for transfer training should include wheelchair push-up exercises. *The client should adhere to sternal precautions* (Abramson et al, 2012).
7. _F_ A client with a LVAD and good recovery can generally resume taking a bath at approximately 8 to 10 weeks. *The equipment cannot get wet, and the client cannot be immersed in water* (Abramson et al., 2012; Padmanabhan & Thankachan, 2011; Wilson et al., 2009).
8. _T_ Clients with an implanted nonpulsatile VAD may not have a palpable pulse (Wells, 2013).
9. _F_ The OT should instruct the client to wear elastic-waist pants over the driveline. *Kinks or pressure that obstruct the line may impede blood flow* (Abramson et al., 2012; McIntyre, 2007).
10. _F_ For a client with a VAD, a noncontact sport, such as swimming, is generally recommended to help with reconditioning *The equipment cannot get wet and the client cannot be immersed in water* (Abramson et al., 2012; Padmanabhan & Thankachan, 2011; Wilson et al., 2009).
11. _T_ The traditional method of assessing blood pressure may not be reliable with a client with a VAD (Wells, 2013; Wilson et al., 2009).
12. _T_ Clients with a VAD and/or their caregivers must be able to distinguish between different types of alarms associated with the particular device. *The devices have various auditory and visual alarms that signal specific problems, such as low batteries, pump failure, or malfunction* (Casida & Peters, 2009; Wilson et al., 2009).
13. _F_ For a client with a VAD, it is preferable that the client have a posterior pelvic tilt when in a seated position. *This position may cause kinks or pressure that might obstruct the driveline and impede blood flow* (Abramson et al., 2012; McIntyre, 2007; Wells, 2013).
14. _T_ To better accommodate the LVAD driveline, the OT might recommend the use of button-down shirts when dressing. *The abdomen upper quadrant is where the driveline exits the body* (Abramson et al., 2012).
15. _F_ Clients whose lives were saved with a VAD are not considered at risk for anxiety or depression because they are generally happy to be alive. *Clients may have significant concerns about their medical condition, occupational changes, possible power failure, ability to manage the device, and self-image, for example* (Casida & Peters, 2009; McIntyre, 2007; Padmanabhan & Thankachan, 2011; Shepherd & Wilding, 2006; Wilson et al., 2009).

Worksheet 9-8: Skilled Nursing Facility

1. D. Memory difficulty is an early sign for people with Alzheimer's disease (Alzheimer's Association, 2009). Although an individual in the early stages may still be able to operate a car, a big concern is that the person may not be able to do this safely. The person may have problems with following the rules of the road, spatial orientation, reaction time, or may easily get lost, creating significant safety concerns. Family education and other measures (e.g., taking away keys, disabling car) should be put in place to help keep an unsafe person from operating a motor vehicle.
2. A. A client functioning at Allen Cognitive Level 3 has poor problem-solving skills and diminished capacity for new learning, particularly when a device is unfamiliar, such as a sock assist. For this client, the OT's time would probably be better spent working on other aspects of dressing in which the client can better participate.
3. C. A seat alarm would not restrain Mary, but would alert staff if she begins to stand. As Mary has poor fine motor skills, a seat belt with buckle and a lap board are considered restraints if the client is unable to open or remove them.
4. D. For clients with unilateral neglect, it is useful for an occupational therapy practitioner to incorporate activities that involve having the client use both upper extremities, such as using a rolling pin (symmetrical task) or holding toothpaste in one hand and applying it to a toothbrush held in the other hand (asymmetrical task). Applying lotion to the neglected side can help bring attention to it. The call bell should always be placed where the client can attend to it if needed. In this situation, it should be placed at Mary's right side, not the left.

5. A. A client functioning at Allen Cognitive Level 2 has severe cognitive impairment (Allen, 1985). Reality orientation would not be effective. Answers B, C, and D are techniques that can be used with a caring approach to minimize the client's apparent emotional discomfort (Hellen & Padilla, 2012).
6. D. The client is sleepy. She is at risk for a burn if she falls asleep holding the cup and spills the hot beverage onto herself. The client wishes to consume her tea, so the OT should alert the nursing staff to the safety hazard and ask them to supervise the client drinking it.
7. A. Orthodox Christians typically celebrate Christmas on January 7 (Timeanddate.com, 2014). It is also not unusual for clients who have been hospitalized (or even healthy adults) to be off by a day or so when stating the date. As long as the client is very close to the actual time frame, it is generally not cause for concern.
8. B. The OT must adhere to HIPAA guidelines. The other choices would violate confidentiality. The client's companions may not be aware of his diagnosis, hospitalization, or rehabilitation. When encountering a client in the community, it is best to allow the client to make the initial contact or explanation of how you two know each other.
9. B. CIMT entails restraining the nonaffected upper extremity during selected tasks so that the affected upper limb is actively used during functional activities (Gillen, 2011).
10. D. (www.cms.gov)

Worksheet 9-9: Speech and Language

Resource: American Speech-Language-Hearing Association (www.asha.org).

1. _*_ dysarthria
2. ___ dysphagia
3. ___ dystonia
4. _*_ dysphonia
5. _*_ cadence
6. ___ dysrhythmia
7. ___ aspiration
8. _*_ intelligibility
9. ___ shuttering
10. _*_ intonation
11. _*_ apraxia of speech
12. ___ hemianopsia
13. _*_ aphasia
14. _*_ dysphasia
15. _*_ fluency
16. _*_ articulation
17. ___ dysthymia
18. _*_ anomia
19. ___ dysesthesia
20. _*_ pitch

Worksheet 9-10: Wheeled Mobility

References: Fairchild, 2013; Frazier Rehab Institute, 2009.

1. D. This option would allow for independent wheeled mobility for desired occupational roles, although other types of cushions could also be appropriate. The client is able to manage a joystick control and the tilt in space component would provide pressure relief. Leona's weight does not warrant a heavy-duty (bariatric) wheelchair.
2. C. A sports wheelchair would allow this athletic client to play adaptive sports such as basketball. His weight does not warrant a heavy-duty (bariatric) wheelchair, and he is able to use a manual wheelchair independently for general mobility.
3. A. Because this client has upper extremity function and is able to transfer and shift positions, she does not require tilt in space or sip and puff components. A one-arm drive wheelchair requires manual propulsion, which would still cause fatigue. A power mobility scooter would be the most practical option for occupational participation.
4. B. This option would allow the client to propel and steer the wheelchair using only his unaffected upper extremity. The client's weight and condition do not warrant a heavy-duty (bariatric) wheelchair, special lightweight wheelchair, or a power wheelchair.
5. A. The rear wheel axles are in a more posterior position to stabilize the wheelchair and compensate for the lost leg weight (Fairchild, 2013).

6. D. Fall injury prevention programs strive to prevent falls and injuries while minimizing the use of restraints.
7. D. Toggle brake locks can get in the way during sliding transfers. A different type of brake lock, called scissor locks, are attached under the seat front and do not impede sliding transfers. To prepare for the transfer, the wheelchair front rigging with attached leg rest should be swung away/removed in addition to removing the wheelchair armrest (Fairchild, 2013; Frazier Rehab Institute, 2009).
8. C. A lap belt with a loop Velcro closure will help keep the client from sliding forward, yet allow him to use gross movement to put his hand and wrist through the loop and pull it to unfasten it. Although an alarm can alert staff, it will not directly assist with the physical aspect of keeping this client upright in the wheelchair. Keeping the legs separated with an abduction wedge also will not help with upright positioning. A lap tray may be considered a restraint as the client will not likely be able to remove it himself.
9. A. Fairchild, 2013; Frazier Rehab Institute, 2009.
10. C. The client needs to engage (lock) the toggle brake and unlock the front rigging to swing it away.

Worksheet 9-11: Amputation Levels

Reference: Murphy, 2014.

F	Transfemoral amputation (AKA) *Comprises 85% of all lower extremity amputations; desirable when BKA will not heal.*
C	Chopart amputation *Removal of navicular, cuboid, cuneiforms, metatarsals, and phalanges*
A	Transcarpal amputation *Intact forearm supination and pronation and flexion and extension of the wrist*
E	Pirogoff amputation *Between tibia and calcaneous*
G	Partial hand amputation *Fingers and or part of the thumb*
H	Transhumeral amputation *Best results when the deltoid insertion is maintained*
I	Transradial amputation *Best lever arm when radial length is no shorter than 2 centimeters above the wrist*
D	Scapulothoracic amputation *Removal of entire arm and scapula*
B	Hip disarticulation *Removal of entire leg*

Worksheet 9-12: Prosthetic Devices

Reference: Murphy, 2014.

1. T
2. T
3. F. Three types of hand prosthesis include the passive prosthetic device, body-powered devices, and externally driven devices.
4. T
5. F. Maintaining the knee in extension is necessary to prevent flexion contractures, which will impair functional ambulation. The quadriceps will not maintain knee extension unaided.
6. F. Ideally, a hand prosthesis will allow for a spherical grasp, a gross grasp, a lateral pinch, pincer grasp. and three-jaw chuck grasp.

7. T
8. F. Phantom limb pain occurs in approximately 85% of those with amputations. Clients report stinging, ripping, and cutting pains.
9. T
10. T
11. T
12. T

Worksheet 9-13: Dysphagia

Reference: National Dysphagia Diet Task Force, 2002.

Diet levels include the following.

NDD Level I

Dysphagia—Pureed

1. Homogenous
2. Very cohesive
3. Pudding-like, smooth
4. Requiring no chewing ability

NDD Level II

Dysphagia—Mechanically Altered

1. Cohesive, minimal texture
2. Moist, soft
3. Semisolid foods (e.g., meats are ground/minced and moist)
4. Requiring some chewing

NDD Level III:

Dysphagia—Advanced

1. Soft foods requiring more chewing ability

Regular: all foods allowed (including hard, solid, and textured foods)

Proposed levels of liquid viscosity are:

- Thin: no alteration
- Nectar-like: slightly thicker than water; the consistency of unset gelatin
- Honey-like: a liquid with the consistency of honey
- Spoon-thick: a liquid with the consistency of pudding

Worksheet 9-14: Feeding and Eating Terms

Reference: Adapted from AOTA, 2007.

1.	Adaptive feeding equipment	Equipment used to assist with the ability to eat, typically used to compensate for such difficulties as poor coordination, weakness, impaired, range of motion, or suboptimal positioning.
2.	Airway protection	The prevention of accidental introduction of liquids, food, or medications into the trachea during eating or drinking.
3.	Aspiration	Secretions, fluids, food, or any foreign object entering the lungs. Can be fatal due to the development of pneumonia.
4.	Bolus	An orally processed mass of food or liquid that is swallowed.
5.	Enteral feeding	Tube feedings where nutrients are placed in and absorbed in the intestinal tract.
6.	Esophageal phase	Swallowing phase in which the bolus of food travels along the esophagus and into the stomach.
7.	Mendelsohn maneuver	A swallowing technique that results in keeping the upper esophageal sphincter open longer to allow bolus passage.
8.	Oral phase	Swallow phase in which the bolus of food is moved to the pharynx by the tongue.
9.	Oral preparatory phase	Swallowing phase in which the bolus of food is chewed and manipulated by the lips, cheek, and tongue to create the bolus that is the correct texture for swallowing.
10.	Oral stage function	"Includes bolus intake and containment, bolus formation, bolus transit and clearing time, velar function, behavioral components, base of tongue contact to pharyngeal wall, residue post swallow" (AOTA, 2007, p. 696).
11.	Pharyngeal phase	Swallow phase where the actual swallowing response is initiated.
12.	Pocketing	Food erroneously remains between the teeth and cheek.
13.	VitalStim	A United States Food and Drug Administration–cleared method to of neuromuscular electrical stimulation that promotes swallowing by strengthening and re-educating muscles.
14.	Upper aerodigestive tract	The organs and tissues of the respiratory tract and the upper part of the digestive tract.
15.	Total parenteral nutrition	The provision of nutrients through an intravenous tube.
16.	Therapeutic feedings	Food delivery techniques used to facilitate therapeutic outcomes of improved feeding, eating, and swallowing ability; should not be used as a primary source of nutrition or hydration.
17.	Supraglottic swallow	"A swallowing technique used for airway protection where the client is told to take a breath and hold it while swallowing and then coughs after the swallow; results in the voluntary closure of the vocal folds before, during, and after the swallow" (AOTA, 2007, p. 696).
18.	Silent aspiration	The leakage of food into the lungs without overt coughing or choking; may indicate a motor or sensory deficit (AOTA, 2007).
19.	Self-feeding	The ability of the individual to set up food and bring to mouth without assistance (AOTA, 2007).
20.	Secretion management	"The ability to retain, manipulate, and swallow one's own saliva" (AOTA, 2007, p. 696).
21.	Preoral phase	The phase of eating where food or drink is brought to the mouth either by a feeder or the person himself or herself.
22.	Double/multiple swallows	Two or more attempts are used to swallow food (AOTA, 2007).

Worksheet 9-15: Low-Vision Rehabilitation

Reference: Warren, 2008.

1. C. Professionals with baccalaureate or master's degrees have been eligible for orientation and mobility certification after taking an approved university program
2. B. Visual resonance is not an actual part of vision.
3. C. The need to constantly move to adjust the focus of the device is not an advantage
4. B
5. D. Moving about with the community can be hazardous and requires training by a specialist to ensure client safety.

Worksheet 9-16: Low-Vision Basics

Resource: Warren, 2008.
True or false:

1. _F_ Low vision visual deficits are permanent and cannot be corrected with surgery.
2. _T_
3. _T_
4. _F_ Medicare has only covered occupational therapy services for low vision since 2012.
5. _T_
6. _T_ (Visual acuity, visual field, contrast sensitivity, glare modulation, visual perception)
7. _T_
8. _F_ A cataract is cloudiness of the lens of the eye.
9. _T_
10. _F_ Optical devices can only make objects appear bigger and therefore more readily identifiable.
11. _F_ A low-vision specialist who is an OT must understand how all optical devices work to ensure they are being used correctly by clients.
12. _T_
13. _T_
14. _T_
15. _F_ It is well within the scope of practice of an occupational therapy practitioner to recommend voice-activated and audio-output devices to assist a person with difficulty reading to participate in occupations.

Chapter 9 References

Abramson, M., Harvey, J., Greenfield, M., Lauman, S., & Metzler, D. (2012). Partners in the journey: A case study of OT intervention for a recipient of a left ventricular assist device. *Advance for Occupational Therapy Practitioners 28*(16), 16. Retrieved from http://occupational-therapy.advanceweb.com/Web-extras/Online-Extras/Partners-in-the-journey.aspx

Allen, C. K. (1985). *Occupational therapy for psychiatric diseases: Measurement and management of cognitive disabilities*. Boston: Little, Brown and Company.

Alzheimer's Association. (2009). 10 Early signs and symptoms of Alzheimer's. Retrieved from http://www.alz.org/alzheimers_disease_10_signs_of_alzheimers.asp

American Occupational Therapy Association. (2007). Specialized knowledge and skills in feeding, eating and swallowing in occupational therapy practice. *American Journal of Occupational Therapy, 61*, 686–700.

Casida, J. M., & Peters, R. M. (2009). Self-care demands of persons living with an implantable left-ventricular assist device. *Research and Theory for Nursing Practice: An International Journal, 23*, 279–293.

Centers for Medicare & Medicaid Services. (2003a). *Medicare Benefit Policy Manual* (Pub. 100-02: Ch. 7, Section 30.1.1). Baltimore: Centers for Medicare & Medicaid Services. Retrieved from http://www.cms.gov/Regulations-and-Guidance/Guidance/Manuals/Downloads/bp102c07.pdf

Centers for Medicare & Medicaid Services. (2003b). *Medicare Benefit Policy Manual* (Pub. 100-02: Ch. 7, Section 30.1.2). Baltimore: Centers for Medicare & Medicaid Services. Retrieved from http://www.cms.gov/Regulations-and-Guidance/Guidance/Manuals/Downloads/bp102c07.pdf

Centers for Medicare & Medicaid Services. (2011). *Medicare Benefit Policy Manual* (Pub. 100-02: Ch. 7, Section 40.2.1). Baltimore: Centers for Medicare & Medicaid Services. Retrieved from http://www.cms.gov/Regulations-and-Guidance/Guidance/Manuals/Downloads/bp102c07.pdf

Centers for Medicare & Medicaid Services. (2012). *Outcome and Assessment Information Set: OASIS-C Guidance Manual* (chap. 1). Baltimore: Centers for Medicare & Medicaid Services. Retrieved from http://www.cms.gov/Medicare/Quality-Initiatives-Patient-Assessment-Instruments/HomeHealthQualityInits/HHQIOASISUserManual.html

Centers for Medicare & Medicaid Services. (2013). Medicare hospice data. Retrieved from http://www.cms.gov/Medicare/Medicare-Fee-for-Service-Payment/Hospice/Medicare_Hospice_Data.html

Fairchild, S. L. (2013). *Pierson and Fairchild's principles & techniques of patient care* (5th ed.). St. Louis: Saunders.

Frazier Rehab Institute. (2009). Spinal Cord Medicine Handbook for Patient and Family. Louisville, KY: Frasier Rehab and Neuroscience Center. Retrieved from https://www.jhsmh.org/LinkClick.aspx?fileticket=PTR0IWI0wEg%3D&tabid=332

Gateley, C. A., & Borcherding, S. (2012). *Documentation manual for occupational therapy: Writing SOAP notes* (3rd ed.). Thorofare, NJ: SLACK Incorporated.

George, A. H. (2013). Infection control and safety issues in the clinic. In H. M. Pendleton & W. Schultz-Krohn (Eds.), *Pedretti's occupational therapy: Practice skills for physical dysfunction* (7th ed., pp. 140–156). St. Louis: Mosby.

Gillen, G. (Ed.). (2011). *Stroke rehabilitation: A function-based approach* (3rd ed.). St. Louis: Elsevier Mosby.

Hellen, C. R., & Padilla, R. (2012). Working with elders who have dementia and Alzheimer's disease. In R. L. Padilla, S. Byers-Connon, & H. L. Lohman (Eds.), *Occupational therapy with elders: Strategies for the COTA* (3rd ed., pp. 275–289). Maryland Heights, MO: Elsevier Mosby.

McIntyre, M. (2007). Keeping VAD patients functional. *ADVANCE for Occupational Therapy Practitioners, 23*(5), 43. Retrieved from http://occupational-therapy.advanceweb.com/Article/Keeping-VAD-Patients-Functional-1.aspx

Morreale, M. J. (2015). *Developing clinical competence: A workbook for the OTA*. Thorofare, NJ: SLACK Incorporated.

Morreale, M. J., & Borcherding, S. (2013). *The OTA's guide to documentation: Writing SOAP notes* (3rd ed.). Thorofare, NJ: SLACK Incorporated.

Murphy, D. (2014). *Fundamentals of amputation care and prosthetics*. New York: Demos Medical.

National Dysphagia Diet Task Force (2002). *National dysphagia diet: Standardization for optimal care*. Chicago, IL: American Dietetic Association.

Oakes, C. E. (2014). Safety and support. In K. Jacobs, N. MacRae, & K. Sladyk (Eds.), *Occupational therapy essentials for clinical competence* (2nd ed., pp. 137–148). Thorofare, NJ: SLACK Incorporated.

Padmanabhan, K., & Thankachan, S. (2011). Occupational therapy in cardiac care: left ventricular assistive devices. *OT Practice, 16*(22), 15–20.

Shepherd, J., & Wilding, C. (2006). Occupational therapy for people with ventricular assist devices. *Australian Occupational Therapy Journal, 53*(1), 47–49.

Siegel, J. D., Rhinehart, E., Jackson, M., Chiarello, L., and the Healthcare Infection Control Practices Advisory Committee. (2007). 2007 Guideline for isolation precautions: Preventing transmission of infectious agents in healthcare settings. Retrieved from http://www.cdc.gov/hicpac/pdf/isolation/Isolation2007.pdf

Timeanddate.com (2014). Orthodox Christmas Day in United States. Retrieved from http://www.timeanddate.com/holidays/us/orthodox-christmas-day

Warren, M. (Ed.). (2008). *Low vision: Occupational therapy evaluation and intervention with older adults* (rev. ed.). Bethesda, MD: AOTA Press.

Wells, C. L. (2013). Physical therapist management of patients with ventricular assist devices: Key considerations for the acute care physical therapist. *Physical Therapy,* 93,266–278.

Whyte, J. (2011). Rancho Los Amigos Scale. In *Encyclopedia of clinical neuropsychology* (p. 2110). New York: Springer.

Wilson, S. R., Givertz, M. M., Stewart, G. C., & Mudge, G. H. (2009). Ventricular assist devices: The challenges of outpatient management. *Journal of the American College of Cardiology*, 54,1647–1659. doi: 10.1016/j.jacc.2009.06.035

Wilson, B. A., Shannon, M. T., & Shields, K. M. (2014). *Pearson nurse's drug guide.* Upper Saddle River, NJ: Pearson Education.

Chapter 10

Implementing Pediatric Assessments and Interventions

Occupational therapy practitioners working with children require specialized knowledge and skills unique to that practice area, such as an understanding of typical development and the various physical and psychosocial factors and conditions that can have an impact on occupational participation. Pediatric settings can include neonatal intensive care units (NICUs), hospitals, schools, rehabilitation centers, day care, after-school and community programs, clinics, institutions, and the child's home. Early intervention services address the needs of infants and young children with (or at risk for) developmental delay, including the contexts that hinder or support development. Occupational therapy in educational settings focuses on activities and occupations that the child needs to succeed in school. Interventions may include recommendations (such as sensory strategies or assistive technology) to minimize challenges in the classroom/school environment, or therapeutic activities designed to remediate the student's underlying weaknesses that hinder educational performance. The worksheets and learning activities in this chapter focus on the knowledge and skills therapists need to assess children, understand models of practice, and implement appropriate interventions in various settings. Answers to worksheet exercises are provided at the end of the chapter.

Contents

Morreale, M. J., & Amini, D.
The Occupational Therapist's Workbook for Ensuring Clinical Competence (pp. 357-388).

Worksheet 10-1

Theories Guiding Pediatric Practice

As in all areas of practice, occupational therapists working in pediatric settings subscribe to various models of practice, also known as frames of reference, to approach intervention from a theoretically sound and evidence-based foundation. This exercise, along with Worksheet 10-2, will allow you to assess your own knowledge of several major models used in pediatric practice.

Match the name of the model with its description.

______ Motor learning and skill acquisition
______ Social skills training
______ Systems approach
______ Cognitive orientation to daily occupational performance (CO-OP)
______ Neurodevelopmental theory
______ Sensory integration
______ Adaptation and compensation
______ Coping model
______ Developmental approaches

1. The occupational therapist is a facilitator in the development and mastery of life skills and the ability to cope with life's expectations.
2. An approach that seeks to provide a child with opportunities for sensory experiences in the form of proprioception, vestibular, and tactile input within the context of meaningful activities.
3. An approach primarily indicated for children with cerebral palsy that historically focused on underlying postural reactions needed for development of normal movement. It now considers motor learning and dynamic systems theory as well as meaningful, contextually appropriate activities in treatment.
4. Building skills through goal-directed functional actions. Movement, balance, and control that occur within occupations are important considerations.
5. Used in mental health settings with children and adolescents to assist with the development of positive coping strategies through involvement with others and safe interactive experiences.
6. A model addressing psychosocial functioning that uses strategies and resources to help the child deal with the stressors of life occurring within the environment.
7. Used to ensure the ability to participate in meaningful activities and occupations when remediation of the underlying disability or performance skill limitation is not possible or indicated.
8. A top-down approach to intervention, in which the child learning motor skills is involved in learning the relevant aspects of the task, understanding how they are currently completing the task, identifying why they are not successful, thinking about solutions and trying out the solutions.
9. The therapist gains an understanding of environmental, family, and child factors that affect performance. Activities are selected on the basis of the complexity and interaction of the person, the environment, and the desired occupation.

Worksheet 10-2

Match the Model of Practice

Match the model of practice to the correct scenario.

Motor learning and skill acquisition
Social skills training
Systems approach
Cognitive orientation to daily occupational performance (CO-OP)
Neurodevelopmental theory
Sensory integration
Adaptation and compensation
Coping model
Developmental approaches

1. Latasha is a 9-year-old child with left hemiparetic cerebral palsy. She participates in an age-appropriate classroom in the local elementary school, where she has been receiving occupational therapy for school-related activities since she was 5 years old. Latasha is independent in most school and home-related tasks, but does take extra time to eat lunch and use the restroom because of the moderate limitations in her left hand movement. The occupational therapist (OT) has decided to frame intervention around an approach in which Latasha will be asked to participate in the activities that she finds difficult. While participating, Latasha will be asked to consider the activity, how she is completing it, and what factors are causing her difficulties. She will then brainstorm with the OT on ways to improve her abilities.

   This is an example of a/an ________________________ model of occupational therapy.

2. Following administration of the Sensory Integration and Praxis Test (SIPT), the therapist creates an intervention plan for 5-year-old Micca (a preschool student) that includes activities such as jumping on a small trampoline, creeping through a maze tunnel, throwing and catching a playground ball, playing in a ball pit, and playing with magic sand at a table. The activities will provide proprioceptive, vestibular, and tactile input.

   This is an example of a/an ________________________ model of occupational therapy.

3. Geneva, a 16-year-old girl, sustained a severe traumatic brain injury (TBI) 1 year ago when she was in a head-on collision. Geneva is living with her parents, who provide mod/max assist for all activities of daily living (ADL) and instrumental ADL (IADL) activities. She is alert most of the day and is able to follow two-step commands. Geneva and her parents would like to see her able to turn her television and radio on and off independently because these are activities that bring her pleasure during the day. The OT explores several environmental control units with Geneva's parents; they decide to purchase a scanning unit to be operated with a leaf switch attached to Geneva's bedside.

   This is an example of a/an ________________________ model of occupational therapy.

4. Jacque is an 8-year-old boy with the diagnosis of athetoid type cerebral palsy. He is receiving occupational therapy services to improve coordination and control of his upper extremities to facilitate computer use in the classroom. The OT provides many activities for Jacque that involve weight-bearing, stabilization, and physical prompting while he completes typical school-based activities, such as accessing a tablet, coloring with crayons, and participating in music class.

   This is an example of a/an ________________________ model of occupational therapy.

5. Joshua is a 12-year-old male attending a typical middle school and participating in age-level class. Joshua has the diagnosis of pervasive developmental disorder. He is high-functioning, but has experienced difficulties with social participation with his peers. Joshua's mother obtained a referral to a local OT who runs a group program for children aged 10 to 19 years who have similar concerns. Joshua attends the group experience twice weekly, where the group members hold discussions, engage in role-plays, and complete tasks such as game play, cooking, and major crafts together.

   This is an example of a/an ________________________ model of occupational therapy

Worksheet 10-3

Typical Development

1. What is the typical sequence of gross movements for a 12-month-old child who is transitioning from a sitting position on the floor to standing?
   A. Half-kneeling, kneeling, weight shift backward, squatting and rising with symmetrical lower extremity extension
   B. Kneeling, half-kneeling, shifting weight backward, squatting and rising with asymmetrical lower extremity extension
   C. Kneeling, half-kneeling, shifting weight forward, squatting and rising with symmetrical lower extremity extension
   D. Twelve-month-old children have not typically gained the ability to stand without a surface to pull up on

2. Which of the following is *not true* of a typical 7-month-old child?
   A. Landau is increasing
   B. Does not like supine
   C. Pulls self to stand
   D. Assumes sitting from quadruped

3. At which age has the typical child started cruising?
   A. 12 months
   B. 11 months
   C. 9 months
   D. 6 months

4. A typically developing child who is just learning to stabilize himself or herself in a more complex position (such as sitting), will do which behavior when a desired activity requires more support?
   A. Ask Mom or Dad for help
   B. Revert to more stable postures
   C. Use the finer patterns even if it means tipping over
   D. A child who has not gained stability in all patterns will not do any other activities

5. At which age have equilibrium reactions been established in all positions except for walking?
   A. 12 months
   B. 10 months
   C. 8 months
   D. 6 months

6. A child who rises to standing through kneeling and half-kneeling while holding on to a surface is most likely how old?
   A. 10 months
   B. 12 months
   C. 8 months
   D. 7 months

Worksheet 10-3 (continued)

Typical Development

7. At what age will a child start to lower himself from standing instead of letting go and dropping down from cruising?
   A. 10 months
   B. 12 months
   C. 6 months
   D. 8 months

8. Which of the following is the method of locomotion where the body is quadruped with trunk and pelvis above the floor and arms and legs moving reciprocally?
   A. Crawling
   B. Walking
   C. Bear walking
   D. Creeping

9. The child who is able to sit independently on the floor, but may tip over if he moves too far from midline is likely how old?
   A. 1 to 2 months
   B. 3 to 4 months
   C. 5 to 6 months
   D. 7 to 8 months

10. Which of the following describes physiological flexion?
    A. The ability of the 12-month-old to grasp an object from the floor and bring it to her mouth when holding onto furniture
    B. A normal reflex observed in a child who is between 4 and 5 months old; useful as the child gains the ability to sit independently
    C. A state of muscle tension found in the newborn in which limbs rest in a flexed position; dissipates during the first and second months of life
    D. The state of muscle tension found in the 6-month-old allowing her to grasp toes while in supine without rolling onto her side; dissipates when the child is able to stand independently.

Worksheet 10-4

Typical and Atypical Development

Indicate true (T) or false (F) for each of the following statements.

1. ______ A 15-month-old child has typically not yet developed a fine pincer grasp.
2. ______ When a 12-month-old begins to walk independently, the child's legs move in a "stride" pattern (hip forward flexion, knee extension, and full heel strike).
3. ______ Pelvic stability is needed for the child to gain the ability to walk correctly.
4. ______ To have *good* fine motor skills, proximal stability of the scapula is essential.
5. ______ An 11-month-old child can typically stand up independently from a squatting position.
6. ______ Twelve months of age is within the normal range for beginning independent walking.
7. ______ If a 10-month-old child in prone hyperextends his neck with shoulder flexion and extended arms, but is unable to maintain head in midline or bear weight on forearms, he is demonstrating a typical pattern of development.
8. ______ A 16-month-old child with a diagnosis of cerebral palsy who has obligatory head and neck asymmetry is likely to be dominated by an asymmetrical tonic neck reflex (ATNR).
9. ______ When significant winging of the scapula and poor trunk endurance are seen in a school-age child, the primary concern is that trunk and scapular stability have not developed.
10. ______ A child with a lack of abdominal stability with an anterior pelvic tilt may require assistive devices to walk.
11. ______ Sitting is the most functional and versatile position for the 7-month-old.
12. ______ When the 10-month-old is walking with hands held, he typically requires the person assisting to move him in a forward motion.
13. ______ When sitting, a 5-month-old has no trunk control and will flop over.
14. ______ Neck righting refers to the position that the child assumes when prone in the ninth month.
15. ______ At approximately 2 months of age, a child is in a period of development known as "astasia abasia."
16. ______ The rooting reflex is of concern if it is observed in a child older than 1 month of age.
17. ______ An obligatory suck/swallow reflex extending beyond 3 months of age can affect the development of normalized eating and swallowing.
18. ______ Children will typically be able to secure an object in their hand and bring to their mouth before the sixth month of life.
19. ______ Children begin to hold a crayon and make scribbles after demonstration as early as 5 months old.
20. ______ When sitting with both knees flexed and soles of feet touching, a child is said to be "pretzel sitting."

Worksheet 10-5

Determining Chronological Age

Many normed assessment tools used in pediatric practice require the use of the chronological age of the child to determine the most accurate scoring. This worksheet provides you an opportunity to practice your skills for finding the chronological age of children.

Following is a formula for determining chronological age:

Always start with the date. If the number for today is less than the number for the birthday, borrow 30 days from the month column (remember to use the number of the month) and subtract. Next, subtract the birth month from today's month. If today's month is smaller than the birth month, borrow 12 months from the year and add to the month (do not forget that when you borrow you lose a year). Next, subtract the birth year from this year. You now have an accurate chronological age.

Example:

	Year	**Month**	**Date**
Today	2015	January (1)	13
Birthday	2008	March (3)	30
Age	6 years	9 months	13 days

1. Amy was born on July 15, 2005. Today is December 5, 2015. How old is Amy?
2. Zack was born on August 30 in 2013. Today is January 1, 2016. How old is Zack?
3. Today is November 15, 2015; Patish was born on January 31, 2011. How old is Patish?
4. Mora was born on January 23, 2008; today is January 5, 2016. How old is Mora?
5. Today is March 3, 2016; Hamed was born on the 30th of November in 2015. How old is Hamed?
6. What is your birthday? What is today's date? How old are you today?

Worksheet 10-6

Pediatric Assessments

The use of reliable assessment tools to determine the status of the child's occupational participation as well as performance skills, patterns, and client factor functioning are paramount to the creation of the OT plan of care. In addition, tools that address the context and environment and the interests and desires of the child also help to ensure a comprehensive, occupation-based and client-centered approach to intervention. This worksheet will provide you the opportunity to recall popular tools seen in pediatric practice.

Respond to the following multiple-choice questions:

1. An assessment created as a diagnostic tool to distinguish between typical children and those with sensory integrative and learning deficits. Indicated for children 4 to 9 years of age, the assessment takes approximately 3 hours to administer and score.
   A. Sensory Performance Analysis (SPA)
   B. DeGangi-Berk Test of Sensory Integration (TSI)
   C. Clinical Observations of Motor and Process Skills (COMPS)
   D. Sensory Integration and Praxis Test (SIPT)
2. An assessment based on interview and observation that is appropriate for individuals age 2 years to adult. The assessment measures the quality of social interactions with persons the client typically sees in natural context of life tasks that normally involve social communication.
   A. Evaluation of Social Interaction, 2nd edition (ESI)
   B. Children's Assessment of Participation and Enjoyment (CAPE)
   C. Assessment of Preschool Children's Participation (APCP)
   D. Social Profile
3. This tool is the 3rd edition of a visual perception measure originally created by Marianne Frostig in 1961. This assessment is a paper-and-pencil task–based tool and is appropriate for children ages 4 through 12. The assessment takes approximately 20 minutes to administer and 20 minutes to score.
   A. Developmental Test of Visual Perception-Adolescent and Adult (DTVP-A)
   B. Motor Free Visual Perception Test (MVPT, 3rd)
   C. Perceptual-Motor Assessment for Children; Emotional/Behavioral Screening Program (P-MAC/ESP)
   D. Developmental Test of Visual Perception (DTVP-3)
4. This tool is based on the Model of Human Occupation (MOHO) and is used to obtain an overview of the child's occupational performance, identifying strengths and barriers to participation. The tool is appropriate for all conditions and can be used with children as young as 6 months to 21 years of age.
   A. Children's Assessment of Participation and Enjoyment (CAPE)
   B. Short Child Occupational Profile (SCOPE)
   C. Performance Skills Questionnaire
   D. Perceived Efficacy and Goal Setting System (PEGS)
5. This tool assesses daily living skills function of children and identifies those who may be intellectually disabled or emotionally disturbed. The valid and reliable questionnaire-based tool is appropriate for children aged 6 to 18 years and takes less than 30 minutes to administer.
   A. Adaptive Behavior Assessment System, 2nd edition (ABAS-II)
   B. Disabilities of the Arm, Shoulder and Hand Outcome Measure (DASH)
   C. Asperger Syndrome Diagnostic Scale (ASDS)
   D. Adaptive Behavior Inventory (ABI)

Worksheet 10-6 (continued)

Pediatric Assessments

6. This is an assessment created in 2014 by OTs to evaluate the performance of ADLs and IADLs within the natural environment. The tool is a performance-based checklist appropriate for children 5 to 8 years of age. In addition to determining areas of strength or challenge, the tool assists with goal writing.
   A. Do-Eat Assessment
   B. Assessment of Motor and Process Skills, 7th edition (AMPS)
   C. Arnadottir OT-ADL Neurobehavioral Evaluation (A-ONE)
   D. Kohlman Evaluation of Daily Living Skills, 3rd edition (KELS)
7. Tool designed to assist with planning appropriate educational programs for children with special needs. Used to monitor a child's nonacademic functional performance within the school setting. The tool is appropriate for children from kindergarten to Grade 6 with a variety of disabilities. The tool is questionnaire-based, rated by one or more school professionals who are familiar with the child and his or her performance capabilities.
   A. School Function Assessment (SFA)
   B. Educational Assessment of School Youth for Occupational Therapists (EASY-OT)
   C. Kindergarten Readiness Test—Larson (KRT—Larson)
   D. FirstSTEp Screening Test for Evaluating Preschoolers
8. This assessment tool measures spontaneous organization of play and includes cognitive play behaviors. Preacademic problems are identified through the observation of play behaviors that can be discriminated as typical vs nontypical.
   A. Revised Knox Preschool Play Scale (RKPPS)
   B. Child-Initiated Pretend Play Assessment (ChIPPA)
   C. Play History (PH)
   D. Test of Environmental Supportiveness (TOES)
9. A performance-based observation checklist that examines gross motor maturation in infants from birth to 18 months of age. Used to identify motor delay and evaluate motor development over time.
   A. Bayley Scales of Infant and Toddler Development, 3rd edition: Motor Scale (Bayley-III Motor Scale)
   B. Bruininks Motor Ability Test (BMAT)
   C. Alberta Infant Motor Scale (AIMS)
   D. Fugl-Meyer (FM) assessment
10. A checklist based on observation and task performance designed to chart the development of prehension and describe the hand skills of children from birth to 6 years of age. The tool is also used to identify gaps in developmental sequences in older children and adults to indicate the need for in-depth assessment.
    A. Infant-Toddler Developmental Assessment (IDA)
    B. Erhardt Developmental Prehension Assessment, Revised (EDPA)
    C. Hawaii Early Learning Profile (HELP)
    D. Miller Assessment for Preschoolers (MAP)

Worksheet 10-7

Choosing Pediatric Assessments

Match the assessment tool to the case scenario for which it will be most appropriate.

a. Sensory Integration and Praxis Test (SIPT)
b. Evaluation of Social Interaction, 2nd edition (ESI)
c. Developmental Test of Visual Perception (DTVP-3)
d. Short Child Occupational Profile (SCOPE)
e. Adaptive Behavior Inventory (ABI)
f. Do-Eat Assessment
g. School Function Assessment (SFA)
h. Child-Initiated Pretend Play Assessment (ChIPPA)
i. Alberta Infant Motor Scale (AIMS)
j. Erhardt Developmental Prehension Assessment, Revised (EDPA)

1. Marlia is a 6-month-old girl who was born 1 month premature. Her parents have noticed that she is not able to maintain her head in midline while in supported sitting as her 5-month-old cousin can. The pediatrician recommended an occupational therapy evaluation. Which tool would the OT use to evaluate the motor development of Marlia? ____________________
2. Cason is a first-grader in a typical classroom. His teacher has noticed that he is having difficulty managing fasteners on his clothing, holding his pencil, and manipulating small items during math and art classes compared with his peers. His teacher consults with the OT, who uses which tool to assess Cason's developmental hand function? ____________________
3. In addition to the tool used above, Cason's OT decides to conduct another assessment because of his teacher's concerns for his ability to complete self-care activities needed for school, such as opening containers at lunch, managing clothing for toileting, going outside in cold weather, and getting on and off the bus without assistance. Which tool does he select? ____________________
4. Joey is an 11-year-old boy with the diagnosis of spastic diplegia. He is ambulatory with Lofstrand crutches but needs extra time to go from classroom to other areas of the school. Although he is high-functioning academically, his teachers do have concerns that his motor challenges may be affecting his overall success in school. The school principal, on the recommendation of his teachers, calls in an OT to assess Joey. The therapist decides to use an assessment that is distributed to all of Joey's teachers to get a clear picture of his functional abilities in the school setting. ____________________
5. Marcus is 13 years old and started attending middle school this year. He met with his school psychologist last week to talk to her about concerns that he is having with being bullied and called a "nerd" by other children. He explains that he does not have a lot of friends and prefers to stay home in his room playing video games rather than interacting with other kids in the neighborhood. After contacting Marcus's parents and finding that they also have concerns, the psychologist asks for the school OT to conduct an evaluation to see whether there are areas that require intervention. The OT uses two assessment tools during the evaluation. ____________________ and ____________________

Worksheet 10-8

Pediatrics—Early Intervention

1. Which of the following choices is correct regarding the developmental sequence of prehension from earlier to later?
   A. Raking grasp, radial digital grasp, inferior pincer grasp
   B. Raking grasp, palmar grasp, developmental scissors grasp
   C. Radial digital grasp, radial palmar grasp, three-jaw chuck
   D. Inferior pincer grasp, developmental scissors grasp, radial digital grasp

2. Under the Individuals with Disabilities Education Act (IDEA), the term *least restrictive environment* refers, in part, to which of the following conditions?
   A. Minimizing clutter in the home to allow for motor development
   B. Avoiding the use of restraints for positioning
   C. A therapy room that has adequate space for required therapy tasks, such as sensory integration equipment
   D. Placing atypical children in settings with typical children with opportunities to interact and learn together

3. Derek, a 7-month-old infant diagnosed with cerebral palsy, is unable to roll over independently and also does not demonstrate spontaneous use of the left upper extremity. The OT should recommend that the parents place the child in which of the following positions during supervised play to best facilitate spontaneous left arm function?
   A. Standing to push a toy shopping cart
   B. Supine to reach for a mobile
   C. Supported right side-lying to reach for a rattle
   D. Prone to reach for a rattle

4. Which of the following clients would not currently be eligible for early intervention services under Part C of IDEA?
   A. Three-month-old infant born with low birth weight to a mother who abuses alcohol
   B. Six-year-old child diagnosed with Duchenne muscular dystrophy
   C. A-year-and-a-half-old child diagnosed with failure to thrive
   D. Thirty-month-old child diagnosed with lead poisoning

5. An OT at a preschool is working with a 4-year-old child diagnosed with a developmental delay. The therapist asks the child to identify alphabet letters written on a blackboard and painted on blocks. The therapist also has the child pick out magnetic letters to spell the child's name. The underlying prewriting skill that is not being specifically addressed with these tasks is which of the following?
   A. Visual closure
   B. Form constancy
   C. Visual memory
   D. Visual discrimination

Worksheet 10-9

Play as an Occupation

The occupation of play is important for the development of motor, process/cognitive, and social interactive skills in the child. This worksheet outlines four types of play (pretend/symbolic, constructive, rough-and-tumble/physical play, and social play) in which preschool children participate (Case-Smith & O'Brien, 2010). Sort the list of play activities that follow into the type of play that best describes them.

Play Activities: Jumping, puzzle building, participate in circle time, swinging, puzzle building, parallel play activities, imitates adults, build structures with building blocks, tell stories, games with a winner, participates in dress up, plays with stuffed animals to create stories, sliding, running, singing and dancing in groups, plays house, creates arts and crafts projects, interactive games, takes on a particular role in play drama, sport activities

Pretend/symbolic play

1.
2.
3.
4.

Rough-and-tumble/physical play

1.
2.
3.
4.
5.

Constructive play

1.
2.
3.

Social play

1.
2.
3.
4.
5.
6.
7.

Learning Activity 10-1: Play Performance Skills

Based on the list of play activities in Worksheet 10-9, choose an activity from each of the four play groups. For each activity, identify the performance skills (motor, process/cognitive, and social interactive) that you can use in that type of activity to develop specific skills in a preschool-aged child.

Example:

Constructive play: *Building structures with building blocks:*
Motor skills

Reach: reaches for blocks from floor

Bend: bends at waist to reach blocks

Manipulate: turns blocks into correct orientation for building with hands

Coordinate: uses two hands together to manipulate blocks

Constructive Play:

Social Play:

Pretend/Symbolic Play:

Rough and Tumble/Physical Play:

Worksheet 10-10

Pediatrics—School Setting

1. An OT is observing a first-grade student, Olivia, to ascertain the prehension pattern that Olivia uses for writing. The therapist observes that as Olivia is completing a homework assignment, she is holding the pencil tightly with her right thumb, index, long, and ring fingers together and using entire arm movements when forming the letters. The therapist should document that Olivia is using what kind of grasp?
   A. Static tripod grasp
   B. Static quadrupod grasp.
   C. Dynamic quadrupod grasp
   D. Static ulnar digital grasp

2. Steven is a second-grade student who has decreased pinch strength in his dominant right hand. As a result, he exhibits difficulty with handwriting and reports that his hand gets tired. Steven's Individualized Education Program (IEP) delineates that an occupational therapy consultative model will be used to address these deficits. To implement the IEP, which of the following actions should the OT take?
   A. Work with Steven directly in the occupational therapy room to address fine motor skills using media such as therapy putty and clothespins.
   B. Work with Steven directly in the classroom to address fine motor skills using media such as clay and a pegboard.
   C. Suggest to the teacher that Steven use clay at play time and 1-inch pom-poms to erase a picture he drew on a small whiteboard
   D. Cotreat with the physical therapist (PT) to improve Steven's fine motor skills more quickly.

3. In a school setting, which of the following would not likely be a goal established in an IEP for a 14-year-old female student diagnosed with autism and dyspraxia?
   A. Ability to get from one class to another on time
   B. Ability to apply makeup independently
   C. Ability to manage feminine hygiene independently
   D. Ability to select and insert proper denomination of coins to use in a cafeteria vending machine

4. An OT is working in a school setting with Evan, a second-grade student who exhibits poor attention and fidgets frequently while seated at his desk. Which of the following is least appropriate for the therapist to recommend to Evan's teacher?
   A. Have Evan sit directly under the bright overhead lighting to allow him to see better and improve concentration
   B. Have Evan use headphones to reduce ambient noise during independent tasks
   C. Have Evan help to move a stack of books or classroom furniture
   D. Allow Evan to use a "fidget," such as a small squeeze ball when seated at his desk

5. An OT is working in a school setting with a 12-year-old student named Daisy who is diagnosed with cerebral palsy. During today's OT session, Daisy begins to sob and states that her classmates are saying mean things about her on the Internet. What primary action should the therapist should take?
   A. Tell Daisy she is overreacting and should ignore the other student's comments
   B. Call the other children's parents
   C. Notify the police
   D. Ask Daisy for specific examples

Learning Activity 10-2: School Occupations

For each of the following student challenges in performance skills or client factors, list three educationally related activities that may be affected by those challenges in a school setting. Examples are provided for each category.

Specific Factor/Skill Creating Challenges for Student	***Educationally Related Activity That May Be Impacted in a School Setting***
Tactile sensory processing	*Completing an art class project using glue*
	1.
	2.
	3.
Organizational skills	*Writing down all homework assignments and developing appropriate timeline for completion*
	1.
	2.
	3.
Proprioception	*Regulating the appropriate amount of pressure to avoid breakage of pencil or crayon when writing or coloring*
	1.
	2.
	3.
Time management	*Consistently getting to next class in allotted time frame*
	1.
	2.
	3.
Fine motor skills	*Managing fastenings on clothing when changing for gym class*
	1.
	2.
	3.

Specific Factor/Skill Creating Challenges for Student	***Educationally Related Activity That May Be Impacted in a School Setting***
Grip strength	*Carrying a full lunch box*
	1.
	2.
	3.
Standing balance/tolerance	*Standing in line to purchase lunch in cafeteria*
	1.
	2.
	3.
Shoulder range of motion (ROM)	*Hanging clothing on hook in locker*
	1.
	2.
	3.
Upper extremity strength	*Carrying books to class*
	1.
	2.
	3.
Eye-hand coordination	*Opening combination lock on locker*
	1.
	2.
	3.
Crossing midline	*Turning pages in a large book when reading in class*
	1.
	2.

Specific Factor/Skill Creating Challenges for Student	***Educationally Related Activity That May Be Impacted in a School Setting***
Spatial relations	*Fastening buckle on school bus seat belt*
	1.
	2.
	3.
Bilateral integration	*Washing hands after toileting*
	1.
	2.
	3.
Visual-motor	*Copying notes from the blackboard*
	1.
	2.
	3.
Categorization	*Sorting school papers according to subject*
	1.
	2.
	3.
Calculation skills	*Calculating cost of two items at school bake sale and determining the change back from $1*
	1.
	2.
	3.
Emotional regulation	*Walking in a line going to the cafeteria or school bus and remaining calm when accidentally getting bumped by a classmate*
	1.
	2.
	3.

Adapted from Morreale, M. J. (2015). *Developing clinical competence: A workbook for the OTA*. Thorofare, NJ: SLACK Incorporated.

Learning Activity 10-3: Positioning Equipment

Positioning is an important part of facilitating occupational participation. When children are not able to maintain positioning of their body because of muscle weakness, limited movement, abnormal tone, or movement patterns, using a device to maintain their body in a functional position is beneficial. Positioning equipment can also be used when working on specific client factors, such as reducing muscle tone through weight-bearing or increasing ROM by positioning a joint in a lengthened position. Skills such as reaching and manipulating objects are enhanced when proximal stability is maintained with an appropriate positioning device.

The following chart provides you an opportunity to consider the use of several common positioning devices. Fill in the squares after considering possible ages, diagnoses, positions, occupations, and client factors and skills that could be addressed with the equipment listed. Some resources for specialized pediatric positioning equipment include www.adaptivemall.com and www.pattersonmedical.com.

	Population: Age/Diagnosis	***Positions to Be Achieved***	***Occupations to Be Facilitated***	***Client Factors and Skills to Be Addressed***
Standing table	*Devices come in many sizes. Children as young as 10 months could be placed in an appropriately sized stander. Diagnosis: cerebral palsy, spinal bifida, ataxia*	*Standing*	*All occupations that can be completed at a tabletop and that do not require moving from place to place (e.g., eating, completing school work, participating in class activities, completing upper body grooming)*	*Lower extremity tone and strengthening, trunk strengthening, coordination of upper extremities through improved proximal support offered by stander*
Corner chair				
Bolsters				
Wedges				
Scooter board				
Wheelchair				
Balance board				

	Population: Age/Diagnosis	***Positions to Be Achieved***	***Occupations to Be Facilitated***	***Client Factors and Skills to Be Addressed***
Therapy balls				
Suspension slings/nets				
Bolster swing				
Tadpole (Vinyl-coated foam system for small children)				
T-stool				
Peanut balls				
Supine stander				
Prone stander				
Wooden chair with multiple adjustments				

Worksheet 10-11

Autism

Autism has become a common condition treated by occupational therapy practitioners in early intervention and within the school system. The following questions are based on the description of autism and diagnostic criteria described in the *Diagnostic and Statistical Manual of Mental Disorders, Fifth Edition* (DSM-5) (American Psychiatric Association, 2013).

Mark true (T) or false (F).

1. ______ Initially described in 1946, autism was considered a syndrome of communication deficits combined with repetitive and stereotypical behaviors that had an early childhood onset.
2. ______ In previous versions of the DSM, other conditions, such as Rhett syndrome and Asperger disorder, were delineated. These conditions have now been combined with autism.
3. ______ Autism is now considered a neurodevelopmental syndrome and is termed *autism syndrome disorder.*
4. ______ Autism can be diagnosed later in childhood than outlined in previous versions of the DSM due to the understanding that young children have few observable social demands and parents can give support to decrease the need for social interaction.
5. ______ Characteristics of autism may include deficits in social-emotional reciprocity, ranging from abnormal social approach and failure of normal back-and-forth conversation.
6. ______ Social characteristics of autism may also include nonverbal sharing of interests and emotions.
7. ______ Children with autism may have completely absent facial expressions.
8. ______ When diagnosing autism according to the DMS-5, a severity scale is used. One aspect of the severity criteria involves insistence on sameness with inflexible adherence to routines or ritualized verbal or physical behaviors.
9. ______ Severity can also be a factor of sensitivity to sensory input. Individuals with autism are always hyporeactive to sensory input and seldom react to physical touch.
10. ______ Intellectual disability is always associated in some way with autism, which was part of the reason for disagreement among theorists when redefining this diagnosis for the DSM-5.

Learning Activity 10-4: Cerebral Palsy

Cerebral palsy (CP) occurs at a rate of 1 to 2 cases per 1,000 births and results from trauma to the brain before, during, or shortly after birth. Cerebral palsy can present in several ways, including location and type of motor control limitations, depending on the location and severity of damage to the brain. Secondary concerns of cerebral palsy include intellectual disability, seizure disorders, and functional limitations that vary from significant to minor (Case-Smith & O'Brien, 2010).

The following table provides an opportunity to recall the various types of cerebral palsy, their presentation and tone, as well as the opportunity to consider various treatment options for possible functional limitations.

Type of CP	**Description of Tone**	**Presentation**	**Describe a Functional Limitation**	**Identify a Treatment Model and Describe a Treatment**	**Describe an Adaptation**
Example: Athetoid	*Fluctuating between spastic and low tone*	*quadriplegia*	*Child unable to feed self due to inability to hold utensil securely and bring hand to mouth in coordinated manner.*	*Neurodevelopmental treatment (NDT)-Bobath* *Engage child in a reaching activity while in supported quadruped position. This position provides weight-bearing to upper extremities. Weight-bearing is used to improve cocontraction of shoulder and elbow to facilitate coordinated movements for activities in sitting such as feeding.*	*Universal cuff to secure fork in hand. Positioning device to ensure upright positioning, and trunk stability.*

Learning Activity 10-5: Pediatric Case Study

In the following case study, you will find information about Jack, a young school-age boy with Down syndrome. Read the case and complete a plan of care as instructed. Use a professional format to formulate proper goals that contain all the necessary elements. A useful goal format is the COAST method, which stands for client, occupation, assist level, specific conditions, timeline (Gateley & Borcherding, 2012; Morreale & Borcherding, 2013). When you are done creating your plan, share it with a fellow occupational therapy student and discuss your ideas using the following questions:

- Are the assessment tools appropriate for Jack's age, diagnosis, and your hypothesis regarding areas of delay or challenge?
- Is your plan relevant for school-based practice?
- Are your goals measurable and occupation-based?
- Do your goals contain all components identified in the COAST method?
- On which frame of reference or practice model is your intervention plan based?
- Are the activities going to work on the goals effectively?
- Are the activities appropriate for school-based practice?
- Are you aware of the evidence to support your treatment activity choices?

Jack is a 10-year-old boy with a diagnosis of Down syndrome. Jack has an IQ score of approximately 65. He attends public school and is in an inclusive classroom. He receives assistance from a resource teacher for several of his academic classes. Recently, an occupational therapist was called in to evaluate Jack based on some concerns of his regular classroom teacher.

Jack is having difficulty writing in class; he is slow and seems to have to rest his entire trunk on the table to stabilize his hand. He holds his pencil much like a 1-year-old does. Jack has difficulty in the lunchroom carrying his tray and opening some milk cartons and plastic containers. On the playground, other children do not invite Jack to play because he is not well-coordinated for sport activities; he cannot catch or kick balls as well as his peers. Jack also has trouble with other activities because of possible hypotonia in his hands and coordination difficulties. He cannot close or open fasteners such as buttons, snaps, and zippers. This makes it difficult for him to don and doff his pants for toileting and for putting on outerwear on cold or rainy days.

Your mission is to identify three relevant assessment tools to assist you in determining Jack's functional abilities, skills, and client factor functioning. You should then identify at least three problems that you find most significant based on the information reported by his teacher, your observations, and the results of standardized testing. *It is important to remember that in school-based practice, the problems and goals should all relate to school functioning.* Once the problems are identified, write out long-term goals that indicate each problem has been solved (the desired outcomes) and then 2 short-term goals for each long-term goal. You should then chose one short-term goal from each problem area and describe activities that you will do to accomplish the goals and eradicate the problem. If you decide to provide a piece of adaptive equipment, you must describe the process of educating the child with that equipment.

Assessment tools: ____
____
____

Functional problem 1 ____

Occupation-based long-term goal 1 ____

Short-term goal 1a ____

Short-term goal 1b ____

Learning Activity 10-5: Pediatric Case Study (continued)

Functional problem 2 ____________________

Long-term goal 2 ____________________

Short-term goal 2a ____________________

Short-term goal 2b ____________________

Functional Problem 3 ____________________

Long-term goal 3 ____________________

Short-term goal 3a ____________________

Short-term goal 3b ____________________

Activity 1 (based on short-term goal ______)

Activity 2 (based on short-term goal ______)

Activity 3 (based on short-term goal ______)

Worksheet 10-12

Specialized Area of Practice: Neonatal Intensive Care Unit

The American Occupational Therapy Association (AOTA) asserts that practice within the Neonatal Intensive Care Unit (NICU) is not representative of entry-level practice and that additional expertise and competence is required of the practitioner who desires to work with this practice area (AOTA, 2006). The following multiple-choice questions and Worksheet 10-13 reinforce the knowledge required of those interested in pursuing this area.

1. Infants within the NICU are often physiologically fragile and easily affected by environmental conditions. Because of the fragile nature of these children, practitioners must be aware that:
   A. Parents will often refuse to allow the medical team to interact with their child.
   B. All interventions should be reserved for a time when it is apparent that the child has adapted to his or her surroundings.
   C. Interactions and interventions that may appear minor can result in instability and can risk the life of the newborn.
   D. Neurodevelopmental interventions and sensory integration strategies have no place in the NICU.
2. OTs working in the NICU must also be concerned with the families of the infants and their abilities to bond with the baby. Which one of the following is not a concern of families that occupational therapy practitioners should initially consider?
   A. The stress of the uncertain outcome of the infant's medical status
   B. Possible maternal complications after birth
   C. The stress associated with knowing that the infant will have disabilities
   D. The sense of helplessness associated with being in a highly technical environment
3. According to AOTA, occupational therapy practitioners should have experience and expertise in all but one of the following before deciding to seek employment in the NICU.
   A. Longitudinal care for children who have been in the NICU
   B. Typical development of all children, especially young children
   C. Communication with parents and other care providers
   D. Working with children with multiple diagnosis including childhood cancers
4. As a critical area of care, an OT working within this setting should possess many specific personal and professional attributes. Identify the one attribute from the following list that is not necessary for an OT to possess.
   A. Understanding of one's communication skills and style and the ability to modify them in response to the needs of others
   B. Interest in and ability to bring about changes in the social and physical environments
   C. The interest and ability to obtain specialty certification in pediatric practice
   D. Insight into one's professional knowledge and skills
5. Occupational therapy within the NICU requires the therapist to support the infant's medical and physiological status to do which one of the following:
   A. Enhance infant neurobehavioral organization
   B. Facilitate social participation of the family with the health care team
   C. Enhance the ability of the child to feed self from a bottle
   D. Ensure that the child is able to indicate when he or she is hungry

Worksheet 10-13

Neonatal Intensive Care Unit Basics

Indicate whether the following statements are true (T) or false (F).

1. _____ A child born 14 days ago to a woman at 35 weeks of pregnancy has a gestational age of 37 weeks.
2. _____ A child weighing 2,800 grams at birth is considered to have low birth weight.
3. _____ A child born before 37 weeks of pregnancy is considered preterm.
4. _____ When encouraging parents to take pictures of their preterm baby to facilitate bonding, the OT should document this intervention in the chart as phototherapy.
5. _____ Environmental factors can cause infants to lose heat through evaporation, radiation, convection, and conduction.
6. _____ Because it is important to minimize ambient noise for a preterm infant, the OT should recommend that the parents not verbalize directly to the child.
7. _____ When bathing a preterm infant, immersing the child in water with swaddling is generally more soothing than sponge bathing.
8. _____ Having the parent hold the child with skin-to-skin contact is called "kangaroo care."
9. _____ Signs of distress that an OT might observe in a preterm infant may include yawns, startles, or hiccups.
10. _____ Fortified formula is generally better than breast milk for a preterm infant's nutrition.
11. _____ An example of nonnutritive sucking is using a pacifier.
12. _____ For extremely preterm infants who have hypotonia, the OT should generally include upper extremity orthotic devices as part of the intervention plan.
13. _____ When facilitating feeding, the health team should work toward the infant achieving the typical mature suck-swallow-breathe pattern of 2:1:2.
14. _____ During intervention, the OT must be careful to protect the infant from heat destabilization.
15. _____ To stimulate alertness for a preterm baby, it is preferable that the OT use bright overhead lights during intervention.

Answers to Chapter 10 Worksheets

Worksheet 10-1: Theories Guiding Pediatric Practice

References: Bly, 2011; Case-Smith & O'Brien, 2010.

__4__ Motor learning and skill acquisition
__5__ Social skills training
__9__ Systems approach
__8__ Cognitive orientation to daily occupational performance (CO-OP)
__3__ Neurodevelopmental theory
__2__ Sensory integration
__7__ Adaptation and compensation
__6__ Coping model
__1__ Developmental approaches

Worksheet 10-2: Match the Model of Practice

References: Bly, 2011; Case-Smith & O'Brien, 2010.

1. CO-OP
2. Sensory integration
3. Adaptation and compensation
4. Neurodevelopmental theory
5. Social skills training

Worksheet 10-3: Typical Development

References: Bly, 2011; Case-Smith & O'Brien, 2010.

1. C
2. A
3. C
4. B
5. A
6. A
7. A
8. D
9. C
10. C

Worksheet 10-4: Typical and Atypical Development

References: Bly, 2011; Case-Smith & O'Brien, 2010.

1. *False:* A 15-month-old child has typically not yet developed a fine pincer grasp.

   Children typically develop a fine pincer grasp by 12 months of age.
2. *False:* When a 12-month-old begins to walk independently, the child's legs move in a "stride" pattern (hip forward flexion, knee extension, and full heel strike).

   A newly walking child will not be able to shift weight effectively to unweight a hip for flexion. The 12-month-old will quickly shift weight side to side and appear to "toddle."
3. *True:* Pelvic stability is needed for the child to gain the ability to walk correctly.
4. *True:* To have *good* fine motor skills, proximal stability of the scapula is essential.

5. _True:_ An 11-month-old child can typically stand up independently from a squatting position.
6. _True:_ Twelve months of age is within the norm range for beginning independent walking.
7. _False:_ If a 10-month-old child in prone hyperextends his neck with shoulder flexion and extended arms, but is unable to maintain head in midline or bear weight on forearms, he is demonstrating a typical pattern of development.

   A child should be able to cocontract flexors and extensors of the neck for midline dynamic head stability. Cocontraction of the shoulder and arm musculature should provide dynamic stability for weight shifting for reaching and maintaining prone on forearms.
8. _True:_ A 16-month-old child with a diagnosis of cerebral palsy who has obligatory head and neck asymmetry is likely to be dominated by an asymmetrical tonic neck reflex (ATNR).
9. _True:_ When significant winging of the scapula and poor trunk endurance are seen in a school-age child, the primary concern is that trunk and scapular stability have not developed.
10. _True:_ A child with a lack of abdominal stability with an anterior pelvic tilt may require assistive devices to walk.
11. _True:_ Sitting is the most functional and versatile position for the 7-month-old.
12. _True:_ When the 10-month-old is walking with hands held, he typically requires the person assisting to move him in a forward motion.
13. _False:_ When sitting, a 5-month-old has no trunk control and will flop over.

    A 5-month-old can sit unsupported using arms to prop as needed and when not moving too far from midline.
14. _False:_ Neck righting refers to the position that the child assumes when prone in the ninth month.

    Neck righting is a reflex that may be present until the child is 9 months old where the shoulders and trunk turn toward the position of head when it is rotated to one side.
15. _True:_ At approximately 2 months of age, a child is in a period of development known as "astasia abasia."
16. _False:_ The rooting reflex is of concern if it is observed in a child older than 1 month of age.

    The rooting reflex can be elicited until the child is 3 to 4 months of age.
17. _True:_ An obligatory suck/swallow reflex extending beyond three months of age can impact the development of normalized eating and swallowing.
18. _True:_ Children will typically be able to secure an object in their hand and bring to their mouth before the sixth month of life.
19. _False:_ Children begin to hold a crayon and make scribbles after demonstration as early as 5 months old.

    Children begin to hold a crayon and make scribbles between 12 and 24 months
20. _False:_ When sitting with both knees flexed and soles of feet touching, a child is said to be "pretzel sitting."

    This position is ring sitting.

Worksheet 10-5: Determining Chronological Age

1. Amy is 10 years, 4 months, and 20 days old.
2. Zack is 2 years, 4 months, and 1 day old.
3. Patish is 4 years, 9 months, and 14 days old.
4. Mora is 7 years, 11 months, and 12 days old.
5. Hamed is 3 months and 3 days old.
6. Today you are ______ years, ______ months, and ______ days old.

Worksheet 10-6: Pediatric Assessments

Reference: Asher, 2014.

1. D	3. D	5. D	7. A	9. C
2. A	4. B	6. A	8. B	10. B

Worksheet 10-7: Choosing Pediatric Assessments

Reference: Asher, 2014.

1. I
2. J
3. F
4. G
5. B, D

Worksheet 10-8: Pediatrics—Early Intervention

1. A. (Edwards, Buckland, & McCoy-Powlen, 2002)
2. D. (Küpper, 2012; U.S. Department of Education, n.d.) Part C of IDEA provides services to eligible children under age 3 years. *Least restrictive environment* (LRE) means that a child with a disability should have the opportunity to interact and be educated with peers who are not disabled and have access to the same programs to the greatest extent possible.
3. C. Placing the child lying on the right side would limit motion of the uninvolved arm and, thus, best encourage spontaneous use of the affected left arm to reach for and grasp the rattle. In supine or prone, the child would likely attempt reaching for a mobile or rattle with the favored right arm, so choice B and D are not the best answers (although the therapist or parent could certainly guide and encourage use of the involved arm). At 7 months, the child would not yet have the ability to walk.
4. B. Under Part C of IDEA, early intervention services are provided from birth up to age 3 for children with, or at risk for, a disability and their families. However, under IDEA Part B, related services and special education can be extended to age 21 (Küpper, 2012; U.S. Department of Education, n.d.).
5. A. Visual closure involves the identification of a letter or figure when it is incomplete. This is a skill needed to form letters when writing, but, in this situation, the letters are already complete (Pendzick & Rockwell, 2009).

Worksheet 10-9: Play as an Occupation

Reference: Case-Smith & O'Brien, 2010.

Pretend/symbolic play
Imitates adults
Plays with stuffed animals to create stories
Plays house
Takes on a particular role in play drama

Rough-and-tumble/physical play
Jumping
Swinging
Sliding
Running
Sports activities

Constructive play
Building structures with building blocks
Creates arts and crafts projects
Puzzles

Social play
Participate in circle time
Participates in dress-up
Parallel play activities
Singing and dancing in groups
Plays games with a winner
Interactive games
Tell stories

Worksheet 10-10: Pediatrics—School Setting

1. B. (Edwards, Buckland, & McCoy-Powlen, 2002)
2. C. Occupational therapy practitioners using a consultative model provide direct recommendations to the teacher and other education staff to implement with a particular student, such as strategies or activities the student would benefit from in the classroom. A direct service model provides designated therapy services to the child either inside the classroom or as pullout services performed outside the classroom (Steva, 2014). The two models are not always mutually exclusive. OT services may be provided individually or in a group and must support specific occupations needed in the school environment. Interventions may include a variety of methods, such as compensatory techniques, sensory integration activities, exercises for postural control, gross and fine motor tasks, and instruction in assistive technology, for example.

3. B. Goals in an IEP must relate to the skills a student needs to function within the school environment. Toileting skills, feminine hygiene, ability to get to class, and cafeteria functions, such as carrying a tray, purchasing lunch/snacks (e.g., using a school vending machine) are all related to the educational setting. Although the student may desire to be able to apply makeup independently, that is not an educationally related task.
4. A. A child with poor attention would benefit more from calming strategies, such as dim lighting and the strategies in answers B, C, and D (Gallagher, 2015).
5. D. Harassment, intimidation, and bullying [HIB] is a serious matter that should not be taken lightly. Schools strive to create a welcoming and safe environment for students. Policies are created to prevent HIB of students, and a variety of resources are available (New Jersey Department of Education, 2010; Ohio Department of Education, 2014). An OT working in a school setting has a duty to report such behavior to help ensure the child's safety and emotional well-being. The OT should ask the child about the general nature of the comments (e.g., teasing vs direct threat of bodily harm) and follow the protocol that the school district has in place for handling these situations.

Worksheet 10-11: Autism

Reference: American Psychiatric Association, 2013.

1. _T_ Initially described in 1946, autism was considered a syndrome of communication deficits combined with repetitive and stereotypical behaviors that had an early childhood onset.
2. _T_ In previous versions of the DSM, other conditions, such as Rhett syndrome and Asperger disorder, were delineated. These conditions have now been combined with autism.
3. _F_ Autism is now considered a neurodevelopmental syndrome and is termed *autism syndrome disorder.*

   Autism is now considered to be spectrum and is termed autism spectrum disorder, *which is a neurodevelopmental disorder.*
4. _T_ Autism can be diagnosed later in childhood than had been outlined in previous versions of the DSM because of the understanding that young children have few observable social demands and parents can give support to decrease the need for social interaction.
5. _T_ Characteristics of autism may include deficits in social-emotional reciprocity, ranging from abnormal social approach and failure of normal back and forth conversation.
6. _F_ Social characteristics of autism may also include nonverbal sharing of interests and emotions. *Social characteristics of autism may include a lack of sharing of interests and emotions.*
7. _T_ Children with autism may have completely absent facial expressions.
8. _T_ When diagnosing autism according to the DMS-5, a severity scale is used. One aspect of the severity criteria involves insistence on sameness with inflexible adherence to routines or ritualized verbal or physical behaviors.
9. _F_ Severity can also be a factor of sensitivity to sensory input. Individuals with autism are always hyporeactive to sensory input and seldom react to physical touch. *Individuals with autism may demonstrate hyper- or hyporeactivity to sensory input.*
10. _F_ Intellectual disability is always associated in some way with autism, which was part of the reason for disagreement among theorists when redefining this diagnosis for the DSM-5. *The diagnosis of autism can be made with either accompanying intellectual impairment or no intellectual impairment.*

Worksheet 10-12: Specialized Area of Practice: Neonatal Intensive Care Unit

Reference: AOTA, 2006.

1. C. Infants in the NICU are sensitive to even small changes in their physical and social environment. Answer A is not correct because there is no evidence to suggest that parents refuse care in the NICU. Although it is important for a child to adapt to her or her surroundings, treatment is not withheld until this ongoing process is complete, so choice B is incorrect. Choice D is also not the correct answer because many treatment philosophies can be indicated for infants with the NICU and must be administered with care and caution.
2. C. Not all infants will have permanent disabilities despite being candidates for the NICU after birth. Although stress may be due to the unknown, it is not always associated with the certainty of disability.

3. D. It is more important for the therapist to understand and have experience working with very young children who have motor, cognitive, and social concerns. Childhood cancers are rare and are not linked with the NICU experience.
4. C. Specialty certification is not required for work with the NICU.
5. A. Occupational therapy within the NICU requires the therapist to support the infant's medical and physiological status to enhance infant neurobehavioral organization. Answer B is not the best choice because even though good communication is important between the family and the health care team, participating in outside activities is not indicated. Answer C is not correct because infants within the NICU are not candidates for self-feeding; this is a skill developed later in the first year of life. Understanding that an infant is hungry (answer D) is the role of the caregiver, not the child

Worksheet 10-13: Neonatal Intensive Care Unit Basics

Reference: Hunter, 2010; World Health Organization, 2011.

1. F A child born 14 days ago to a woman at 35 weeks of pregnancy has a gestational age of 37 weeks. *Gestational age is the number of weeks in utero. In this situation, the infant's gestational age is 35 weeks.*
2. F A child weighing 2,800 grams at birth is considered to have low birth weight. *Low birth weight is considered less than 2,500 grams (5.5 pounds)* (WHO, 2011).
3. T A child born before 37 weeks of pregnancy is considered preterm (WHO, 2011).
4. F When encouraging parents to take pictures of their preterm baby to facilitate bonding, the OT should document this intervention in the chart as phototherapy. *Phototherapy is light therapy, such as is used to treat jaundice.*
5. T Environmental factors can cause infants to lose heat through evaporation, radiation, convection, and conduction (Hunter, 2010).
6. F Because it is important to minimize ambient noise for a preterm infant, the OT should recommend that the parents not verbalize directly to the child. *Soft, soothing parental interaction with the infant is encouraged to facilitate bonding* (Hunter, 2010).
7. T When bathing a preterm infant, immersing the child in water with swaddling is generally more soothing than sponge bathing (Hunter, 2010).
8. T Having the parent hold the child with skin-to-skin contact is called "kangaroo care" (Hunter, 2010; WHO, 2011).
9. T Signs of distress that an OT might observe in a preterm infant may include yawns, startles, or hiccups (Hunter, 2010).
10. F Fortified formula is generally better than breast milk for a preterm infant's nutrition (WHO, 2011).
11. T An example of nonnutritive sucking is using a pacifier (Hunter, 2011).
12. F For extremely preterm infants who have hypotonia, the OT should generally include upper extremity orthotic devices as part of the intervention plan. *It is typical that extremely premature infants exhibit hypotonia. While splints may be used in certain instances, they may hinder movement or cause pressure areas on fragile skin* (Hunter, 2010).
13. F When facilitating feeding, the health team should work toward the infant achieving the typical mature suck-swallow-breathe pattern of 2:1:2. *The typical rhythm is 1:1:1* (Hunter, 2010).
14. T During intervention, the OT must be careful to protect the infant from heat destabilization (Hunter, 2010).
15. F To stimulate alertness for a preterm baby, it is preferable that the OT use bright overhead lights during intervention. *Because the preterm infant's visual system is not fully developed, bright light is not tolerated well* (Hunter, 2010).

Chapter 10 References

American Occupational Therapy Association. (2006). Specialized knowledge and skills for occupational therapy practice in the neonatal intensive care unit. *American Journal of Occupational Therapy, 60*, 659–668.

American Psychiatric Association. (2013). *Diagnostic and statistical manual of mental disorders* (5th ed.). Arlington, VA: American Psychiatric Association.

Asher, I. E. (Ed). (2014). *Asher's occupational therapy assessment tools: An annotated index* (4th ed.). Bethesda, MD: AOTA Press.

Bly, L. (2011). *Components of typical and atypical motor development.* Laguna Beach, CA: Neuro-Developmental Treatment Association.

Case-Smith, J., & O'Brien, J. (2010). *Occupational therapy for children* (6th ed.). Maryland Heights, MO: Mosby.

Edwards, S. J., Buckland, D. J., & McCoy-Powlen, J. D. (2002). *Developmental & functional hand grasps.* Thorofare, NJ: SLACK Incorporated.

Gallagher, S. (2015). A third-grader with attention deficit hyperactivity disorder. In K. Sladyk & S. E. Ryan (Eds.), *Ryan's occupational therapy assistant: Principles, practice issues, and techniques* (5th ed., pp. 204–221). Thorofare, NJ: SLACK Incorporated.

Gateley, C. A., & Borcherding, S. (2012). *Documentation manual for occupational therapy: Writing SOAP notes* (3rd ed.). Thorofare, NJ: SLACK Incorporated.

Hunter, J. G. (2010). Neonatal intensive care unit. In J. Case-Smith & J. O'Brien (Eds.), *Occupational therapy for children* (6th ed., pp. 649-680). Maryland Heights, MO: Mosby.

Küpper, L. (Ed.). (2012). The basics of early intervention: 9 key definitions in early intervention (Section 3 of Module 1). *Building the legacy for our youngest children with disabilities: A training curriculum on Part C of IDEA 2004.* Washington, DC: National Dissemination Center for Children with Disabilities. Retrieved from http://nichcy.org/laws/idea/legacy/partc/module1

Morreale, M. J. (2015). *Developing clinical competence: A workbook for the OTA.* Thorofare: NJ: SLACK Incorporated.

Morreale, M. J., & Borcherding, S. (2013). *The OTA's guide to documentation: Writing SOAP notes* (3rd ed.). Thorofare, NJ: SLACK Incorporated.

New Jersey Department of Education. (2010). *Harassment, intimidation, & bullying (HIB).* Trenton, NJ: Author. Retrieved from http://www.state.nj.us/education/students/safety/behavior/hib

Ohio Department of Education. (2014). *Anti-harassment, intimidation and bullying resources.* Retrieved from http://education.ohio.gov/Topics/Other-Resources/School-Safety/Safe-and-Supportive-Learning/Anti-Harassment-Intimidation-and-Bullying-Resource

Pendzick, M. J., & Rockwell, D. L. (2009). Interventions for education. In J. V. DeLany & M. J. Pendzick, *Working with children and adolescents: A guide for the occupational therapy assistant* (pp. 265–289). Upper Saddle River, NJ: Pearson Education.

Steva, B. J. (2014). Interventions to enhance occupational performance in education and work. In K. Jacobs, N. MacRae, & K. Sladyk (Eds.), *Occupational therapy essentials for clinical competence* (2nd ed., pp. 347–365). Thorofare, NJ: SLACK Incorporated.

U.S. Department of Education. (n.d.). *Building the legacy: IDEA 2004.* Retrieved from http://idea.ed.gov

World Health Organization. (2011). Optimal feeding of low birth-weight infants in low- and middle-income countries. Geneva: World Health Organization. Retrieved from http://www.who.int/maternal_child_adolescent/documents/9789241548366.pdf

Chapter 11

Demonstrating Managerial Skills

The worksheets and learning activities presented in this final chapter address a variety of areas applicable to managing an occupational therapy department and implementing client interventions. These areas include billing and reimbursement, budget, quality improvement, marketing, clinical reasoning, creative problem solving, and the appropriate handling of client situations. Answers to worksheet exercises are provided at the end of the chapter.

Contents

Morreale, M. J. & Amini, D.
The Occupational Therapist's Workbook for Ensuring Clinical Competence (pp. 389-414).

Worksheet 11-1

Billing and Reimbursement

1. An occupational therapist (OT) provides 30 minutes of therapy to a 50-year-old outpatient client who is recovering from a shoulder fracture. The therapist is unsure what the proper billing codes are for therapeutic exercise and ADL retraining. Which of the following would be the most useful resource?

   A. International Classification of Diseases (ICD) manual

   B. Medicare Benefit Policy Manual

   C. Current Procedural Terminology (CPT) manual

   D. Minimum Data Set

2. A 75-year-old client who receives outpatient rehabilitation has Medicare B as his primary health insurance. The OT and physical therapist (PT) work together with the client for 30 minutes to instruct the client in safe transfers. The PT plans to bill Medicare for 2 units of therapy. How many units should the OT bill Medicare for this cotreatment?

   A. 0

   B. 1

   C. 2

   D. 3

3. A client in a skilled nursing facility has Medicare B as his primary health insurance. An OT works with the client in occupational therapy, providing 20 minutes of activities of daily living (ADL) training. How many units can the OT bill Medicare for the therapy provided?

   A. 1

   B. 2

   C. 5

   D. 20

4. An OT is working in an acute care hospital with a 65-year-old inpatient who is a retired businessman. Of the following choices, the third-party payer for the client's health care is most likely which of the following?

   A. TRICARE

   B. Medicare Part A

   C. Medicare Part B

   D. Medicare Part D

5. An OT is working on an acute psychiatric unit with a 72-year-old client who is a retired factory worker. The client has Medicare as his primary health insurance. The facility will most likely be reimbursed through which of the following?

   A. Medicare Part A Prospective Payment System

   B. Medicare Part B Physician Fee Schedule

   C. Medicare Part D Rehabilitation Fee Schedule

   D. Medicare Part B Therapy Cap

Worksheet 11-1 (continued)

Billing and Reimbursement

6. An OT is working in an outpatient clinic. A client in occupational therapy is 45 years old and has private insurance that pays 80% of health care costs after a $150 deductible is met. The client's occupational therapy evaluation last week cost $100 and today is the client's first treatment session that costs $70. The client has not had any other health services this calendar year. How much money out-of-pocket will the client have to pay for today's session?
   A. $20
   B. $54
   C. $56
   D. $70

7. Which of the following is a mandatory insurance that businesses pay to cover the health costs of workers who are injured on the job?
   A. TRICARE
   B. Unemployment Insurance
   C. Medicare Part C
   D. Worker's Compensation

8. Which of the following does not meet the Medicare criteria to be classified as durable medical equipment?
   A. Wheelchair
   B. Commode
   C. Tub seat
   D. Quad cane

9. A 14-month old child with a developmental delay would most likely receive OT services resulting from which legislation?
   A. Omnibus Budge Reconciliation Act (OBRA)
   B. Individuals With Disabilities Education Act (IDEA) Part B
   C. IDEA Part C
   D. Health Insurance Portability and Accountability Act (HIPAA)

10. Which of the following choices is most likely the third-party payer for health care for an unmarried 28-year old female who has been unemployed for 12 months, is pregnant, and has no assets?
   A. Unemployment insurance
   B. Supplemental Security Insurance
   C. Worker's Compensation
   D. Medicaid

Worksheet 11-2

Medicare Billing and Reimbursement

1. A client in a busy outpatient setting has Medicare B as his primary insurance. An occupational therapy aide works with that client for 23 minutes to instruct the client in a home exercise program using exercise bands. How many units of therapy should an OT bill Medicare for that service?

   A. 23

   B. 2

   C. 1

   D. 0

2. A client with Medicare has been paying the supplemental monthly premium. He was admitted to a skilled nursing facility for rehabilitation following a cerebrovascular accident (CVA). Depending on his inpatient length of stay at that facility, the client's occupational therapy may be reimbursed through which of the following for covered services?

   A. Medicare A

   B. Medicare B

   C. Medicare A or B

   D. Medicare D

3. Anna, a 68-year-old woman with Medicare B, sustained a Colles fracture and was referred to outpatient occupational therapy. According to Medicare guidelines, which of the following must an OT document as part of the initial evaluation process?

   A. G Codes

   B. D Codes

   C. J Codes

   D. A Codes

4. A home care client with Medicare would benefit from occupational therapy skilled maintenance services and meets the eligibility requirements. These services are not reimbursable if which of the following conditions are present?

   A. An OT provides maintenance therapy

   B. The client's condition is not expected to functionally improve

   C. Another discipline is providing maintenance services concurrently

   D. An occupational therapy aide provides the maintenance therapy

5. An outpatient who requires an orthosis has Medicare B as his primary insurance. According to the Healthcare Common Procedure Coding System (HCPCS), which of the following should an OT use to bill Medicare for fitting and issuing the orthosis, not counting the time needed to educate the client regarding use and care of the orthotic device?

   A. CPT codes

   B. Level II L codes

   C. Minimum Data Set

   D. Outcome Assessment Information Set

Learning Activity 11-1: Billing Codes

Current procedural terminology (CPT) are standard billing codes that are part of the Healthcare Common Procedure Coding System (HCPCS) and used to bill insurance companies for individual skilled health services, such as outpatient occupational therapy (Centers for Medicare & Medicaid Services [CMS], 2011). Billing for some therapy procedures is based on units of time (in 15-minute increments). Other procedures are considered untimed and billed only 1 unit regardless of the time provided for that service (CMS, 2011). Use a CPT manual (found at a library, fieldwork site, or online) to find the correct billing codes for the following OT interventions. Determine what general intervention category the specific tasks come under, if it is considered a timed service, and whether constant attendance or one-on-one care by the OT practitioner is required. An example is provided.

OT Intervention Implemented	***Billing Category***	***Is This Intervention Considered Timed or Untimed?***	***Is This Intervention Considered as Only a Supervised Modality or Is It Classified as Requiring Constant Attendance or One-On-One With an OT Practitioner?***	***CPT Billing Code***
Example: *Upper extremity coordination exercises*	*Neuromuscular reeducation*	*Timed*	*One-on-one intervention*	*97112*
Teaching use of a buttonhook				
Measuring a client for a wheelchair				
Instruction and practice using worksheets to improve sequencing and problem solving				
Using a hot pack				
Checking and modifying a splint				
Assessing upper extremity strength				
Teaching compensatory techniques for cooking				
Educating a client in sliding board transfers				
Hand strengthening using a hand gripper and therapy putty				
Assessing a client's home for safety				
Teaching coping strategies to a client who abuses alcohol				
Teaching a client how to propel and use a wheelchair				
Paraffin treatment				

Reprinted with permission from Morreale, M. J. (2015). *Developing clinical competence: A workbook for the OTA*. Thorofare, NJ: SLACK Incorporated.

Learning Activity 11-2: Diagnosis Codes

The World Health Organization (WHO) maintains a standard, universal listing of codes for diseases and conditions, called the *International Classification of Diseases* (ICD), which is periodically revised (WHO, 2013). The United States shifted from using version ICD-9 to the use of ICD-10, effective October 1, 2015, as mandated by the United States Department of Health and Human Services (American Academy of Professional Coders [AAPC], 2014a). For the following conditions, use a current ICD manual to look up each of the diagnosis codes. Realize that the condition may be listed as a synonym in the ICD manual.

1. Parkinson's disease ______________________________
2. A cut to the index finger ______________________________
3. Marfan syndrome ______________________________
4. Middle cerebral artery subarachnoid hemorrhage ______________________________
5. Cubital tunnel syndrome ______________________________
6. Down syndrome ______________________________
7. Failure to thrive (child) ______________________________
8. Schizophrenia ______________________________
9. Glaucoma ______________________________
10. Ulnar shaft open fracture ______________________________

Worksheet 11-3

Department Management

Occupational therapy practitioners planning to establish a private practice therapy program or clinic must first create a sound business plan, carefully considering factors such as the potential client base, likely funding sources (e.g., Medicare, Workers' Compensation, Early Intervention, private insurance, client self-pay), and available budget. Reimbursement from third-party payers is normally contingent on meeting strict criteria to be able to bill that insurer for therapy (such as becoming a Medicare-certified agency or being part of an insurer network). In addition, there are many legal and logistical factors involved with owning or managing a program or clinic. As a creative exercise, imagine that you have decided to open up a private outpatient therapy clinic. Consider the following factors in regard to this endeavor:

1. **Vision**

   Determine what your vision is for this new program and decide on a name for the program or facility. Consider the geographic area (e.g., county, entire state, multiple states) and client population that the clinic will likely serve (infants, school-age children, adults, elderly). Decide on the specific types of services that will be offered (e.g., health and wellness, adult rehabilitation, sensory integration, driver rehabilitation, low vision, hand therapy). Looking toward the future, consider whether your plans would include eventually expanding the clinic or establishing other sites.

   Vision for private practice:

   a. Name of facility: ______________________

   b. Geographic area: ______________________

   c. Type of practice area: ______________________

   d. Population served: ______________________

   e. Services offered: ______________________

   f. Likely funding sources: ______________________

   g. Future plans: ______________________

2. **Space**

   Besides the cost, determine at least 10 criteria to consider when looking for a suitable space to rent (or buy):

   1.
   2.
   3.
   4.
   5.
   6.
   7.
   8.
   9.
   10.

3. **Equipment and supplies**

   Assume you have rented empty space and now need to purchase all the equipment and supplies for this clinic. Brainstorm a list of items that will be needed. Prioritize the items into three categories: items that are essential for day 1, items that are needed but do not have to be purchased immediately, and a "wish list" of items that will be purchased as revenue increases. Do not include professional expenses such as insurance, building permits, and licensing fees in this list.

Worksheet 11-3 (continued)

Department Management

Category	***Essential Items***	***Needed but Can Be Deferred***	***Wish List***
Safety			
Office furniture			
Office equipment			
Office supplies			
Evaluation tools			
General supplies			
Exercise equipment			
ADL equipment			
Adaptive equipment			
Physical agent modalities (PAMs)			
Upper extremity orthotic supplies			
Other:			
Other:			

4. **Staff and Professional Services**

   Besides possibly hiring other occupational therapy practitioners, list at least eight other disciplines or services you may need to pay for when starting or owning a private practice. Do not include other rehabilitation disciplines such as physical or speech therapy.

   1.
   2.
   3.
   4.
   5.
   6.
   7.
   8.

Worksheet 11-4

Budget

Indicate whether the following statements are true (T) or false (F).

1. ______ A fiscal year goes from January 1 to December 31.
2. ______ An example of an occupational therapy capital budget expenditure is a tub seat.
3. ______ Revenue equals total income minus expenses.
4. ______ An example of a fixed cost is rent.
5. ______ Accounts receivable include the money due from an insurance company.
6. ______ An example of variable expenses are office supplies.
7. ______ Nonprofit means that the organization does not meet its expenses.
8. ______ Total costs subtracted from revenue equals profits.
9. ______ An OT department budget always contains money for staff to attend continuing education seminars to maintain National Board for Certification in Occupational Therapy (NBCOT) certification.
10. ______ Costs for items ordered, but not paid for are considered accounts payable.
11. ______ Bandages, lotions, and paraffin are considered direct use supplies.
12. ______ Cash flow consists of pending money due from third-party payers.
13. ______ Expenses that are fixed, such as salaries and equipment leases, are called *overhead*.
14. ______ Productivity refers to the amount of billable services that an individual provides.
15. ______ A piece of capital equipment that is depreciating is considered an asset.

Reprinted with permission from Morreale, M. J. (2015). *Developing clinical competence: A workbook for the OTA*. Thorofare, NJ: SLACK Incorporated.

Learning Activity 11-3: Mission Statements

Choose two health-related facilities in your community, such as a hospital, doctors' group, or outpatient rehabilitation clinic. One facility should be classified as a not-for-profit organization and the other a for-profit organization. Using the company websites, locate the mission statements for both facilities and compare and contrast them.

	Not-for-Profit Health Facility	***For-Profit Health Facility***
Name of facility/organization		
Is this facility part of a larger network or organization? If so, describe.		
Overall philosophy (e.g., religious, philanthropic, social justice)		
Population served (geographic area and/or types of diagnoses)		
List three primary services provided to the community it serves	1. 2. 3.	1. 2. 3.
List five words from the mission statement that best convey the values of the organization	1. 2. 3. 4. 5.	1. 2. 3. 4. 5.
Stated vision for the future		

Reprinted with permission from Morreale, M. J. (2015). *Developing clinical competence: A workbook for the OTA*. Thorofare, NJ: SLACK Incorporated.

Learning Activity 11-4: Quality Improvement

Describe an issue that has a negative impact on client satisfaction, safety, or care that you have either (a) personally experienced while receiving health services or (b) that you have observed on fieldwork or on the job at a health facility/agency. For example, perhaps you find that you have to wait at your doctor's office for at least an hour before you are seen for a scheduled appointment; your department is out of certain essential supplies when you need them; or that your outpatient clients forget to bring their orthotic devices to their follow-up therapy sessions. Once you have identified an issue needing quality improvement, use the following worksheet to develop an action plan to address the issue.

1. Identified problem: ____________________

   ____

   ____

2. Describe why this is a problem (e.g., safety concern, client satisfaction):

   ____

   ____

   ____

3. Brainstorm possible solutions:
   a.
   b.
   c.
   d.
   e.

4. Choose one idea from your list that you think will be the best solution:

   ____

5. Develop an action plan. List the steps needed to implement your plan, the staff member(s) who will be responsible (e.g., rehab aide, secretary, OT, nursing), and possible factors limiting implementation (cost, staff time, etc.):

Action Plan Steps	*Staff Member(s) Responsible*	*Factors Limiting Implementation*

6. Identify a method to evaluate, measure, or track the effectiveness of your intended plan:

   ____

   ____

   ____

Worksheet 11-5

Marketing

An occupational therapy manager scheduled a staff meeting to elicit ideas for marketing the hospital's outpatient OT program. During the brainstorming session, the OTs and OTAs suggested the following ideas. Critique each idea and explain the rationale for why it may or may not be feasible to execute. Discuss factors that would affect implementation, such as specific costs, personnel requirements, and ethical or legal considerations. Create two additional marketing ideas to critique also. Develop a marketing plan for the idea you think would work out the best.

1. Host a breakfast or lunch for a group of physicians to explain the unique value of occupational therapy.
2. Contact potential referring physicians and offer a referral bonus for each client that the physician refers to the OT department.
3. Develop an informational brochure about the OT department and send it to physicians in the surrounding area.
4. Create a commercial for the local TV station.
5. In the lobby or next to the hospital cafeteria, host an OT event, such as an exhibition of adaptive equipment or wellness activities.
6. Write an article for the local newspaper about occupational therapy and the specific OT services provided at the hospital.
7. Provide educational sessions to local organizations such as support groups for individuals with arthritis, Alzheimer's disease, or Parkinson's disease.
8. Provide free occupational therapy screenings to members of the community.
9. Other:
10. Other:

Worksheet 11-6

Creative Problem Solving

One of the most important skills of an occupational therapy practitioner is the ability to creatively problem-solve all challenging situations. To help you practice this skill, fill in the blanks after each scenario. It is important to remember that each client is unique and has individual circumstances. A therapist must always use clinical judgment to determine which interventions are appropriate and safe to use with a "real" client.

1. As part of a home visit, you are addressing self-feeding skills with a client diagnosed with CVA. The client needs a solution to keep the plate from sliding on the table, but you did not bring any nonslip matting (e.g., Dycem [Dycem, Ltd]) with you. List four items commonly found in a home that you may be able to substitute at this time.
   a. ______
   b. ______
   c. ______
   d. ______
2. You are working in an outpatient setting with a client diagnosed with Parkinson's disease. Because the client has balance deficits, you recommend that the client use a tub seat for safety while bathing. The client tells you he cannot afford to purchase a tub seat. Besides possibly helping the client to obtain financial assistance or donated/borrowed equipment, what other practical solutions could you offer for this problem?
   a. ______
   b. ______
3. You are working with an outpatient client who is diagnosed with rheumatoid arthritis. She has decreased range of motion (ROM) in both shoulders and impaired fine motor skills. The client takes great pride in her appearance, but reports difficulty putting on and removing jewelry. What are some practical suggestions you can offer for this occupation?
   a. ______
   b. ______
   c. ______
   d. ______
   e. ______
   f. ______
4. You have issued an orthotic device that has a complex set of straps to position the client's extremity properly. Besides verbal and written instructions and actual practice, what can you do to make it easier for the client to apply the correct sequence and position of the straps?
   a. ______
   b. ______
   c. ______
   d. ______
5. You are working in a hospital with a client who will be going home with an indwelling catheter in place. The client needs instruction in lower body dressing and managing clothing for toileting. He plans to remain at home until the catheter is removed next week. What recommendations could you offer?
   a. ______
   b. ______
   c. ______
   d. ______
   e. ______

Worksheet 11-6 (continued)

Creative Problem Solving

6. You receive a phone call from the OTA that you are supervising. The OTA, who works in a rural skilled nursing facility, is concerned because a client with a partial gross grasp of her dominant hand is being discharged to home unexpectedly. The client is able to feed herself at the facility with an adapted fork and spoon, but has no equipment for home use. Without these devices, she will no longer be independent in this ADL. What could you recommend to the OTA?
   a. ____________________
   b. ____________________
   c. ____________________
7. Two hours ago, you created a dynamic flexion orthosis for a client who underwent a zone 2 flexor tendon repair 3 days ago. The referring physician calls you stating that the client phoned her office reporting that the orthosis was uncomfortable. It is 30 minutes from the end of the business day. What do you do?
   a. ____________________
   b. ____________________
   c. ____________________
   d. ____________________
   e. ____________________
8. You have recently started your first job in an outpatient rehabilitation department. Today you will be evaluating a client with Huntington disease who has been referred to OT due to increasing difficulty with self-care ADLs. You plan to measure hand strength, ROM, and fine motor coordination but cannot locate the appropriate tools (dynamometer, goniometer, and nine-hole peg test). How will you complete your evaluation without these tools?
   a. ____________________
   b. ____________________
9. Knowing that you are an OT, your neighbor asks your opinion about her 8-year-old son. Although he is healthy, she is concerned because he is not able to write his name legibly, takes more than an hour to complete his homework, and requires physical assistance to set up his lunch and fasten clothing after toileting at school. What can you do to assist your neighbor?
   a. ____________________
10. You are working in a community-based "clubhouse" serving individuals with persistent mental illness. As part of the life skills program, the members of the clubhouse work at the fund-raising consignment shop located on the property. Today, one of the members came to see you with a report that another member treated him badly. What steps would be appropriate for you to take as a staff member?

Learning Activity 11-5: Problem Solving

OTs encounter situations not taught in school that can affect a client's ability to participate in desired occupations. One of the most important skills of an occupational therapy practitioner is the ability to creatively problem-solve all challenging situations. Read the following scenarios and write out ways that you could assist the client in overcoming the obstacle described. Be as detailed as possible because several situations require more than one step to solve the problem. Remember that OTs are members of the health care team and should feel free to call in the expertise of other professionals as needed. If completing this activity with classmates, you will find that there are several ways to solve these problems

1. Ray is an 80-year-old male who has permanent cauda equina syndrome with urinary incontinence. He uses an indwelling catheter and external bag. At home, he is ambulatory with a cane, but prefers to use a wheelchair as his primary means of mobility when he is out of the house. Ray is planning to attend the wedding of his great granddaughter next month, but does not want the catheter bag to be visible to others. He also plans to wear a tuxedo, as he would not be comfortable at a formal wedding wearing regular trousers. What can you recommend for Ray? If necessary, what/how will you teach Ray to do what you recommend?

2. Reba, a 39-year-old client who sustained a zone 2 flexor tendon laceration (flexor digitorum profundus and flexor digitorum superficialis) with repair 6 days ago has told you that she must return to work as an administrative assistant, but is unable to type with the dorsal protective orthosis that you have fabricated. How can you facilitate the ability of this client to return to work while preserving the integrity of her healing tendons?

3. Jose is a Gulf War veteran who lost both arms in combat many years ago. Jose is not a candidate for prosthetic devices because of the level of his amputations, but has used assistive aids and techniques to complete his self-care, work, and other activities independently through the years. Jose is about to become a grandfather for the first time and would like to hold and play with his grandchild. What could you suggest or provide for this client to facilitate his ability to interact with his grandchild?

4. Marta, a 75-year-old client with severe rheumatoid arthritis with limitations in ROM of all upper extremity joints insists on living independently within her one-story home. She reports that her greatest challenges are with medication management, food preparation, and securing various items from cabinets throughout her home. How can you help to ensure that Marta will be able to age in place?

5. An elderly couple live in the second story of a Cape Cod style home. The only access to the apartment is a steep outside staircase. The wife is nonambulatory due to a cerebellar stroke. Her husband is in his 80s and has several medical concerns, such as history of myocardial infarction, hypertension, and type 2 diabetes. The couple is not interested in moving to an accessible residence. What can you suggest or implement in the event of an emergency where the couple must be evacuated?

Handling Situations Appropriately

An occupational therapy practitioner must perform professional duties competently, such as selecting and implementing appropriate interventions, documenting client care, and completing departmental tasks within acceptable time frames. In addition, OTs and OTAs must "expect the unexpected" and be prepared to handle unpredictable situations that may occur during the course of the workday. It is essential that an occupational therapy practitioner demonstrate good clinical judgment and respond swiftly and appropriately when faced with emergency situations, difficult client behaviors, safety issues, unusual occurrences, and ethical concerns (AOTA, 2010, 2015). As you complete Learning Activities 11-6 and 11-7, consider the following suggestions in Box 11-1 for managing various clinical situations.

Box 11-1.

Tips for Handling Situations Appropriately

- Remain calm
- Exercise prudence
- Obtain help as needed
- Use good clinical reasoning
- Demonstrate professionalism and sensitivity
- Incorporate therapeutic use of self
- Maintain client dignity
- Do what is in the best interest of the client
- Make safety a priority
- Know relevant emergency procedures and undergo training for first aid/CPR
- Use proper infection control techniques
- Understand liability issues
- Keep current with legislation influencing OT practice
- Complete documentation requirements
- Adhere to facility policies and procedures
- Follow-up as needed
- Notify your supervisor, and others as appropriate, according to facility policy and relevant laws
- Implement preventative measures
- Learn from the experience
- Maintain healthy habits and manage your own stress level for optimal work performance

Reprinted with permission from Morreale, M. J. (2015). *Developing clinical competence: A workbook for the OTA*. Thorofare, NJ: SLACK Incorporated.

Learning Activity 11-6: Handling Situations Appropriately

Indicate how you would respond appropriately with professionalism and sensitivity to the following actual clinical situations that various occupational therapy practitioners have encountered (any identifying details have been changed). Consider what you would say to the clients, the immediate action you would take, and any follow-up that may be required.

1. Marge, a 75-year-old client in a skilled nursing facility, is 10 days status post-pinning for a right femoral neck fracture. When you arrive at her room to bring her to therapy, Marge is lying in bed. Marge states that she just fell out of bed, but was able to get back in by herself. She starts to cry and states, "I should not have told you I fell. I'm OK now. Please do not tell anyone what happened or they will put a restraint on me."

2. You are transferring a client from the hospital bed to a chair. The client is wearing only a hospital gown and is a little groggy from just waking up. As you are providing moderate assistance to transfer the client from sit to stand, the client suddenly becomes incontinent of feces, most of which lands directly on your shoe. The client does not appear to realize what just happened.

3. There are several clients present in the therapy room. As they are performing their exercises, they are making small talk and joking around. As the conversation turns to the topic of an upcoming election, the clients get into a very heated discussion and begin yelling at each other and using profanity.

4. A man receiving occupational therapy after a carpal tunnel release has been carrying a briefcase to each session. He typically asks for copies of his treatment notes and evaluations and places them in the briefcase. One day, when his treatment session has ended and the OT is leaving the clinic to go to the OT office, the client calls the OT back and says, "Look what I forgot to leave in my car." He then pulls out a handgun from the briefcase and turns it over several times to allow the OT a good look.

5. You are working in a skilled nursing facility with Harold, a 78-year-old client diagnosed with moderate stage Alzheimer's disease and a recent shoulder fracture. When you enter Harold's room to bring him to therapy, you discover that Harold has completely disrobed and is wandering around the room.

Learning Activity 11-6: Handling Situations Appropriately (continued)

6. A man is sent to occupational therapy directly from the physician's office for fabrication of a volar resting pan orthosis. The client underwent surgery 2 days earlier to repair a lacerated extensor indicis tendon and had his surgical dressing removed moments ago. The OT realizes this appointment is urgent and squeezes the client into the therapist's busy, full work schedule today. However, the OT only has enough time to fabricate the orthosis and provide minimal instruction until the next day when the client will be scheduled for a full evaluation and follow-up orthotic check. The man is fitted with the orthotic device and told not to remove it until he sees the OT tomorrow. However, the client does not show up the next day for his appointment. The OT calls to reschedule, but the client misses each appointment. Finally, after 2 weeks the client reappears complaining that his hand smells. The OT removes the orthosis and observes that the client's volar hand is severely macerated and the splint is soggy and odorous. When asked why this is, the client reported that he followed the OT's instruction not to remove his orthosis until he was seen back in therapy. In the meantime, the client had bathed every day with the orthosis on, not removing it to dry his skin.

7. An OT working in an outpatient clinic fabricated a finger orthosis 2 days ago for a client. When the client arrives today for a follow-up splint check, he reports that he accidentally flushed the orthosis down the toilet yesterday when washing his hands after toileting.

8. You are working in an outpatient clinic with a client who has a neurological condition. You transfer the client to the mat table to work on upper extremity exercises with the client positioned in supine. As the client initiates the exercises, you suddenly notice that the client was incontinent of urine, resulting in his pants and the mat getting wet. The client does not mention what just occurred.

9. You are an OT providing home care services to a young male client with a diagnosis of traumatic brain injury (TBI). Today, you are alone in his basement apartment working with him on a dressing activity. Suddenly, the client reaches and grabs your breast.

10. You are working in an outpatient therapy clinic. One day you are sitting at a table with a client who is performing fine motor activities. Suddenly you notice that your client is slumped over and appears to be turning blue.

Learning Activity 11-7: Handling Situations Appropriately—More Practice

Indicate how you would respond appropriately with professionalism and sensitivity to the following actual clinical situations that various occupational therapy practitioners have encountered (any identifying details have been changed). Consider what you would say to the clients, the immediate action you would take, and any follow-up that may be required.

1. Joe, a 55-year-old male client, has undergone hand surgery and is receiving outpatient OT. He has an outgoing personality, likes to make people laugh, and enjoys being the center of attention. Today, there are five other middle-aged clients in the therapy clinic. Joe begins to loudly tell a joke that has sexual overtones.

2. A client is receiving outpatient occupational therapy following a shoulder fracture. The client has deep religious beliefs and always brings a holy book to read in the clinic waiting room and during his hot pack treatments. Today, the client inquires about the therapist's religious affiliation, which is very different from that of the client. The client states that the therapist is misguided and begins to proselytize. The client then asks the therapist to look at a passage in the holy book.

3. An OT is working with Stanley, a 75-year-old male who exhibits left hemiplegia and severe left neglect. As the therapist is walking past Stanley's hospital room, Stanley calls out excitedly for her to come into his room right away. The therapist goes in the room and observes that Stanley is beaming. Stanley begins lifting his *unaffected* right arm and leg up and down vigorously while saying, "Look, look—it's a miracle! I can now move my arm and leg!"

4. An OT working in a skilled nursing facility is covering for a colleague who is on vacation this week. He has been delegated a client diagnosed with chronic obstructive pulmonary disease (COPD). Today, the client makes several derogatory remarks regarding the vacationing therapist's ethnicity (or religion) and then states, "Do I have to work with that OT? I would prefer to just work with you."

5. An OT working in home care has been delegated a client, Eva, who is recovering from a hip fracture. Eva lives with her spouse and currently requires contact guard assistance to ambulate with a walker. As the therapist arrives at the client's home and is ringing the doorbell, she can see Eva through the glass door panels. The therapist then observes that as Eva starts to get up out of her chair unattended, she trips and falls to the floor. The client did not lose consciousness in the fall and calls out for help.

Answers to Chapter 11 Worksheets

Worksheet 11-1: Billing and Reimbursement

Suggested resources for billing and reimbursement: Morreale & Borcherding, 2013; Thomas, 2011.

The AOTA website (www.AOTA.org) has useful information about public policy and reimbursement of OT services. Further information about Medicare can be found at (www.medicare.gov) and information about Medicaid can be found at (www.medicaid.gov). The Centers for Medicare & Medicaid Services (CMS) manuals can be found online at (www.cms.gov). Publication 100-02: Medicare Benefit Policy Manual Chapter 15, Section 220 delineates the criteria for reimbursement of outpatient OT services and Chapter 7, Section 40.2 delineates the criteria for home care. Publication 100-04: Medicare Claims Processing Manual Chapter 5 delineates coding requirements and claims procedures.

1. C. Current Procedural Terminology (CPT) are billing codes for health care services provided. ICD-10 contains diagnosis codes. The Minimum Data Set is an assessment tool used in skilled nursing facilities. The client is likely not eligible for Medicare.
2. A. According to the CMS guidelines for cotreating, the total units billed by both disciplines cannot exceed the allowable units based on time. Thirty minutes equals 2 units. The OT and PT can each bill 1 unit or *either* the OT or PT can bill the entire 2 units (CMS, 2009).
3. A. According to CMS, 1 unit of a timed service equals 8 to 22 minutes (CMS, 2011).
4. B. Medicare Part A covers inpatient acute stays, although there are some out-of-pocket expenses.
5. A. Inpatient hospital stays using Medicare Part A is reimbursed through the Prospective Payment System, which pays a predetermined per-diem rate.
6. B. The client has to pay the full cost of the deductible before the insurance provides any reimbursement. To meet the deductible, the client has to pay in full for the evaluation ($100), plus $50 for the second visit. For the remaining $20 owed for the second visit, the insurance pays 80% ($16), and the patient must pay the remaining $4. Thus, the total out-of-pocket cost for the second visit is $54 ($50 + $4).
7. D. TRICARE is health insurance for military members and their family. Unemployment insurance covers some lost wages, but does not reimburse health care costs. Medicare is a separate program.
8. C. Answers A, B, and D are classified as durable medical equipment (DME). Items such as tub seats, grab bars, reachers, sock aids, and the like are not because they are considered self-help or hygienic devices and are not considered medical in nature (CMS, 2005).
9. C. IDEA Part C covers children under 3 years of age. IDEA Part B covers preschool and school aged children (National Dissemination Center for Children With Disabilities, 2011).
10. D. Medicaid covers health care costs for eligible individuals who meet low income guidelines. Unemployment insurance, Supplemental Security Insurance, and Worker's Compensation are separate programs that do not cover health care costs.

Worksheet 11-2: Medicare Billing and Reimbursement

The American Occupational Therapy Association (AOTA) website (www.AOTA.org) has useful information about public policy and reimbursement of OT services. Further information about Medicare can be found at (www.medicare.gov). The Centers for Medicare & Medicaid Services (CMS) manuals can be found online at (www.cms.gov). Publication 100-02: Medicare Benefit Policy Manual Chapter 15, Section 220 delineates the criteria for reimbursement of outpatient OT services and Chapter 7, Section 40.2 delineates the criteria for home care.

1. D. Medicare guidelines state that occupational therapy services must be provided by a qualified therapist or appropriate support personnel (OTA) and meet the criteria for skilled care. Services of an aide do not meet those criteria (AOTA, 2014; CMS, 2014b).
2. C. Medicare A benefits cover limited lengths of stay in a skilled nursing facility. Medicare B provides some additional coverage for SNF stays when Medicare A benefits are used up (www.medicare.gov).

3. A. G-codes are used to meet Medicare B requirements for functional reporting at the start of care and at specified intervals (CMS, 2012).
4. D. Medicare guidelines delineate eligibility requirements for skilled maintenance services and specify that an OT provide the skilled maintenance care (CMS, 2014a). Coverage does not require that the client demonstrate functional improvement, only that skilled care is necessary for the client's condition (CMS, 2014a).
5. B. Level II codes are used to bill Medicare for medical equipment/supplies such as DME, orthotics, and prosthetics and also some specific services (e.g., ambulance) (AAPC, 20014b). Providers use Level II L-codes to bill Medicare for orthotics and fitting (Marchand, 2011). CPT codes are considered Level 1 codes, which are used in occupational therapy to bill for specific skilled interventions (procedures), such as ADL retraining, orthotic training, and therapeutic exercises.

Worksheet 11-3: Department Management

Suggested resources: Ellexson, 2011; Giles, 2011.

Space: Here are suggestions when choosing a space, but you may come up with others:

1. Meets requirements for local zoning and building codes
2. Available client base in area
3. Proximity to competitors in area
4. Wheelchair accessibility
5. Parking
6. Space adequate for types of services to be provided/number of rooms
7. Outdoor facilities/space if required (e.g., playground equipment for sensory integration or gross motor tasks)
8. Bathroom facilities present in space or building
9. Adequate electrical outlets and supply
10. Adequate water supply for hand hygiene, orthotic fabrication, etc.
11. Overhead lighting

Equipment/Supplies: The specific equipment and supplies required will depend on the type of practice setting, space, and available budget. Some considerations are noted below.

- Safety—personal protective equipment (e.g., gloves, gown, mask), fire extinguisher, smoke detector, soap and paper towels, first aid kit, wheelchair, etc.
- Office furniture—chairs, desk, table, mat, plinth, etc.
- Office equipment—computer, phone, fax, copier, file cabinets, washer/dryer, etc.
- Office supplies—pens, paper, toner, envelopes, stapler, paper clips, folders, etc.
- Evaluation tools—specific formal/informal assessments, goniometer, tape measure, dynamometer, pinch meter, volumeter, specific sensory tests, etc.
- General supplies—bandages, treatment table paper, pillows, pillowcases, towels, crayons, toys, lotion, etc.
- Exercise equipment—putty, weights, exercise bands, pegboard, cones, hand grippers, etc.
- ADL equipment—refrigerator, stove, microwave, coffee maker, laundry basket, pots/pans, utensils, etc.
- Adaptive equipment—reachers, buttonhooks, long shoehorns, built-up utensils, etc.
- PAMs—Paraffin unit, paraffin, hydrocollator, hot packs, cold packs, terry cloth covers, tongs, timer, etc.
- Upper extremity orthotic supplies—splint pan, heat gun, thermoplastics, hook-and-loop fastener, scissors, spatula, prefabricated splints, etc.

Possible staff or professional services needed (noninclusive list):

1. Accountant
2. Attorney
3. Janitor/handyman
4. Cleaning person
5. Electrician/plumber/carpenter (will depend on renovations required)

6. Engineering service/technician to calibrate or repair medical equipment
7. Billing service
8. Secretary
9. Marketing professional/web designer
10. Information technology specialist
11. Landscaper/snow removal
12. Rehabilitation aide
13. Laundry service

Worksheet 11-4: Budget

References: Ellexson, 2011.

1. T___ F _*_ A fiscal year goes from January 1 to December 31. *(An organization determines its own fiscal time frame consisting of a 1-year period, such as October 1 to September 30.)*
2. T___ F _*_ An example of an occupational therapy capital budget expenditure is a tub seat. *(A capital expense is a larger cost item (such as items >$1,000) that can be considered an asset and usually depreciated. A tub seat comes under the category of general equipment and supplies and does not meet those criteria.)*
3. T___ F _*_ Revenue equals total income minus expenses. (*Revenue equals total income before expenses.)*
4. T_*_ F___ An example of a fixed cost is rent. *(Fixed costs are steady for a period of time and not affected by volume of services.)*
5. T_*_F___ Accounts receivable include the money due from an insurance company.
6. T_*_F___ An example of variable expenses are office supplies.
7. T ___F _*_ Nonprofit means that the organization does not meet its expenses.
8. T_*_F___ Total costs subtracted from revenue equals profits.
9. T___ F _*_ An OT department budget always contains money for staff to attend continuing education seminars to maintain NBCOT certification.
10. T_*_ F___ Costs for items ordered, but not paid for are considered accounts payable.
11. T_*_F___ Bandages, lotions, and paraffin are considered direct use supplies.
12. T___ F _*_ Cash flow consists of pending money due from third-party payers. *(Cash flow is the money that actually comes in and out and is available for use.)*
13. T_*_ F___ Expenses that are fixed, such as salaries and equipment leases, are called *overhead.*
14. T_*_ F___ Productivity refers to the amount of billable services that an individual provides.
15. T_*_ F___ A piece of capital equipment that is depreciating is considered an asset.

Worksheet 11-5: Marketing

Here are some suggestions, although you may come up with others. As you can see by the answers that follow, some ideas should not be implemented because they may be impractical or unethical.

Marketing Idea	*Costs Incurred*	*Tasks/Personnel Needed*	*Other Considerations*
Host a breakfast or lunch for a group of physicians to explain the unique value of occupational therapy	Food and beverages Paper goods Invitations/postage Staff time	Create list of potential referral sources Create and send out invitations Keep track of responses Order and setup food and beverages Host event	Costs may not be reflected in department budget Participating staff will not be able to implement client interventions during this time Determining a mutually agreeable time and suitable space

Marketing Idea	***Costs Incurred***	***Tasks/Personnel Needed***	***Other Considerations***
Contact potential referring physicians and offer a referral bonus for each client that the physician refers to the OT department	—	—	*This is unethical* because anti-kickback laws are in place regarding federal funds such as Medicare and Medicaid (U.S. Department of Health and Human Services, n.d.)
Develop an informational brochure about the OT department and send it to physicians in the surrounding area	Cost of preparing brochure/postage Services of a marketing professional or IT professional Staff time	Create brochure Create list of potential referral sources Mail or e-mail brochure	Costs may not be reflected in department budget
Create a commercial for the local TV station	Cost of ad time Services of a marketing professional, videographer, actors	Coordinate with the facility's public relations/marketing department Create ad Purchase air time	Costs probably not reflected in department budget Suitable space and time for filming Obtain releases from persons in ad
In the lobby or next to the hospital cafeteria, host an OT event such as an exhibition of adaptive equipment, wellness activities, etc.	Decorations Giveaways or prizes Poster boards Brochures/copies of marketing materials Staff time	Determine agenda Reserve space Setup and host event Create poster boards or marketing materials	Costs may not be reflected in department budget Participating staff will not be able to implement client interventions during this time Determine suitable time frame and space
Write an article for the local newspaper about occupational therapy and the specific OT services provided at the hospital	Staff time Photographer	Write article Collaborate with facility public relations/marketing department Contact newspaper Take pictures	Obtain releases from persons in pictures
Provide educational sessions to local organizations such as support groups for individuals with arthritis, Alzheimer's disease, or Parkinson's disease	Staff time Transportation costs if offsite Handouts, brochures/copies of marketing materials	Collaborate with facility public relations/marketing department Contact appropriate agencies Create handouts or PowerPoint presentations	Participating staff will not be able to implement client interventions during this time Determine if these sessions will be pro bono or not

Marketing Idea	Costs Incurred	Tasks/Personnel Needed	Other Considerations
Provide free occupational therapy screenings to members of the community	Cost of particular assessments or materials used Transportation costs if offsite Handouts, brochures/copies of marketing materials Staff time	Collaborate with facility public relations/marketing department Schedule appointments if needed Setup event/screening area Administer screenings	Participating staff will not be able to implement client interventions during this time Obtain suitable space Privacy concerns That state's OT practice act regarding OT screenings

Worksheet 11-6: Creative Problem Solving

1. Here are several suggestions, but you may come up with others.
   - *A piece of shelf liner*
   - *A flat rubber jar opener disc*
   - *A dampened dish towel or washcloth*
   - *Nonslip placemat*
2. Here are several suggestions, but you may come up with others. The therapist must ensure that methods used are appropriate and safe for the particular client.
   - *Place commode in tub*
   - *Place a plastic lawn chair and rubber mat in tub*
3. Here are several suggestions, but you may come up with others. Some alternate jewelry clasps/necklace extenders are readily available in craft stores and the items below can also be found by doing an Internet search.
   - *Consider larger/bulkier jewelry that may be easier to manage*
   - *Adapt or purchase jewelry with alternate fastenings, such as magnetic clasps, toggle, or "s" loop closures*
   - *Use larger length necklaces that can slip over the head (can extend existing necklaces with extra loops/necklace extender kits)*
   - *Elastic bracelets and watch bands (not too tight)*
   - *Watchband with a hook and loop closure*
   - *Use a bracelet fastening tool*
   - *A jeweler can adapt rings with adjustable/expandable ring shanks so that the rings can go over enlarged joints*
   - *Use extra large earring backs*
   - *Use French wire earrings without backs*
   - *If indicated, warm up hands and perform ROM exercises prior to task*
4. Here are several suggestions, but you may come up with others.
   - *Color-code the straps and corresponding Velcro tabs*
   - *Number the straps and corresponding Velcro tabs*
   - *Take a picture of the correct placement of straps while client is wearing orthotic device*
   - *Use rivets to secure one end of each strap to the orthotic device*
5. When moving an attached catheter bag (such as threading it through garments) or hanging it when the client is resting, keep it below the level of the bladder to avoid backflow (Fairchild, 2013; George, 2013). Do not place the bag on the floor. Also, ensure that the catheter bag is moved accordingly during transfers, ambulation,

and other concerns to avoid tension at the insertion site. Here are some suggestions for managing lower body clothing with a catheter in place (Malecare, 2014):

- *Wear boxer shorts*
- *Wear athletic type shorts or loose fitting shorts*
- *Wear looser pants, such as sweatpants or pants with a drawstring closure*
- *Wear basketball type pants with side snaps or zippers*
- *Wear a dress or skirt*
- *When resting at home, use a hospital gown, nightgown/nightshirt, short pajamas, or a bathrobe*

6. Because this is an important activity for the client, you and the OTA must create a solution that is agreed on by the client and her family, and is within reimbursement and facility guidelines. Options include the following:
   - *Offering to order large-handled utensils from an adaptive equipment catalog on behalf of the client, having spouse complete the payment section*
   - *Provide the family with a list of local medical supply stores or specialty kitchen stores that sell appropriate products.*
   - *Provide the family with an adaptive equipment catalog with the appropriate equipment identified*
   - *Suggest that family purchase cylindrical pipe insulation at the local hardware store to place on the handles of the utensils*
7. Regardless of the time of day, steps must be taken to ensure that the client is not at risk for skin break down because of an ill-fitting orthosis or tempted to remove the orthosis (due to the diagnosis) because of discomfort. Consider the following options:
   - *Immediately phone the client, explain that you heard from the physician and request more details regarding her concerns.*
   - *Ask the client to return to the office to have the orthosis assessed and adjusted. You will arrange to stay at the office until the client can return.*
   - *If the client is unable to return to the office, consider appropriate methods to increase comfort through the night. For example, ask the client if resting the arm relieves discomfort. Ask if placing a bandage or soft material, such as cotton, under the orthosis will relieve pressure. If so, explain in detail how the orthosis should be removed and redonned.*
   - *Consider a video conference session if available; check your state practice act to ensure that this is not against your practice act. Do not bill for this follow-up.*
   - *Schedule the client for a visit first thing in the morning.*
8. Consider a top-down approach to your assessment. Ask which psychometrically sound, normed, or criteria-based assessment tools that your facility has available.
   - *Choose to complete a function-based assessment, such as the Canadian Occupational Performance Measure (COPM), to determine which areas of ADLs are becoming difficult.*
9. The issues described by your neighbor sound as if they may be having an impact or will have an impact on her son's ability to be successful in school. Because she stated that the pediatrician has never noted any medical concerns:
   - *You may suggest that your neighbor make an appointment with her son's classroom teacher to discuss her concerns. If the teacher agrees, she can recommend an occupational therapy evaluation.*
10. The clubhouse model provides individuals with a physical space where clients are afforded respect and varied opportunities to pursue valued and chosen occupations that hold meaning and purpose. Clubhouses accredited and run by staff and clients following Clubhouse Standards published by the International Center for Clubhouse Development (ICCD). If a member reports that they were not treated with respect, the OT should:
    - *Ask the client to bring this issue to the next clubhouse meeting for group discussion.*

Chapter 11 References

American Academy of Professional Coders. (2014a). *In the news.* Retrieved from http://www.aapc.com/index.php/2014/05/in-the-news

American Academy of Professional Coders. (2014b). *What is HCPCS?* Retrieved from http://www.aapc.com/resources/medical-coding/hcpcs.aspx

American Occupational Therapy Association. (2010). Standards of practice for occupational therapy. *American Journal of Occupational Therapy, 64*(Suppl. 6), S106–S111.

American Occupational Therapy Association. (2014a). Guidelines for supervision, roles, and responsibilities during the delivery of occupational therapy services. *American Journal of Occupational Therapy, 68*(Suppl. 3), S16–S22.

American Occupational Therapy Association. (2015). Occupational therapy code of ethics (2015). *American Journal of Occupational Therapy,* 69 (Suppl. 3), 6913410030. http://dx.doi.org/10.5014/ajot.2015.696S03.

Centers for Medicare & Medicaid Services. (2005). *Medicare National Coverage Determinations (NCD) Manual* (Pub. 100-03: Ch. 1, section 280.1). Baltimore: Centers for Medicare & Medicaid Services. Retrieved from http://www.cms.gov/Regulations-and-Guidance/Guidance/Manuals/Internet-Only-Manuals-IOMs-Items/CMS014961.html

Centers for Medicare & Medicaid Services. (2009). 11 Part B billing scenarios for PTs and OTs. Retrieved from http://www.cms.gov/Medicare/Billing/TherapyServices/downloads/11_Part_B_Billing_Scenarios_for_PTs_and_OTs.pdf

Centers for Medicare & Medicaid Services. (2011). *Medicare claims processing manual* (Pub. 100-04: Ch. 5, section 20.2). Baltimore: Centers for Medicare & Medicaid Services. Retrieved from http://www.cms.gov/Regulations-and-Guidance/Guidance/Manuals/downloads//clm104c05.pdf

Centers for Medicare & Medicaid Services. (2012). Medicare Learning Network: Preparing for therapy required functional reporting implementation in CY 2013. Retrieved from http://www.cms.gov/Outreach-and-Education/Outreach/NPC/Downloads/FunctionalReportingNPC.pdf

Centers for Medicare & Medicaid Services. (2014a). *Medicare benefit policy manual* (Pub. 100-02: Ch. 7, Section 40.2.1). Baltimore: Centers for Medicare & Medicaid Services. Retrieved from http://www.cms.gov/Regulations-and-Guidance/Guidance/Manuals/downloads/bp102c07.pdf

Centers for Medicare & Medicaid Services. (2014b). *Medicare benefit policy manual* (Pub. 100-02: Ch. 15, Section 230.2). Baltimore: Centers for Medicare & Medicaid Services. Retrieved from http://www.cms.gov/Regulations-and-Guidance/Guidance/Manuals/Downloads/bp102c15.pdf

Ellexson, M. T. (2011). Financial planning and budgeting. In K. Jacobs & G. L. McCormack (Eds.), *The occupational therapy manager* (5th ed., pp. 113–125). Bethesda, MD: American Occupational Therapy Association, Incorporated.

Fairchild, S. L. (2013). *Pierson and Fairchild's principles & techniques of patient care* (5th ed.). St. Louis: Saunders.

George, A. H. (2013). Infection control and safety issues in the clinic. In H. M. Pendleton & W. Schultz-Krohn, (Eds.), *Pedretti's occupational therapy: Practice skills for physical dysfunction* (7th ed., pp. 140–156). St. Louis: Mosby.

Giles, G. M. (2011). Starting a new program, business, or practice. In K. Jacobs & G. L. McCormack (Eds.), *The occupational therapy manager* (5th ed., pp. 145–166). Bethesda, MD: American Occupational Therapy Association.

Malecare, Inc. (2014). Clothing. Retrieved from http://malecare.org/clothing

Marchand, S. (2011). *Coding and billing for therapy and rehab.* Brentwood, TN: Cross Country Education.

Morreale, M. J. (2015). *Developing clinical competence: A workbook for the OTA.* Thorofare, NJ: SLACK Incorporated.

Morreale, M., & Borcherding, S. (2013). *The OTA's guide to documentation: Writing SOAP notes* (3rd ed.). Thorofare, NJ: SLACK Incorporated.

National Dissemination Center for Children With Disabilities. (2011). Part C of IDEA: Early intervention for babies and toddlers. Retrieved from http://nichcy.org/laws/idea/partc

Thomas, V. J. (2011). Reimbursement. In K. Jacobs & G. L. McCormack (Eds.), *The occupational therapy manager* (5th ed., pp. 385–405). Bethesda, MD: American Occupational Therapy Association.

U.S. Department of Health and Human Services. (n.d.). *Guidance on the Federal Anti-Kickback Law.* Retrieved from http://bphc.hrsa.gov/policiesregulations/policies/pal199510.html

World Health Organization. (2013). *Classifications: International Classification of Diseases (ICD) information sheet.* Geneva: Author. Retrieved from http://www.who.int/classifications/icd/factsheet/en/index.html

Index

For Product Safety Concerns and Information please contact our EU representative GPSR@taylorandfrancis.com Taylor & Francis Verlag GmbH, Kaufingerstraße 24, 80331 München, Germany

Batch number: 10733534

Printed by Printforce, the Netherlands